Community Preparedness and Response to Terrorism

COMMUNITY PREPAREDNESS AND RESPONSE TO TERRORISM

II The Role of Community Organizations and Business

Edited by
James A. Johnson, Michael H. Kennedy, and
Nejdet Delener

General Editors
James A. Johnson, Gerald R. Ledlow, and Mark A. Cwiek

PRAEGER PERSPECTIVES

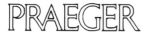

Westport, Connecticut
London

Library of Congress Cataloging-in-Publication Data

Community preparedness and response to terrorism / James A. Johnson, Gerald R.
  Ledlow, and Mark A. Cwiek, general editors.
    p. cm.
  Includes bibliographical references and index.
  Contents: v. 1. The terrorist threat and community response / edited by Gerald R.
Ledlow, James A. Johnson, and Walter J. Jones—v. 2. The role of community
organizations and business / edited by James A. Johnson, Michael H. Kennedy, and
Nejdet Delener—v. 3. Communication and the media / edited by H. Dan O'Hair,
Robert L. Heath, and Gerald R. Ledlow.
    ISBN 0–275–98366–8 (set : alk. paper)—ISBN 0–275–98365–X (v. 1 : alk. paper)—
ISBN 0–275–98369–2 (v. 2 : alk. paper)—ISBN 0–275–98373–0 (v. 3 : alk. paper)
    1. Terrorism—United States—Prevention. 2. Emergency management—United
States. 3. Civil defense—United States. 4. Community organization—United States.
5. Terrorism and mass media—United States. 6. Preparedness—United States.
I. Johnson, James A., 1954– II. Ledlow, Gerald R. III. Cwiek, Mark A.
HV6432.C654 2004
363.34'97–dc22   2004042290

British Library Cataloguing in Publication Data is available.

Library of Congress Catalog Card Number: 2004042290
ISBN: 0–275–98366–8 (set)
        0–275–98365–X (Volume I)
        0–275–98369–2 (Volume II)
        0–275–98373–0 (Volume III)

First published in 2005

Praeger Publishers, 88 Post Road West, Westport, CT 06881
An imprint of Greenwood Publishing Group, Inc.
www.praeger.com

Printed in the United States of America

The paper used in this book complies with the
Permanent Paper Standard issued by the National
Information Standards Organization (Z39.48–1984).

10 9 8 7 6 5 4 3 2 1

Contents

Acknowledgments

The editors wish to thank the contributors for their wisdom, creativity, and extraordinary work ethic for bringing this volume to a successful conclusion. The tight deadlines and requested revisions were met with professionalism and promptness that exceeded expectations. We are deeply grateful to our families for giving up private time, especially over weekends and holidays, so that we could devote attention to this project. We thank Hilary Claggett and Sarah Coe from Praeger Publishing for their masterful expertise in helping us bring this volume to publication. Finally, thanks go to Aamna Qamar, Bolanle Oyefesobi, and Olawaale Adjenor for developing the index, to Ritva Carlson of Capital City Press for her outstanding editorial guidance, and to Cheryl Reen for her invaluable administrative support throughout the project.

Introduction

James A. Johnson

I was working in New York City the day the *9/11 Commission Report* was released. On that day, not only did I acquire a copy of the report, I also chose to visit the World Trade Center site. While standing there looking at that dust covered hole in the ground, I was reminded once again of just how unpredictable terrorism is. Only a few years ago, my wife and I stood on top of the Trade Center building looking out across the beautiful, peaceful New York skyline. I remember feeling not just the grandeur of the scene but also the sense of permanence the building evoked under our feet. As with any place of prominence in any community anywhere, we had the feeling it would be there forever, and our children and their children someday would stand on the same spot. We all yearn for a time when it was easier to assume such things. However, after September 11, 2001, no one can have such comforting assumptions, no matter where they live. As a medical social scientist having worked in countries around the globe, I have always carried the message to any who would listen: "Disease respects no borders." We have seen this with AIDS, West Nile Virus, and Mad Cow Disease (the list goes on). Now, it seems I can make the same frightful statement about terrorism. In fact, one can look at terrorism as a social disease, by which all populations are potentially susceptible, whether they be large countries or small ones, big cities or rural farming communities. Additionally, the victims, as with disease, include all ages, all races, and all nationalities. In short, the "disease" of terrorism has the potential to spread to any person on this planet. For some, it is simply being in the wrong place at the wrong time, for others they are a symbolic target. Either way, death or harm can come to those who do not expect it.

This book seeks to enlighten community and business leaders about the many threats of terrorism and the preparedness needed to address the challenge. It is imperative in today's environment for everyone to be better informed and to actively participate in making each community safer.

Community leaders need to take responsibility for addressing concerns about the possibility of terrorist activity. Awareness is the key. Leaders should inform all their key stakeholders, including the public, that preventive as well as responsive policies and programs are underway. This may be in the form of briefings, in-service workshops, simulations and mock exercises, security enhancements, and coordination with local, state, and federal agencies. Many communities will want to develop "disaster plans" that help victims and their families remain in the information loop or in some cases to evacuate. If the threat level is high for a given organization within the community, a security audit by an outside firm might be in order.

Several "critical success factors" for all communities to consider when addressing the challenge might include the following:

training (i.e., a well informed workforce);

the mitigation of confusion;

time management (time is critical);

building a response capacity;

economic constraints;

coordination with local health agencies; and

mitigation of fear and panic.

TRAINING IS ESSENTIAL

This could be in the form of awareness enhancement or, for businesses at greater risk, actual training in disease or threat detection and early intervention. Additionally, the training of at least one "disaster coordinator" or "health coordinator" would be important. This individual can serve as a resource person, advisor, counselor, and organizer. They also could have the responsibility for staying informed and maintaining contact networks with local agencies. Ideally, this coordinator would receive continuing education through national organizations that provide periodic updates on skills and knowledge needed to be effective in that role.

MITIGATION OF CONFUSION

This is a critical success factor in managing any crisis. The natural tendency of humans in a state of confusion is to panic. If this occurs, more harm can result. Training, preparedness, and discussion within the community and businesses of a range of possibilities and response scenarios all help to mitigate confusion. Fast, clear communications to all personnel is essential, too. No one should be left in the dark on these matters. Lastly, some organized protocol for testing and prophylaxis in the case of bioterrorism will help provide much needed reassurance that the business or agency cares for its people and is taking steps to be prepared.

TIME MANAGEMENT

Time is critical in all matters pertaining to infectious disease. Early signs, early diagnosis, early warning to the uninfected, and early intervention all have positive implications for the spread and eventual impact of disease. Time management can be equally important in the case of chemical and radiation exposure. Timeliness by first responders becomes key to saving lives and preventing further injuries.

RESPONSE CAPACITY

This may be in the form of trained personnel along with needed equipment and proper training. It also includes working with local agencies to develop a quick response to a crisis. There are financial considerations such as cost of training, supplies, equipment, and down time that should be part of the capacity building within the business or community. In the case of biological threats, some might even consider a "bioterrorism crisis reserve" for contingency planning. Another major consideration is the ratio in a community between pre-identified community members given vaccinations and other prophylaxis versus the potentially 'infected' population in the community. Pre-identified members should be health care givers and support personnel, firefighters and law enforcement personnel, sanitation workers, utility workers, and other individuals considered essential for community functions and maintenance to respond to the potential crisis.

MITIGATION OF FEAR AND PANIC

There is no better way to decrease stress and anxiety in anticipation of a possible terrorist attack, and likewise no better way to control panic after an attack, than putting in the requisite time and resources to properly train the workforce and larger community. The more people are told in the beginning, the less anxiety there will be. Often, the greatest fear comes from uncertainty.

As you read this volume, it is my wish that you utilize the many tools, examples, and recommendations of the various authors to develop or enhance your own preparedness efforts. Terrorism will continue to evolve, as will its methods and creative modes of destruction. It is indeed a pathogen that has been around a long time. It is not likely to come to an end anytime soon, and as mentioned previously, none of us are immune from its potential threat. As stated by General Wesley Clark, "In the wake of 9/11, Americans are seeing themselves in a new way. And we are looking at each other differently, seeking a community with greater trust and security." This is a challenge we all face together: every community, every business, and every individual has a part in building a safer world.

1   Overview of Biological Agents and Compounds with Potential Bioterrorism Applications

Joseph N. Inungu

Bioterrorism is defined as the use, or threatened use, of biological agents (bacterial, viral, parasitic, or biological toxin) to promote or spread fear or intimidation upon an individual, a specific group, or the population as a whole for religious, political, ideological, financial, or personal purposes.[1] The use of biological compounds and agents has been well documented throughout history. In the sixth century BC, Assyrians poisoned enemy water supplies with rye ergot, which made their enemies sick and opened their ranks to Assyrian attack. During the siege of Krissa, Solon of Athens used skunk cabbage to poison that community's water supply.[2] In 1346 the Tatar army hurled plague-ridden dead bodies over the walls of the city of Kaffa, forcing the inhabitants to surrender. In 1767 during the French and Indian War, Sir Jeffrey Amherst, the English general, ordered the distribution of smallpox-laced blankets to Indians loyal to the French. The Indians were decimated.[3,4] This may have contributed to the British victory. In Oregon in September 1984, 750 people fell sick from salmonella bacteria intentionally spread by followers of Sri Bhagwan Rajneesh in an effort to influence local elections.[5] In October 2001 anthrax-laden letters were sent to media outlets and two U.S. senators. Five people died and seventeen others were sickened in the attacks. Thousands of people were placed on antibiotics.[6]

To better prepare ourselves to react effectively to any future attack, we must understand the biological agents that may be used as weapons and understand their modes of action.

SELECTED AGENTS AND COMPOUNDS

Anthrax

Causal Factors

Anthrax is an acute infectious disease caused by the spore-forming bacterium *Bacillus anthracis*. The spores can live in soil for years. Humans get infected by handling products from infected animals (cattle, sheep, goats, camels, and antelopes), by eating undercooked meat from infected animals, or by inhaling anthrax spores from contaminated animal products.

Clinical Presentation

Infected individuals may exhibit one of the following three clinical presentations:

1. *Cutaneous.* This is the most common clinical manifestation of anthrax and represents about 95 percent of cases. The infected individual first observes a raised itchy bump, like an insect bite; then the lesion turns into a painless ulcer with a characteristic black necrotic area in the center. The development of secondary regional inflamed lymph nodes is common. About 20 percent of people with untreated cutaneous anthrax die.
2. *Inhalation.* This is the most lethal form of anthrax. The first symptoms resemble those of a common cold—sore throat, mild fever, muscle aches, and general malaise. Several days later, the infected individual develops severe breathing problems and goes into shock.
3. *Intestinal.* This form of anthrax follows the consumption of contaminated meat. The infected individual often experiences nausea, loss of appetite, vomiting, and fever, followed by severe abdominal pain, profuse diarrhea, and vomiting of blood. This form kills 25 to 60 percent of cases.

Methods of Control

For prevention, an effective vaccine against anthrax exists; however, because of possible serious complications, it is primarily given to military personnel and people at high risk (workers in research laboratories that handle anthrax bacteria). The antibiotics (ciprofloxacin and/or doxycycline) used following the exposure are very effective in preventing the development of anthrax disease.

Anthrax can be successfully treated with powerful antibiotics (ciprofloxacin and/or doxycycline). The earlier the treatment, the better the outcome.

Botulism

Causal Factors

Botulism is a muscle-paralyzing disease caused by toxins produced by *Clostridium botulinum*, a spore-forming anaerobic bacterium.

Clinical Presentation

Based on the mode of contamination, we distinguish three main forms of botulism:

1. *Foodborne botulism*. The disease is acquired by ingesting food in which toxins have formed. Toxins are produced in improperly processed or low-acid canned foods and also in non-refrigerated pasteurized foods. Symptoms begin within twelve to thirty-six hours after eating toxin-containing food. The symptoms are visual difficulty (double vision), drooping eyelids, slurred speech, difficulty swallowing, and dry mouth. Vomiting, and constipation or diarrhea may be present. Paralysis of breathing muscles can cause a person to stop breathing and die. This form of botulism kills 5 to 10 percent of cases.
2. *Infant botulism*. This is the most common form of botulism in the United States. The disease affects mainly infants under one year who have ingested spores that then germinate in the infant's intestinal tract. Honey and other foods are the possible sources of spores. Subsequent outgrowth and in-vivo production of toxins produce the disease. The common symptoms of the disease are constipation, lethargy, poor feeding, ptosis, and hypotonia (floppy baby). This form kills about 1 percent of cases.
3. *Wound botulism*. This form occurs when wounds are infected with *C. botulinum* that secretes the toxin.

Method of Control

For prevention, a case of foodborne botulism must trigger a rapid public health investigation, since the contaminated food may still be available to other people.

Intravenous administration of the botulinum antitoxin should be part of the routine treatment. The antitoxin is effective in reducing the severity of symptoms, if administered early in the course of the disease. Antibiotics do not improve the chance of recovery.

Plague

Causal Factors

Plague is an infectious disease caused by *Yersinia pestis* (*Y. pestis*), a bacterium found in rodents, ground squirrels, rabbits, hares, wild carnivores, and domestic cats and their fleas in many areas of the world. Plague remains a threat for humans because of vast areas of persistent wild rodent infection.

The most frequent source of exposure has been the bite of infected fleas (*Xenopsylla cheopis*), which transfer the bacterium to humans.

Clinical Presentation

There are two forms of plague:

1. *Bubonic plague.* This is the initial stage of the disease. The signs and symptoms include fever, chills, malaise, muscle pain, sore throat, headache, and regional inflammation of lymph nodes, especially in inguinal areas (90 percent). The bubonic plague will disseminate to other parts of the body through blood (meninges, lungs). It kills about 50 to 60 percent of cases.
2. *Pneumonic plague. Yersinia pestis* used in an aerosol attack can cause the pneumonic form of plague. The signs and symptoms of this form are fever, weakness, and rapidly developing pneumonia with shortness of breath, chest pain, cough, and sometimes bloody or watery sputum. Nausea, vomiting, and abdominal pain may also occur. Untreated, pneumonic plague leads to respiratory failure, shock, and rapid death in two to four days. Pneumonic plague can be transmitted from person to person.

Methods of Control

Transmission of the bubonic plague is rodent flea-to-human via a bite or by a person handling an infected rodent. Wild rats living in a rural human home might infect their human hosts if they carry plague bacterium–infected rodent fleas. Treatment for the bubonic plague includes immediate treatment with antibiotics such as streptomycin, chloramphenicol, or tetracycline as indicated. Oxygen, intravenous fluids, and respiratory support are additional treatments.

Person-to-person transmission of pneumonic plague occurs through respiratory droplets, which can only infect those who have face-to-face contact with patients. Early treatment of pneumonic plague is essential. Several antibiotics are effective, including streptomycin, gentamycine, tetracycline, chloramphenicol, and fluoroquinolone (such as ciprofloxacin). Prophylactic antibiotic treatment for seven days will protect persons who have had face-to-face contact with infected patients.

Live, attenuated vaccines are used in some countries, but they are not available in the United States.

Smallpox

Causal Factors

Smallpox is a serious infectious disease caused by the *variola* virus. Although the last naturally acquired case of smallpox occurred in 1977, the recent use of anthrax-laden letters has heightened our awareness of the possibility of such an attack. The term *small pockes* (*pocke* means "sac") was first used in England at the end of the fifteenth century to distinguish the illness from syphilis, which was then known as *great pockes*.

Smallpox is transmitted from one person to another through direct and fairly prolonged face-to-face contact. Smallpox can also be transmitted through direct contact with infected bodily fluids or contaminated objects such as bedding or clothing. Humans are the only natural hosts of *variola*. Insects or animals do not transmit smallpox.

Clinical Presentation

About seven to seventeen days after exposure, the first symptoms of smallpox appear. They include fever, chills, headache, nausea, vomiting, and severe muscle aches. These symptoms last two to four days. By the fourth day of illness, the fever drops and the characteristic flat or thickened spots, called macules, appear and quickly progress to raised spots, called papules. These papules continue to enlarge and fill with a clear fluid; at this stage, they are called vesicles. The fluid in the vesicles gradually changes from clear to pus-like, and the lesions are then called pustules. Fever is common at this stage. The pustules start to form into scabs. Over time, the dried scab material falls off of the skin. This entire process takes three to four weeks, and the areas affected can leave permanent scars. There are two clinical forms of smallpox:

1. *Variola major*: the more severe and fatal form of smallpox. It kills about 30 to 50 percent of unvaccinated cases and three percent of vaccinated persons.
2. *Variola minor*: this kills about 1 to 2 percent of unvaccinated individuals.

Methods of Control

There is no proven treatment for smallpox. Infected individuals may benefit from supportive therapy such as intravenous fluids, medicine to control fever or pain, and antibiotics for any secondary bacterial infections.

The vaccine to prevent smallpox was routinely administered in the United States until the early 1970s. Routine vaccination of the civilian population for this disease is not currently recommended by the medical community.

Ricin

Causal Factors

Ricin is a natural highly toxic glycoprotein that comes from castor beans, which are used to make castor oil. Ricin's significance as a potential biological warfare toxin is due in part to its wide availability. Worldwide, about 1 million metric tons of these beans are processed every year. When they are boiled down, the residue is ricin. Ricin can be produced relatively easily and inexpensively in large quantities in a fairly low-technology setting. Ricin was used in the 1978 assassination of Bulgarian dissident Georgi Markov. The author, who had defected to England nine years earlier, was jabbed by the tip of an umbrella while waiting for a bus in London and died four days later.

Ricin is very toxic to cells. It acts by inhibiting protein synthesis.

Clinical Presentation

Signs and symptoms of ricin intoxication depend on the dose and route of exposure. Initial symptoms following inhalation include weakness, fever, cough, dyspnea, nausea, chest tightness, and arthralgia. Sweating, pulmonary edema, and cyanosis follow. Suppurative airway lesions may be noted in conjunction with rhinitis and laryngitis. In untreated patients, respiratory failure and cardiovascular collapse due to inhalation of the agent can lead to death in thirty-six to seventy-two hours.

Ingestion will be followed by rapid onset of nausea, vomiting, abdominal cramps, and severe diarrhea. Other symptoms include fever, thirst, headache, sore throat, and dilation of the pupils. Death may occur on the third day or later, and is usually due to vascular collapse.

Methods of Control

Intoxicated individuals may benefit from supportive therapy such as intravenous fluids and medicine to control fever or pain. For those with pulmonary intoxification, respiratory support may be necessary. Pulmonary edema may need to be treated with positive end expiratory pressure ventilation and diuretics.

Healthcare workers should use standard precautions. Decontaminate exposed skin by washing with soap and water and/or 0.1 percent sodium hypochlorite (one part household bleach added to forty-nine parts water).

Salmonellosis

Causal Factors

Salmonellosis is one of the common causes of food poisoning worldwide. It is an acute infectious disease caused by over 2,000 different types of bacteria called *Salmonella*. Salmonella are widespread in cows, poultry, pigs, pets, and wild animals. The food may be contaminated because the source (animal or bird) was infected. About 50 percent of frozen and fresh chickens contain the bacteria. Infections in dairy herds may lead to the contamination of unpasteurized milk consumed directly or used in the preparation of milk products, such as babies' dried milk.

Clinical Presentation

Within twelve to thirty-six hours of ingestion of contaminated food, the bacteria multiply in the intestines to cause diarrhea, stomach cramps, and sometimes vomiting and fever. Most persons recover without treatment. The elderly, infants, and those with impaired immune systems are more likely to have a severe illness. In these patients, the salmonella infection may spread from the intestines to the bloodstream and then to other body sites, and can cause death, unless the person is treated promptly with antibiotics.

Methods of Control

Individuals with severe diarrhea may benefit from supportive therapy such as intravenous fluids. Antibiotics are not usually necessary, unless the infection has spread to other organs. Ampicillin, gentamicin, trimethoprim/sulfamethoxazole, and ciprofloxacin are the most common antibiotics used. Unfortunately, some salmonella bacteria have become resistant to antibiotics, largely due to the use of antibiotics to promote the growth of feed animals.

Other causes of food poisoning are *Escherichia coli* O157:H7, *Shigella*, and *Vibrio cholerae*.

Tularemia

Causal Factors

Tularemia, or rabbit fever, is a bacterial disease associated with both animals and humans. Although many wild and domestic animals can be infected, the rabbit is most often involved in disease outbreaks.

Tularemia bacteria can be transmitted through many routes. Inoculation of the skin or mucus membranes with blood or tissue while handling infected animals is the most common mode of transmission. The other modes of infection are the bite of an infected tick, contact with fluids from infected deer flies or ticks, and handling or eating insufficiently cooked rabbit meat. Less-common means of spreading the bacteria are drinking contaminated water, inhaling dust from contaminated soil, and handling contaminated animals. Tularemia is not spread from person to person. In aerosol form, it is considered a possible bioterrorism agent. Persons who inhale an infectious aerosol would likely experience severe respiratory illness.

Clinical Presentation

Symptoms of tularemia appear one to fourteen days after exposure and depend on the route of infection. When a person is infected through skin inoculation (from handling an animal carcass), symptoms can include a slow-growing ulcer at the site where the bacteria entered the skin and swollen lymph nodes. If the bacteria are inhaled, a pneumonia-like illness can follow. If the bacteria were ingested, patients may report a sore throat, abdominal pain, diarrhea, and vomiting.

Methods of Control

Streptomycin and gentamicin are the drugs of choice for treating tularemia. Other antibiotics also are effective.

Brucellosis

Causal Factors

Brucellosis is an infectious disease caused by the bacteria of the genus *Brucella* (*Brucella melitensis*, *Brucella suis*, and *Brucella abortus*).

Humans are generally infected in one of three ways: eating or drinking something that is contaminated with *Brucella*, breathing in the organism (inhalation), or having the bacteria enter the body through skin wounds. The most common way to be infected is by eating or drinking contaminated milk products. Wild animals such as deer, elk, and bison may also carry the *Brucella* bacteria. Disease spread from one person to another is rare, but sexual and breastfeeding transmission is possible.

Clinical Presentation

Symptoms of brucellosis include intermittent fever of variable duration, headache, weakness, swollen lymph nodes, profuse sweating, chills, weight loss, and generalized aching. Brucellosis can also cause infection and inflammation of the bones, testicles, and the lining of the heart.

Methods of Control

The treatment is difficult, and recovery may take several weeks, based on the timing of treatment and severity of illness. Doxycycline and rifampin used in combination for six weeks prevent recurring infection.

Avoiding consumption of unpasteurized milk, cheese, or ice cream while traveling may help prevent the infection. Hunters and animal herdsmen should wear rubber gloves when handling the viscera of animals. There is no vaccine available for humans.

Q Fever

Causal Factors

Q fever is an acute infectious disease caused by a species of bacteria called *Coxiella burnetii* (*C. burnetii*). Q fever is a disease contracted from animals.

Cattle, sheep, and goats are the primary reservoirs of *C. burnetii*. Infection has been noted in a wide variety of other animals, including other breeds of livestock and domesticated pets. *Coxiella burnetii* does not usually cause clinical disease in these animals, although abortion in goats and sheep has been linked to infection. The infection of humans usually occurs when they inhale these organisms from air that contains airborne barnyard dust contaminated by dried placental material, birth fluids, and excreta of infected herd animals. This agent could be developed for use in biological warfare and is considered a potential terrorist threat.

Ingestion of contaminated milk, followed by regurgitation and inspiration of the contaminated food, is a less-common mode of transmission. Other modes of transmission to humans, including tick bites and human-to-human transmission, are rare.

Clinical Presentation

The symptoms of acute cases of Q fever include one or more of the following: high fevers (up to 104 to 105°F), severe headache, general malaise, myalgia, confusion, sore throat, chills, sweats, nonproductive coughs, nausea, vomiting, diarrhea, abdominal pain, and chest pain. Most patients usually recover to good health within several months without any treatment. Chronic Q fever, characterized by infection that persists for more than six months, is uncommon, but is a much more serious disease.

Methods of Control

Doxycycline is the treatment of choice for acute Q fever. Antibiotic treatment is most effective when initiated within the first three days of illness. Therapy should be started again if the disease relapses.

Although a vaccine for Q fever has been developed and has successfully protected humans in occupational settings in Australia, it is not commercially available in the United States.

Viral Hemorrhagic Fevers

Causal Factors

Viral hemorrhagic fevers are a group of illnesses that are caused by four distinct families of viruses:

1. *Filoviridae*: Ebola and Marburg viruses
2. *Arenaviridae*: Lassa fever virus
3. *Bunyaviridae*: Crimean Congo hemorrhagic fever virus and Rift Valley fever virus

4. *Flaviviridae*: dengue fever, yellow fever, Omsk hemorrhagic fever, and Kyasanur Forest disease virus

All of these viruses are capable of causing clinical diseases characterized by fever and severe bleeding disorders. Risk factors for these diseases include travel to certain geographic areas where the diseases may naturally occur (such as certain areas of Africa, Asia, the Middle East, and South America), handling of animal carcasses, contact with sick animals or people with the disease, and arthropod bites.

There is the potential for significant morbidity and mortality if hemorrhagic fever viruses were to be disseminated by aerosol dispersal, given the lack of readily available therapy and vaccines. Some of these viruses (namely, Ebola, Marburg, Lassa fever, New World arenaviruses, and Crimean-Congo hemorrhagic fever viruses) are also transmissible from person to person; this characteristic has the potential to amplify disease outbreaks.

Clinical Presentation

Following an aerosol dissemination of any of these viral hemorrhagic fevers, cases would likely appear two to twenty-one days following exposure. Patients would present with fever, rashes, body aches, headaches, and fatigue, and bleeding manifestations could occur later in the course of the disease. Patients with severe cases of viral hemorrhagic fever often show signs of bleeding under the skin, in internal organs, or from body orifices like the mouth, eyes, or ears. Although they may bleed from many sites around the body, however, patients rarely die of blood loss. Severely ill patient cases may also show shock, nervous system malfunction, coma, delirium, and seizures.

Methods of Control

While there is no other treatment or established cure for VHFs, Ribavirin, an antiviral drug, has been effective in treating some individuals with Lassa fever. Treatment with convalescent-phase plasma has been used with success in some patients with Argentine hemorrhagic fever or Ebola. Infected individuals may benefit from supportive therapy.

Other Agents

Emerging Infections

The Institute of Medicine (IOM) in 1992 defined emerging infections as new, re-emerging, or drug-resistant infections whose occurrence in humans has increased within the past two decades, or whose incidence will likely increase in the near future. In addition to increased efforts in the United States, there is a need for an international cooperative effort to monitor, respond to, research, and eradicate newly emerging as well as current infectious disease agents. Influenza, severe acute respiratory syndrome (SARS), tuberculosis, and malaria are few of the emerging infections.

Genetically Engineered Agents

The technology of genetic engineering alters or disrupts the genetic blueprints of living organisms—plants, animals, humans, and microorganisms. Researchers conducting experiments at Michigan State University several years ago found that genetically altering plants to resist viruses can cause the viruses to mutate into new, more virulent forms. Scientists in Oregon found that a genetically engineered soil microorganism, *Klebsiella planticola*, completely killed essential soil nutrients. Environmental Protection Agency whistleblowers issued similar warnings in 1997, protesting government approval of a genetically engineered soil bacterium called *Rhizobium melitoli*.

CONCLUSION

Today, bioterrorism is no longer a threat, but a reality. The tragic events of September 11, 2001, are still fresh in our memories. With the increase of hatred around the world, the likelihood of another biological attack is quite high. Nations around the globe must take the threat of a bioterrorism attack very seriously. Setting up a good surveillance system and promoting cooperation among public health agencies around the world are needed steps to prevent any attack or minimize its effect.

NOTES

1. Arizona Department of Health Services. Definition of bioterrorism. Available from: www.hs.state.az.us/phs/edc/edrp/es/bthistor1.htm. Accessed September 3, 2004.

2. Du J. Bioterrorism: how has it been used? What can it do? How prepared are we? Available from: www.isop.ucla.edu/article.asp?parentid=1352. Accessed September 3, 2004.

3. Amherst J. Letters to Bouquet, Ecuyer, and Croghan [online]. Library of Congress. 1763 June–Aug.

4. Kaye J. Jeffrey Amherst and biological warfare in the Pontiac uprising of 1763. Available from: oprfhs.org/division/history/interpretations/1999interp/Kaye.doc. Accessed September 3, 2004.

5. Markowitz A. Cults and terrorism: understanding indoctrination. Available from: www.cultclinic.org/presentation-terrorist.html. Accessed September 3, 2004.

6. Locy T. FBI fails to re-create anthrax production process. Attempts have produced some leads in attack inquiry. USA Today. 2003 Oct 1. Available from: www.intelmessages.org/Messages/National_Security/wwwboard/messages_03/5704.html.

2 Counterterrorism Training in the Public Sector

Charlane Brown and James O'Keefe

As the nation began to recover from the devastating events that occurred on September 11, 2001, in Pennsylvania, and at the Pentagon and the World Trade Center, American law enforcement, public safety officials, and other first responders employed in public administration immediately inherited a new and ostensibly permanent role—to prevent future acts of international terrorism on American soil.

Prior indications of the international terrorism challenge had been apparent for some time. The U.S. embassy bombings in Kenya and Tanzania in 1998 marked the beginning of a period of heightened awareness. After the U.S.S. *Cole* bombing in 2000, American public officials began to realize seriously that the country faced a specific and, indeed, formidable enemy. "It is clear, and becoming clearer, that the reach and spread of Al Qaeda throughout the world and particularly on the European continent is posing one of the most significant risks to Western democracies" (pp. 102–103).[1] In many ways, international terrorism represented a unique challenge in American history because, since 1968, no more than 1,000 Americans had been killed by terrorist acts in the United States and abroad. Furthermore, no single act of terrorism had ever killed more than 500 people.[2] The terrorist attacks of September 11 established the bloodiest day in America since the 1862 Civil War Battle of Antietam.[3]

For all these reasons, the full recognition and execution of the monumental new task of counterterrorism have now become firmly rooted as a top priority in the mission of public administration. In fact, counterterrorism concerns have triggered the most rapid and dramatic change in the history of U.S. foreign policy. These changes have collectively resulted in the largest and most powerful mobilization of U.S. forces, both military and political, in history.[4] This expansion, and perhaps redefinition, of the public-safety role into counterterrorism is evident in the recent major shifts in agency roles, responsibilities, and organizational structures of many of the organizations even remotely associated with the terrorism fight. Additionally, the rapid enhancement of national legislation, increased staffing levels, and operational funding have all been authorized for the war on terror.

For example, in November 2003, the Department of Homeland Security provided $725 million specifically to enhance counterterrorism security and preparedness levels of urban areas. During that same month, the U.S. government allocated an additional $2.2 billion to support first responders in preparation, response, prevention, and recovery efforts in the war against terrorism.[5] National, state, and local law enforcement agencies have quickly been granted significantly expanded powers in the investigation and interdiction of terrorists through the Uniting and Strengthening America by Providing Appropriate Tools Required to Intercept and Obstruct Terrorism Act (Patriot Act) of 2001. These expanded law enforcement powers include the following:

- Enhanced surveillance procedures
- The International Money Laundering Abate and Antiterrorism Financing Act of 2001
- Improved border protection
- Removing investigative obstacles that involve terrorism
- Funding to provide for the victims of terrorism, public safety officers, and their families
- Increasing information sharing
- Strengthening criminal laws
- Improved intelligence

Clearly, in a relatively short period of time, much about the organizational, operational, legislative, financial, and political components of the war on terror has been accomplished. Much less, however, has been accomplished about the equally compelling responsibility of designing and delivering the appropriate level of education and training required to prepare for the task. Political speeches may set the national tone, and public policy may set the national framework, but only effective education and training can bring about the behavioral changes needed to actually create a safer nation. Public officials involved in law enforcement training have known for years that when a critical incident occurs, public safety officers all rush to the scene and begin saving lives and helping innocent civilians. Because of the way they are trained, they don't stop to consider their own personal safety. They instinctively dash into buildings and up stairs, when everyone else is running out. These typical critical incident scenarios capture the essence of why education and training are so critical to counterterrorism efforts. In a real emergency, public safety officers do exactly what they are trained to do, so it had better be right. Lives literally depend on it.[6]

Associated with the newly expanded role of preventing international terrorism is ensuring that agencies are properly prepared to undertake these new duties and responsibilities that are needed to protect the nation. While some of the tasks can be handled with traditional and well-established law enforcement capabilities, many of the roles and responsibilities are new and counterintuitive to democratic policing.

Some of these newfound roles and responsibilities required to effectively and safely fight the war on terrorism are quite different from traditional law enforcement, and will require quite different training curricula and perspectives. Examples of these broad and innovative education and training challenges include the following considerations:

- Counterterrorism training requires a nontraditional philosophical framework and perspective on what law enforcement in a free society can and should be permitted to do. Traditional law enforcement is trained to promote individual freedoms, while terrorists seek to capitalize on such freedoms.

- Counterterrorism training requires nontraditional education and training that must stress the realization that local, state, and federal law enforcement is no longer a decentralized, isolated occupation, but an interconnected, global one. Effective methods to collect, analyze, and share timely and accurate operational intelligence and interdiction activities must be taught.

- Counterterrorism training requires nontraditional tactics and strategies that must be properly supported by the repetition of training and preparation. It must include a much more thorough and fundamental understanding of the nature of terrorism, including knowledge of the tools and techniques terrorists employ. Effective preparations in the responsibilities and potential issues associated with multiagency first responders are essential. Principles of incident-management systems, and the initial recognition of chemical, biological, cyber, and explosive weapons of mass destruction, are all crucial.

The following does not represent exhaustive coverage of the issues and subject matter appropriate to address in counterterrorism training. Rather, a number of common issues and major considerations will be addressed.

COUNTERTERRORISM AS A GLOBAL ISSUE

Western democracies believe in the sanctity of every human life. They believe in individual freedoms: freedom to say, believe, behave, and move about in total autonomy. International terrorists know this full well, and they focus on these individual freedoms as a strategy of terror. Therefore, among the fundamental objectives to be communicated to emergency responders, and specifically the local law enforcement community, is that addressing terrorism inherently represents the adoption of new roles and responsibilities. In addition to responding to, investigating, and taking summary action for traditional crimes such as robberies, burglaries, and assaults, law enforcement officers will have to learn how to recognize and respond to acts of terrorism.

Training modules addressing this issue should stress that preparing officers to assume this new role will have to involve learning new and nontraditional information and tactics, incorporating traditional practices and tactics, and making an overall change in their daily mindsets. For example, standard patrol practices involving knowledge of a beat and/or patrol area, awareness of current environment and surroundings, and observance of human behavior are just as important in detecting a suspected burglar they are in detecting potential terrorist activity. Visualizing a location and a tactical plan before responding to a scene, or planning tactics while en route to a robbery or fire in progress become even more important en route to a report of suspected terrorist activity. Likewise, police officers should be trained to significantly enhance their intelligence-gathering abilities and properly and promptly report information to agency partners. Just as some existing skills can be beneficial in addressing terrorism threats, officers and first responders will also have to adopt a new mindset to take on the threat posed by terrorism.

On the one hand, when a police officer or other emergency responder arrives on the scene of an incident, many of the same types of traditional duties will still be performed. The first official on site will be expected to secure the scene, establish a command post, initiate communications, assess the scale of overall damage, render first aid to victims, and ensure overall public safety.

On the other hand, however, a terrorist-motivated incident can be significantly different from other emergencies, and therefore responders will have to deal with some new challenges and circumstances.[7] What chiefly distinguishes a terrorist incident from a traditional criminal incident is that the terrorist incident is designed to cause high-profile damage, instill widespread fear, and often to take the lives of many innocent people. By far, terrorist acts transcend the localized danger normally associated with a residential or commercial fire, a street robbery, or a motor vehicle accident. Moreover, many terrorist incidents are not the only to occur, so the initial incident responded to by local authorities may be but one in a series of violent events. In such cases, the first responder is often the target.

Additionally, public safety officials should be educated on the importance of keeping abreast of current world events. Now more than ever, an individual who comes to the attention of a police officer on the streets of New York at 3 a.m. responding to a disturbance may very well be associated with a much broader terrorist plot. Reading the daily newspaper, accessing the Internet on a regular basis, or even incorporating daily events in roll-call officers' briefings can accomplish this. An increased knowledge of global events, current issues, and awareness of how these events can impact a local area, may become an important tool when conducting comprehensive threat assessments or determining whether a terrorist act has occurred. In today's environment, keeping aware of world events is just as important as keeping apprised of local community priorities, agency procedures, and policy changes. The emergency response community must adopt the principle that what happens elsewhere affects what happens here. Now more than ever, public safety officials need to think globally and act locally.

INTERAGENCY COOPERATION

The decisive need for excellent interagency cooperation is another fundamental component of effective counterterrorism education and training. Just as community policing marked a paradigm in law enforcement, where police agencies worked collectively with other agencies and partners to address crime, quality of life, and the fear of crime, so the emergence of counterterrorism training likewise calls for the formation of stronger bonds with all levels of a community, other law enforcement, and emergency responders. Federal reviews undertaken in the aftermath of September 11, 2001, have acknowledged the importance of embedding a firm mechanism for constant communication between all law enforcers and emergency response personnel. Associated with this need is an international recognition that first responders worldwide need to communicate better and exchange ideas and intelligence, methodology, and technology. The overall goals and objectives of any effective counterterrorism training should, therefore, include discussion of this expanded mission of enhanced intra-agency and interagency communication. For example, James Kallstrom, senior advisor on homeland security to New York Governor George Pataki, recently said that "nearly 70,000 cops across New York State who should be used as foot soldiers in the war on terror are out of the loop" when it came to accessing vital intelligence. In municipal policing today, a reliable, accurate, and current briefing and communication system to pass on crucial actionable intelligence to local street cops is still absent.

To further enhance the overall effectiveness of counterterrorism training, at some point in the training curriculum, a working definition of terrorism should be provided. Although there is no universally accepted definition of terrorism, the Federal Bureau of Investigation (FBI) divides the terrorism threat currently facing the United States into two broad categories:

- *Domestic terrorism* is the unlawful use, or threatened use, of violence by a group or individual based and operating entirely within the United States (or its territories) without foreign direction. The domestic terrorist commits its actions against persons or property to intimidate or coerce a government, the civilian population, or any segment thereof to further its political or social objectives.
- *International terrorism* involves violent acts or acts dangerous to human life that violate the criminal laws of the United States or any state, or that would be a criminal violation if committed within the jurisdiction of the United States or any state. These acts transcend national boundaries in the means by which they are accomplished, the persons they appear intended to intimidate, or the locales in which the perpetrators operate.

What the myriad of existing definitions does not underscore, but which should be emphasized in training, is that the foundation of terrorism rests on the ability to communicate and provoke fear.[8] Training should therefore center on efforts of the emergency service community to lessen public fear of terrorism, just as the emergency service community should work to abate fear created by other emergencies or natural disasters.

As recent catastrophic events around the globe have demonstrated, both domestic and international terrorist organizations represent a significant threat to Americans within the borders of the United States. International terrorists have virtually unlimited targets. Targets include government, the commercial/industrial complex, transportation, recreation, and other miscellaneous sites. Potential targets include, but are not limited, to the following:

Government sites

- Law enforcement office buildings and precincts
- Federal, state, and local courthouses
- State and local emergency operating centers
- Military installations
- International embassies
- U.S. Post Office buildings

Commercial/Industrial sites

- Business/corporate centers and banks
- Large office complexes
- Malls and shopping centers
- Hotels and convention centers
- Apartment buildings
- Nuclear power plants
- Water supply plants
- Utilities/power supply systems

Transportation hubs

- Airports
- Subway stations
- Train stations
- Bus terminals and bus stops
- Ferry terminals and seaports
- Tunnels and bridges

Recreational sites

- Sports arenas/stadiums
- Movie theaters
- Concert halls and auditoriums
- Parks

- Museums
- Tourist attractions
- Restaurants/bars/nightclubs

Miscellaneous sites

- Abortion clinics
- Animal research facilities
- Hospitals and medical centers
- Campaign headquarters or political conventions
- Churches, temples, or mosques
- Academic institutions
- Television or newspaper facilities
- Special events, parades, festivals, or celebrations
- Historical buildings, landmarks, or monuments
- Food storage areas (meat packing/processing plants, grain silos, etc.)

DEVELOPMENT AND DELIVERY OF COUNTERTERRORISM TRAINING

Embarking upon a comprehensive counterterrorism education and training curriculum for an agency involves a number of important considerations. These considerations may include the following:

- A significant and genuine commitment from the command staff. Counterterrorism training is labor-intensive, counterintuitive to patrol-allocation models, and expensive. It is a long-term commitment, not the topic of the month.
- A major needs assessment review before training begins. Existing officer capabilities and expertise must be assessed and documented before new training can be developed and delivered.
- A major organizational role assessment should be conducted with the chief of patrol, chief of detectives, chief of counterterrorism, and other key operational commanders. Different public safety organizations have different missions and different priorities and offer unique contributions to the war on terrorism. That is why the operations people, not the training people, must develop any new counterterrorism tactics and strategies. Training directors should develop and offer educational and training experiences that provide the requisite skills to implement approved tactics. Training directors at any level should never get involved in policymaking by default.
- A significant commitment must be made to curriculum development and review. This commitment must incorporate an international review

of the police administration and intelligence community literature, and community threat assessment reports.[9]

- A genuine instructional methodology should be developed around facilitating interagency and interdisciplinary role plays and mock exercises. Traditionally, interagency training has been challenging and awkward to schedule, but these distinctions between agencies can no longer be tolerated.

The educational and training component of counterterrorism is absolutely critical in so many dimensions. Therefore, careful consideration should be given to each of these issues before training can commence.

In assessing an agency's training needs, general considerations should allow for organizational variables such as agency size, operational timetables, available funds, and other training resources. To facilitate this process, the Department of Homeland Security has recently established a number of excellent resources for agencies wishing to embark upon training in this area. Other excellent federal resources are available, such as the State and Local Anti-Terrorism Training Program (SLATT) currently being created to deliver basic terrorism training for all 650,000 American law enforcement personnel.

Before counterterrorism training can begin, prudent consideration must also be given to an agency's mission. For example, it must be determined specifically what role an agency will play in the response to, or detection of, terrorist activities. This is an extremely broad consideration, however, given the scope of the potential terrorism threat. Public safety encounters are possible in the police, fire, ambulance, parks, and many other first-responder services. Existing and prepackaged education and training terrorism materials should be carefully reviewed to ensure that emergency response plans are up to date, operationally appropriate, and consistent with the stated mission of an agency. All related agency policy and procedure guides should be reviewed to determine whether policy determinations have been made concerning agency response to a terrorist threat; for example, whether an agency has a response plan in place to address a biological attack such as the contamination of a water plant. Most agencies are probably aware that a wealth of professional training information is available from the federal government, armed forces, law enforcement, and public health agencies; and they should be viewed as resources in shaping specific training objectives.

INTERAGENCY TRAINING

For many years, interagency training has been seen as a precondition to interagency cooperation. To a large extent, interagency training has never materialized, nor has interagency cooperation. This always has been, and continues to be, a major organizational and operational barrier to the successful fight against terrorism. The crucial need for interagency training parallels the nation's crucial need for increased information sharing between the intelligence community and domestic law enforcement. In addition to this link, other first responders (fire, emergency medical services, etc.) should also consider holding joint training sessions, especially in the area of critical incident command issues. In Maryland, for example, fire and law enforcement response personnel attended an "incident command course" offered by the U.S. Fire Administration. This joint course allowed representatives from the respective agencies to realize and resolve the practical issues that arise in the management of terrorist and other large-scale incidents where multiple agencies are providing services. The course addresses four major areas:

- Overview and historical information concerning the Incident Command System
- Incident assessment and development of incident action plans
- Incident-scene decision-making
- Emergency operations center coordination in which agency representatives collaborate under the direction of a unified incident commander

A review of current counterterrorism curricula suggests that all training should cover, at a minimum, the following topics:

- The history and evolution of international terrorism
- The responder's role vis-à-vis the agency's mission
- Targets and tactics
- Weapons of mass destruction; and chemical, biological, and radiological agents
- Critical incident response and protective equipment

Another issue that constantly arises when addressing terrorism education and training is the importance of identifying and being able to communicate specific acts and behavior based upon the totality of the circumstances.

Special care should be taken to ensure that individuals are not singled out solely due to their religious or political affiliation or identification with a particular group. Hasty decisions in this area will undoubtedly lead to serious problems such as faulty intelligence, insufficient or subsequently excluded evidence, charges of illicit profiling, civil rights abuses, and even the possible disenfranchisement of an entire involved community. In fact, the need to collect vital intelligence chiefly depends on the community that emergency responders defend.

As noted by the Center for Domestic Preparedness, most agencies engaged in emergency response possess the requisite training and equipment to meet the routine challenges called for by their duties. The issue, therefore, becomes the availability of personal protective equipment for additional secondary responders and training resources for this class of personnel.

DEVELOPING AND TEACHING EFFECTIVE INVESTIGATIVE METHODS

All first responders, regardless of whether their primary agency responsibilities involve fire, rescue, hazardous material identification, or public safety, should be aware of "possible indicators" of criminal activity. Any scene can potentially become a crime scene, and any crime scene can potentially be connected to international terrorism.

Therefore, in the fight against terrorism, it is necessary for all emergency responders to understand the fundamental nature of criminal investigation. Important factors such as securing the initial crime scene to facilitate the collection of physical evidence, as well as the need to gather intelligence before, during, and after the occurrence of an act, may become critical to an investigation.

First and foremost, evidence at a crime scene may take the form of physical evidence or even oral statements made by witnesses and/or victims. It should be reinforced that all responders also become part of a crime scene, and may be required to serve as witnesses in a formal proceeding at a later date. Therefore, there is a critical need for training to ensure that all evidence is properly identified, collected, and preserved.

All first responders can aid law enforcement efforts by taking a number of steps to achieve these goals. As a fundamental principle, physical evidence can offer incontestable facts, as opposed to oral statements, which are subject to memories faded by trauma, time, and other causes of ambiguity. So physical evidence also serves to establish a nexus between people and a scene. Both types of evidence, of course, are helpful if a successful prosecution is to occur. First responders should take care when entering an unknown scene and avoid actions that may damage potential physical evidence or compromise an investigation. Such actions may result in the inadmissibility of evidence in court.

Another important point to emphasize during training is that, if in doubt, simply securing a scene and delaying entry may ultimately preserve evidence and allow time for other responders with appropriate equipment and expertise to decontaminate an area.[7]

GATHERING POTENTIAL TERRORIST INTELLIGENCE

First responders should also be trained to identify how to gather and record all possible intelligence with an eye toward noting any potential terrorist activity. First responders sometimes arrive at a scene after receiving a call to the location. At other times, their arrival on the scene of an incident is coincidental and inadvertent. In both cases, the one-time opportunity to obtain and report important intelligence may present itself. In order to provide for the efficient collection, analysis, and timely dissemination of useful criminal information regarding potential terrorism, law enforcement and other responders should be thoroughly trained to observe irregular or suspicious behavior and report the information. Some local law enforcement agencies have established internal intelligence units and joint task forces. Many states and local law enforcement authorities have also established hotlines to report information about terrorist activity. First responders should be armed with these hotline numbers, and know how to immediately report suspicious activity.

Reporting involves obtaining as much information as possible, including names, vehicle descriptions, time of day, and descriptions of persons involved. Even in this day and age of emerging technology, human intelligence and information are the most valuable tools for criminal investigations. The police alone do not solve crime—accurate and timely information solves crime.

A related need is to gather initial information suitable to make complete notifications to an emergency communications center, hospitals, medical personnel, 911 communications personnel, and other key responders. Responders should ensure that all initial information is accurate and timely. In addition to facilitating initial crime scene assessments, accurate and complete information will also reduce the incidence of casualties. The amount of information initially forwarded to communications centers should also be timely and detailed enough to facilitate the centers' efforts to make necessary preparations and deploy the needed resources and response plans.

For critical incident operations to run correctly, it is necessary for 911 dispatchers and operators nationwide to be trained to take quick action when notified of a possible terrorist act or an act involving potential weapons of mass destruction. Communicating basic information requires the ability to distinguish between a terrorist act and a natural catastrophe or hazardous materials (HAZMAT) incident; and to identify the weapons of mass destruction involved, alert responders, and make all the subsequent safety notifications.[7]

Still another essential education and training point to note is that, due to terrorism falling under federal criminal statutes, such acts mandate federal jurisdiction over crisis management. Federal involvement may require standard operating procedures and close coordination with various FBI components, such as field offices and evidence-collection teams. The establishment and joint training of a multiagency liaison or group can prove instrumental in planning and coordinating crime scene stability; and should include EMS personnel, hospitals, the coroner's staff, local law enforcement forensic staff, FBI liaison, and an evidence-response team. Together each of these representatives can incorporate their particular procedures into a comprehensive incident action plan and establish consistency when approaching incidents. Such efforts as the Joint Terrorist Task Forces (JTTF) have been started in each of the FBI field offices throughout the country.

The reality is that when a genuine terrorist incident occurs, the complex issues and contingencies present an enormous number of challenges for first responders. Because of this, the need for major interaction and coordination with key federal, state, and local agencies is crucial, and that reality is effectively communicated through education and training.

When a terrorism incident occurs, an incident commander is designated with the responsibility to deploy all responding personnel. Responders, therefore, should be instructed to plan and prepare to convert from a single-agency to a multiagency, unified command structure. Responders may also be expected to assist coordination with multiple agencies. Naturally, agencies should be continuously cautioned to avoid communication overload.

In any multiagency deployment, the need for familiarizing participants through training with standard agency procedure is paramount. In
addition to communicating standard protocols, personnel can serve for
unilateral observation. This will allow agencies to anticipate and understand how other agencies will respond. Notwithstanding the existence
of standard procedures, incidents involving terrorism will always involve
on-the-spot decisions based on changing conditions. There will always
be areas where discretion is required and that standard operating procedures will not address.

TEACHING THE NATURE OF TERRORISM

Arguably, one of the first substantive topics to be included in a counterterrorism training course is communication of the fundamental principles of terrorism, emphasizing the unique ideology and methodology
of terrorist activity. The fundamentally different, nontraditional, asym-
metrical nature of terrorism truly places the traditional tactics and strategies of law enforcement at a disadvantage. As mentioned earlier, the
implications of terrorism and the intent and motivation of terrorists
require the adoption of a new mindset. The threat that terrorism poses
in a free society and the terrorists' efforts to perpetuate permanent fear
requires careful review of the nature of terrorism. Understanding this
crucial topic is the first step in ensuring preparedness and the provision
of a sound training curriculum.

Readiness presupposes response, and training presupposes readiness.
Any curriculum addressing counterterrorism should begin with an overview of the fundamental nature of terrorism. Just as an understanding
of criminology supports an understanding of why people engage in
crime, an understanding of the causes and conditions that support terrorism promotes understanding about why the resulting activity can
have a devastating and lasting effect on a community. Delivery of this
training may be accomplished by discussing the history and development of terrorist groups, a general description of activities terrorist
groups engage in, and an overview of domestic terrorism as distinguished from international terrorism.

Although one may argue that recent events underscore the dangers
of terrorism, discussions of these topics are important for a number of
reasons. First, offering a historical perspective of terrorism helps classroom participants understand the ideology, tactics, and operations of
terrorist groups. This understanding also facilitates discussion about
why a group or groups select potential targets for their activities.

Through illustration and example, course participants will gain a greater understanding of the threat that terrorism poses to day-to-day existence. Therefore, explaining the fundamental nature of terrorism through real-life examples will increase knowledge of why a local mall or residential building is as much a target as a government building, or why a local elected official or a small town may be as important to developing intelligence as a large city, or why an individual with a strong position on an issue might be as dangerous as an organized group. Laying a proper foundation for first responders and other emergency personnel reinforces the importance of the participants' duties.

One of the first questions often posed concerning a training module addressing an overview and history of terrorism is the amount of time spent on and depth of material. On the one hand, extensive information in this area may bog down the most interested of participants and dilute the importance of the message. On the other hand, significant attention should be paid to this portion of the training because it sets the framework for participants' responses. Although no definite balance has been clearly established, some information in this very important area must be included in counterterrorism curricula.

One way to enhance the interest of participants is to include timely and topical information concerning current events that have an impact upon American interests, both domestically and abroad. Updating curricula in this area is as easy as suggesting that instructors consult their local papers and supplement trainings with current events. Addressing current events also reinforces the need for emergency responders to continue this practice to gain a greater understanding of the importance of connecting emergency incidents with contemporary political and social events.

TRAINING IN THE INITIAL RECOGNITION OF CHEMICAL, BIOLOGICAL, CYBER, AND EXPLOSIVE WEAPONS OF MASS DESTRUCTION

Although it may not be as critical for an emergency responder to immediately recognize that an incident may be related to an act of terrorism, it is critical that an emergency responder *immediately* assess whether the cause of a particular incident stems from one of the common methods employed in warfare. These can be very large and difficult to find, and they create catastrophic, dynamic incidents with large explosions and clouds of smoke. However, many of the weapons typically employed by terrorists are easily concealed and readily obtainable by average people. In addition, as distinguished from incidents involving a natural disaster or a hazardous material spill, use of chemical agents or weapons of mass destruction is clearly intentional and deliberate. The incidents occurring on September 11, 2001, the subsequent reports of anthrax dissemination through the mail system, and the threat to or destruction of domestic nuclear plants are very real and very contemporary examples of the modes utilized to promote terrorism.[7]

Therefore, it is important to augment training with an overview of the various chemical, toxic, incendiary, and other weapons. The FEMA-adopted acronym B-NICE may be familiar to emergency responders and describes the five categories of terrorist incidents: biological, nuclear, incendiary, chemical, and explosive. A presentation of the general background of each of these categories should address the chief characteristics of each, how each may be utilized as a weapon, the potential damage, the general composition of each, how to recognize it, and how these agents are created and where they may be found.

Biological agents such as anthrax, smallpox, and ricin can be rapidly spread, are readily available, pose serious threats, and have the capacity to cause significant casualties. People may be exposed to them by inhalation, injection, or skin absorption. The four most common types of biological agents are bacteria, viruses, rickettsia, and toxins. Terrorists may adapt any of these agents for use as weapons.

Nuclear incidents may result after either the use or detonation of a nuclear bomb or a conventional explosive containing nuclear material. Although most nuclear sites are placed under high levels of security, the potential for compromise should be considered. A nuclear explosive could cripple daily activities and pose extreme long-term health hazards for first responders. It could preclude complete environmental decontamination. Similarly, the detonation of a truck or car bomb near a nuclear site could cause sweeping damage. Possible symptoms of nuclear exposure include skin irritation or burns, nausea, vomiting, and hair loss.

Incendiary devices produce flames that result in burning rather than an explosion. Incendiary devices range in size and complexity limited only by the capacity and creativity of the makers. These devices should be treated like other hazardous materials and require proper handling for safety concerns and the preservation of a crime scene.

Chemical agents are functionally divided, according to their effects, to either incapacitate or be toxic once ingested. In general, military classifications distinguish chemical agents. Federal agencies utilize the military distinctions when discussing these agents; therefore, familiarity with the vocabulary of emergency response is important to ease the flow of interagency communication. There are five types of chemical agents: nerve, blister, blood, choking, and irritating. These agents primarily cripple the respiratory tract and damage body tissue. Because some chemical agents possess a distinct odor, emergency response personnel should be aware of how witnesses or victims describe the odor. It should be noted that because some chemical agents act to damage the respiratory tract, smell might not be the best mode of detection. Sources of chemical agents include chemical plants, food-processing and -storage facilities, gasoline tanks, pesticide manufacturers and distributors, and medical research laboratories. Other points to consider concerning dissemination of chemical agents include downwind hazard predictions, weather, buildings, and terrain.

General knowledge of explosives is particularly important for firefighters, emergency personnel, and law enforcement in their role of first responders in case they encounter a bomb, receive or respond to a bomb threat, or respond in the aftermath of an explosion related to a terrorist act. In addition, terrorists may use explosions to distribute other toxic materials, such as chemical agents.

At a minimum, at the completion of a training module for explosives, the first responder should recognize the potential hazards of explosive devices, understand how these items are constructed, explain the damage that these explosives can cause, and be able to conduct a safe search of an interior/exterior device directed at responders. When presenting material addressing explosive devices, the following minimum objectives are suggested:

- Explain why terrorists use bombs.
- Explain how bombs are used, including suicide and truck bombs.
- Explain how a bomb works and how it causes damage.
- Explain the components of bombs and explosives.
- Explain the procedures to follow upon the notification or discovery of a suspicious package or bomb threat.
- Explain the procedures to follow at the scene of a bombing.
- Explain the general search procedure.
- Explain the measures for safety and self-preservation.

Again, much of the material presented in this training module will incorporate agency standard operating procedures as well as universal safety precautions. If it exists, agency policy on receiving intelligence about bomb threats or discovery of a suspicious package should be repeated to participants. Firefighters and police should be mindful that in their roles as first responders, they may be vulnerable targets; therefore, personal safety is paramount. Discussions concerning bomb components and explosives should emphasize that devices may be created with materials that are readily found in hardware stores or other general locations. Such "household" explosive items can be fashioned from cell phones, thermostats, knives, nails, and balloons. Bombs can be disguised as and/or concealed in many objects, including letters, packages, or briefcases.[10] It is generally helpful to show pictures or diagrams when discussing this module.

Training material should be supplemented to include segments addressing suicide and truck bombings. Domestically, both types of bombing are rare, or have occurred at all in the case of suicide bombings. Suicide bombings are not a new phenomenon. Bomb explosions account for a significant portion of terrorist activity. Truck bombings were cited in the attacks on the World Trade Center attack in 1993 and the Alfred Murrah federal building in Oklahoma City in 1995. Tightened security to thwart incidents of suicide bombings has increased the threat to so-called "soft" targets such as police.[11] An account of the events of both incidents may illustrate the extent of devastation that can occur.

These methods are more often used abroad, however. Suicide attackers and car bombers have attacked military targets. Bombs have been detonated at police stations, causing casualties to officers.[12] In this area, responders should be acquainted with the behavioral and physical indicators and basic information should be included in an explosives training module to increase awareness of these methods.

Among the many documented motives of suicide bombers is revenge, whether religious, ideological or personal. The success of both suicide and truck bombers is contingent upon their maintaining secrecy, conducting extensive surveillance and rehearsals, and receiving support both financial and in kind. Among the resources provided to these terrorists are accommodations, explosive equipment, intelligence, and funds. Indicators include climate-inappropriate dress, anxiety, oblivion to one's immediate surroundings, the presence of chemical burns, missing limbs, and unfamiliarity with the operation of the vehicle or route. Vehicle indicators for truck bombings include few markings, or markings made by hand, tape, or magnet; vehicles transporting spoiled or unproductive loads (produce, waste products, old tires, etc.); noticeably sagging vehicles; and containing unusual items inside.

TEACHING THE USE OF SAFETY EQUIPMENT

When addressing the response to a suspected explosive device, in addition to communicating the need for rendering first aid and protecting the lives of fellow first responders and others at the scene, it is particularly important to maintain evidence integrity by following the well-established law enforcement policy of demarking a large area as crime scene and restricting access of vehicles and personnel into the area. This is of particular importance and warrants discussion when addressing emergency response personnel. Responders associated with law enforcement will be keenly versed in crime-scene preservation and investigation. Emergency management personnel, firefighters, and emergency medical service personnel, on the other hand, may require additional training in this area. All responders should be mindful that response to a scene requires special demands in addition to personal safety. As noted above, incidents involving terrorism or weapons of mass destruction are considered federal crimes, and therefore the areas involved are federal crime scenes; hence, federal agencies assume jurisdiction over crisis management that dictates the need to establish a proper crime scene and preserve evidence.

One critical and essential point to communicate through training in this area is that, notwithstanding the occurrence of a natural disaster, any other incident may simultaneously become a crime scene. Therefore, the first responder will have to coordinate with other responding agencies to ensure the preservation of evidence. A second but equally important point is that first responders to a terrorist incident are also part of the crime scene and are therefore potential witnesses. Consequently, emergency responders may be interviewed by investigative response personnel and required to testify in court or another tribunal.

Therefore, it is critical that personnel maintain notes and take other steps to preserve their recollection of the scene. The description that an emergency responder provides in the early phase of activity can result in a productive investigation and subsequent prosecution. First responders should also disturb as little evidence as possible. Tire treads and boots, for example, can remove or damage evidence.[7] Other suggestions include reporting persons who enter and leave the scene, noting whether these individuals were on foot or in vehicles, noting car descriptions and license plate numbers, and asking bystanders to remain on the scene for investigators. Taking notes and drawing sketches and photographs can be extremely helpful in evidence collection.

FIRST RESPONDER PERSONAL SAFETY

No course addressing the activity of first responders would be complete without a component concerning personal safety and the safety of victims at the scene. Personal safety must be among the primary considerations when responding to a scene of terrorist activity.

Lives would not be saved, subsequent precautionary measures would not be implemented, and investigations would not commence if first responders succumbed to the dangers of a terrorist-ravaged location. Complicating this issue is that a single incident can produce numerous hazards. First responders should be alert for secondary devices and should take care when approaching injured persons. A scene damaged by radioactive, chemical, or biological agents is a contaminated scene; so initial entry should be extremely cautious. In addition, exposure caused by those agents may result in building collapses, fires, explosions, and other risks. First responders should use extreme caution when entering these areas and utilize personal protective equipment (PPE). As illustrated above, in many instances the first responder will have to utilize judgment to distinguish between the safety of individuals at the scene and evidence integrity.

Before embarking on discussions concerning PPE, it may be helpful to discuss hazard recognition and potential damage. Each incident, whether nuclear, biological, or chemical, can present one or many hazards. First responders entering emergency scenes may be subjected to thermal, mechanical, radiological, asphyxiate, chemical, etiological, or psychological damage. For example, biological incidents could cause etiological hazards and result in community public health emergencies such as the spread of smallpox; explosive incidents could create mechanical hazards such as nails or shrapnel and could pose multiple hazards.[7] The potential for harm varies by the type or combination of exposures. Emergency responders should identify and evaluate the risk of harm before devising an appropriate response.

Another important training component involves the proper use of PPE. Different types of PPE exist and offer varying levels of protection. To date, there is no known piece of equipment that provides protection against every agent at every exposure level. Agencies are advised to research the availability of items to ascertain which PPE offers the most protection to what the agents' responders would be most likely to encounter.[7]

It should be noted that the Occupational Safety and Health Administration (OSHA) has outlined guidelines, as the amounts of skin protection and respiratory protection offered by a particular PPE determine the level of protection for the responder.

Some public safety members may already be familiar with the range of PPE equipment available in your agency. Therefore, trainers should offer an overview at a level appropriate to the participants. At a minimum, however, a module addressing PPE should enable participants to identify various types; to identify the equipment components of PPE; and to describe possible psychological and physiological challenges when donning PPE. A practical exercise would involve the responder demonstrating proper procedures for assembling PPE as well as reinforcing familiarity with equipment. Included in this material should also be discussion of self-contained breathing apparatus (SCBA). Responders should be reminded to utilize protective clothing/SCBA and body armor for bombing incidents.

Finally, the Office of Homeland Security color alert should be explained along with what it means to the particular agency. The Department of Homeland Security currently maintains an advisory system that rates threat conditions using a six-color scheme. Each threat condition, from low to severe, represents increasing risk of a terrorist attack. Accompanying each threat condition are recommended protective measures for agencies to implement. The threat levels are as follows:

GREEN = Low risk of terrorist attack

The following measures may be applied:

- Refining and exercising preplanned protective measures
- Providing regularly scheduled training
- Routinely assessing facilities for vulnerabilities and taking measures to reduce them

BLUE = General risk of terrorist attack

In addition to the previously outlined protective measures, the following may apply:

- Checking communications with designated emergency response and command locations
- Reviewing and updating emergency response procedures
- Providing the public with necessary information

YELLOW = Significant risk of terrorist attack

In addition to the previously outlined protective measures, the following may apply:

- Increasing surveillance of critical locations
- Coordinating emergency plans with nearby jurisdictions
- Assessing further refinement of protective measures within the context of available information
- Implementing contingency and emergency response plans as appropriate

ORANGE = High risk of terrorist attack

In addition to the previously outlined protective measures, the following may apply:

- Coordinating necessary security efforts with armed forces and/or law enforcement agencies
- Taking additional precautions, as necessary, at public events

RED = Severe risk of terrorist attack

In addition to the previously outlined protective measures, the following may apply:

- Assigning emergency response personnel and pre-positioning specially trained teams
- Monitoring, redirecting, or constraining transportation systems
- Closing public and government facilities
- Increasing or redirecting personnel to address critical emergency needs

TEACHING THE BASIC PRINCIPLES OF THE "INCIDENT MANAGEMENT SYSTEM"

The Incident Management System was devised in 1970 to respond to a series of wildfires in southern California.[7] This incident resulted in the recognition that increased coordination was required when more than one agency responded to an emergency. The approach that evolved has been applied to a comprehensive response system appropriate for all emergencies. Two key components of the Incident Management System are a cohesive organizational structure and standard management principles. Federal law mandates the use of such a system as a response to HAZMAT incidents. Many states and professional associations, including the International Association of Chiefs of Police and the National Fire Protection Association, use this as their standard. The Incident Management System is also part of the National Interagency Incident Management System (NIIMS).

The Incident Management System (IMS) coordinates effective response of personnel and deployment of resources.[7] It is organized with the recognition that no one agency can take ultimate control to manage an emergency. Therefore, the IMS is organized into five major components: incident command, operations, logistics, planning, and administration. These components form the bedrock of the emergency scene and can range in size from one person and one component to a number of separate management components.

The incident commander directs the command function. This person takes charge of the entire scene and makes assessments, identifies contingencies, deploys resources, and takes action based on a planned organizational structure. Challenges for the incident commander include provision of appropriate protective clothing/SCBA, personnel rotation/deployment, secondary explosive devices, weather, evacuations, location of the incident command post, hazard assessments, communication considerations, crime-scene considerations, media coordination, and response.

The operations section is charged with implementing response activities outlined by the incident commander as well as coordinated section activities, including requesting resources through the incident commander and keeping the incident commander informed of conditions and resource availability.

The logistics section is responsible for providing facilities, materials, and services, including equipment and staff for the incident. The logistics functions are support for the incident responders.

The planning section collects, evaluates, and disseminates information about the development of the incident and the status of resources.

Finally, the administration section tracks incident costs, reimbursement, and accounting.

There are two possible terrorist response scenarios for incident command. Either the terrorist event is warned or it occurs without notice. If the latter, the local emergency response community will undoubtedly arrive through a 911 call. Here, the incident commander must be aware that responders may be initially left to their own devices for several hours. In this instance, local governments and agencies should adopt "stand alone" plans that would be activated until additional resources arrived. Agencies should be reminded that local Offices of Emergency Management will notify the state to request federal assistance.

TEACHING THE STRATEGIES OF MASS DECONTAMINATION

Training should incorporate some discussion concerning the need to decontaminate personnel in the wake of an incident involving a weapon of mass destruction (WMD). Minimum objectives should incorporate the distinction between weapons of mass destruction and HAZMAT decontamination, purposes of decontamination, and emergency decontamination considerations. Again, a practical hands-on exercise in which the responder demonstrates facility with the materials presented is helpful. Trainers may also wish to test knowledge of technical procedure and knowledge of different decontaminants and construction of a decontamination corridor.

Through this material, it should be communicated that responders should decontaminate swiftly to save lives, while being mindful that hasty actions will frustrate the process. Another key point to illustrate is that unlike some HAZMAT scenarios, WMD incidents will involve large numbers of victims. Therefore, there is a need for tracking, crowd control, and triage of mass victims. The increased number of personnel on the scene will also complicate matters and call for a more coordinated response. Responders should be reminded not to damage evidence in the decontamination process, since a WMD incident is also a federal crime.

Ultimately, the safety of responders is foremost, and safety precautions should be reiterated. A few key points to remember when conducting decontamination are

- Responder safety.
- Swift, effective decontamination using water, soap, and/or bleach.
- *Continuous* training to ensure proper readiness to perform decontamination procedures whenever necessary.

CONCLUSION

As recent events around the world have adequately illustrated, the importance of changing the methods and training of law enforcement and first response for fire and emergency services personnel cannot be overstated. The Department of Homeland Security has given a high priority to training when our nation is under the lowest level of threat status. To maximize preparation and resource allocation, counterterrorism training should be ongoing, irrespective of the threat level. In many ways, the local emergency service community occupies the front line in the fight to effectively combat global terrorism. Training in this area must transcend a simple, routine communication of agency policy and should actually translate into a transformation of thinking and performance. Education, training, vigilance, planning, safety, and interagency communication are all crucial components to protecting homeland security.

In the war on international terrorism, failure is not an option. The time-tested and proven strategies for winning the war are effective education and training.

NOTES

1. Simonsen CE, Spindlove J. Terrorism today: the past, the players, and the future. Upper Saddle River, NJ: Pearson Prentice Hall; 2004.

2. Hoffman B. Rethinking terrorism and counterterrorism since 9/11. Studies in Conflict and Terrorism 2002;25:303–16.

3. Taylor FX. Terrorism: U.S. policies and counterterrorism measures. U.S. Foreign Policy Agenda 2001;6(3):7–9.

4. Bennis P. Before and after: U.S. foreign policy and the war on terrorism. New York: Olive Branch; 2003.

5. DHS announces $2.2 billion for state and local first responders source. Available from: www.dhs.gov/dhspublic/index.jsp. Accessed November 14, 2003; U.S. Department of Homeland Security. Understanding the homeland security advisory system. Available from: www.dhs.gov. Accessed December 12, 2003; Securing the homeland: helping our state and local first responders and first preventors. Available from: www.dhs.gov/dhspublic/index.jsp. Accessed November 14, 2003.

6. O'Keefe J. Protecting the republic: the education and training of American police officers. Upper Saddle River, NJ: Pearson Prentice Hall; 2003.

7. Office for Domestic Preparedness, Center for Domestic Preparedness, COBRA. Technical emergency response training responder guide. Emergency response to terrorism self-study. FEMA, U.S. Fire Administration; 1999.

8. Dean J. Examining the president's powers to fight terrorism. 2003. Available from: www.findlaw.com. Accessed December 18, 2003.

9. Flynt B, Olin R. The red, gray, and blue model: a new tool to help law enforcement executives address the transformed security environment. The Police Chief 2002;69:50–8.

10. Pickett M. Explosives: identification guide. Albany, NY: Delmar Publishers; 1999.

11. Suicide bombers strike at 2 U.S. bases, wounding dozens of GI's. New York Times 2003 Dec 10; Attacks go on; kills 6 Iraqi officers. New York Times 2003 Dec 13.

12. Stern J. How America created a terrorist haven. New York Times 2003.

3 Cyberterrorism: A Strategic Perspective

Nejdet Delener

Network security has always been a major concern for information technology (IT) professionals eager to protect the secured information owned by businesses and government agencies. Given the growing dependence of many elements of business and the nation's infrastructure on computers, cyberterrorism has become a primary security issue for every private and public sector since the attack on the World Trade Center in 2001. To understand the consequences that cyberterrorists could bring to our society, we need to know clearly who the cyberterrorists are, what they are able to do, and how they pose threats to the nation and its people. Ultimately, we need to apply effective measures to protect both business and government from future terrorist acts.

Cyberterrorism is simply defined by the Federal Bureau of Investigation (FBI) as "the unlawful use of force or violence against persons or property to intimidate or coerce a [g]overnment, the civilian population, or any segment thereof, in furtherance of political or social objectives."[1] In most cases, cyberterrorism always shows a strong correlation between political attacks and military conflicts. Cyberterrorism can be understood as generally involving the misuse of information technology to hack into computer systems and websites to corrupt, amend, deface, and/or destroy data in order to further a political cause. Cyberterrorist acts such as intruding into government agencies, interrupting online transactions to gather critical information, or even controlling systems at a nuclear power plant, could pose threats to our security. Although there still has been no salient warning for any potential cyberterrorist attacks against American agencies or companies since the September 11 incident, 90 percent of large U.S. corporations and government agencies have detected computer security breaches, according to the FBI and a survey by the San Francisco-based Computer Security Institute. Eighty percent of the affected companies and agencies claimed that the breaches resulted in financial losses, and half of these corporations and agencies said their losses were significant, totaling $456 million.[2] Furthermore, the number of computer security breaches is on the rise. The U.S. Department of Defense, tracked 82,094 incidents in 2002 and 42,586 in just the first quarter of 2003.

The Internet is a vulnerable infrastructure, and criminal activity on it is growing. The FBI reports that on October 21, 2002, all of the thirteen root-name servers that provide the primary road map for almost all Internet communications were targeted in a massive attack. Seven servers failed completely, and two others partially failed.[3] The increasing dependence on computers to manage and operate our critical infrastructures provides a prime target for cyberterrorists.

THE MAJOR THREATS OF CYBERTERRORISM

Technologically prepared terrorists may view cyberterrorism as an effective way to carry out their attacks. The idea of a digital Pearl Harbor, where some great attack sweeps over the nation's IT system, is a concern. Aside from the political message that they would like to spread by defacing websites, cyberterrorists might want to gain control of critical data and facilities in order to prepare destructive terrorist acts. Imagine how cyberterrorists could use electronic fraud—breaking into banking or credit card systems—to finance their operations. At the same time, they also could steal agencies' records to create identities for themselves. There is a concern that likely targets of cyberterrorism will include electric power or water plant facilities, or the banking and financial systems. Experts predict that the most likely targets for a cyberterrorism attack would be in telecommunications, transportation networks, emergency services, government operations, utilities, and the food supply.[4]

Cyberterrorists primarily cause disturbances in digital systems and computer data through a variety of methods such as viruses, worms, Trojan horses, blended threats, spam, pop-up ads, denial-of-service attacks, and identity theft. These methods of destruction, invasion, and intrusion are becoming easier and more accessible to the average computer-literate individual. The skills necessary to operate these forms of terrorism no longer require that sophisticated methods be implemented by their perpetrators. The paragraphs below explain each of the methods cyberterrorists could utilize to accomplish their activities.

The *basic virus* is a software package designed to invade computers and networks through e-mail or Internet connections, where it attaches itself to a file, programs, or the hard drive and then replicates itself. Viruses often present taunting messages, destroy files, or crash computers. An example is Loveletter, which in 2000 caused $8 billion in damage globally. Virus attacks are growing rapidly. In the first half of 2003, a total of 76,404 virus assaults were reported.[5]

Then there is the *worm*, which can spread itself automatically over a network from one computer to the next. Users need not click on their e-mail or open a program to be infected. An example of a worm is Blaster, which infected more than 1 million computers in early August 2003. Welchia, an antidote to Blaster, crashed computers and clogged networks as well.

The *Trojan horse* is a malicious code that masquerades as a benevolent program. This bug does not replicate but instead opens "back doors" in computer systems to allow a hacker to take control of or steal confidential data. An example is the QAZ. In July 2000, the QAZ allowed hackers to view secret Microsoft source code.

More interesting is the *blended threat*, a combination of viruses that tries different ways to infect and spread basic viruses, worms, and Trojan horse techniques. Many attempt to use peer-to-peer file sharing and instant messaging for distribution. An example is Sobig, which hit in mid-August 2003 and, at its peak, infected one of every two e-mails.

Another form of online nuisance to be considered is *spam*. It is relatively inexpensive to create and is an excellent venue for increasing business profits. Anyone can purchase a spam software kit for less than $150. It contains all the information necessary to get the spammer started. For an extra $70, the spammer is able to obtain 100 million e-mail addresses. A spammer working for, say, a pornographic website needs just 10,000 people to respond to a 10 million message campaign to reap between $1,000 and $10,000 in profit, depending on his/her commission.[6] Furthermore, clicking on a "remove me from this list" link also counts as a response by which a spammer can benefit.

Spam may also be used as a way to spread viruses and worms like the plague. Examples are the ILOVEYOU and the Sobig viruses that spread through e-mail. Once Internet users received the spam/virus e-mail and clicked on it, their computers were infected. The virus continued to infect more users. Once opened, it was automatically sent to all of the e-mail addresses in the users' address books.

Spammers may be breaking laws and further strengthening spam's potential use by terrorists who want to create a nuisance for business or individuals. For example, there certainly is a high probability that a spammer sending pornography to millions of names will send a few thousand children under eighteen those e-mails: this is a felony. Advertising prescription drugs without the required disclosures and disclaimers is illegal; so is selling drugs without requiring prescriptions. In addition, sending repeated e-mails after a recipient has asked the sender to stop may be considered harassment. Last, it is considered fraud if a message claims that the user signed up for a list, but s/he did not.

Pop-up advertisements, also known as *pop-up ads*, are another online nuisance. Pop-up ads secretly and silently wait for the unsuspecting Internet user to click on a website, after which a promotional advertisement instantly pops up with information related or unrelated to the site the user is on. Pop-up ads monitor consumer online behaviors. These ads are considered a form of cyberterrorism because they invade and intrude upon the users' privacy by monitoring their actions.

Both spam and pop-up ads have serious implications for business. They are quickly becoming a nuisance and a concern to many consumers: they may cause consumers to lose their patience for, interest in, and loyalty to, corporations. This is serious for companies, because if one loses the consumers' patience, interest, and loyalty, one loses the consumers, and thus revenue. Therefore, businesses should implement ways to limit the amount of e-mail, spam mail, or pop-up ads they send. A manager might simply ask consumers, do you want to receive e-mail from our company, or special ads for upcoming sales? Users can then eliminate spam by opting to receive e-mail only from people who have authenticated their identities. Some companies have included smart cards, or Java cards, in their new computers. These Java cards help authenticate e-mail senders.

Denial of service (DoS) attacks threaten more than do others forms of computer attacks. The primary goal of a DoS attack is to disable the targeted computers, the network, or even the whole organization potentially shutting down a power plant, other utilities, or emergency services. Some DoS attacks can be executed with limited resources against a large, sophisticated site. This type of attack is sometimes called an "asymmetric attack." For example, an attacker with an old computer and a slow modem may be able to disable much faster and more sophisticated machines or networks. A denial of service attack is characterized as an explicit attempt to prevent legitimate users of a service from using the service. Examples include:

- Attempts to "flood" a network, thereby preventing legitimate network traffic.
- Attempts to disrupt connections between two machines, thereby preventing access to a service.
- Attempts to prevent a particular individual from accessing a service.
- Attempts to disrupt service to a specific system or person.

DoS attacks can result in significant loss of time and money for many organizations. Prevention controls could include implementation of router filters, observation of system performance, and routine examination of an organization's physical security.

In addition, the two big threat areas of the future will be wireless routers and hubs. There are still not enough solutions for sophisticated wireless antivirus systems and intrusion detection control systems in both the private and public sectors. Computer software is often functionally deficient and unreliable. In March 2003 hackers capitalized on vulnerability within the Windows system to attack the U.S. Army's web server. Exploitation of this vulnerability was caught by security officials at Microsoft and at the CERT Coordination Center for all Microsoft Windows operating systems, including Windows NT 4.0, 2000, XP, and Server 2003. In response, Microsoft immediately released its latest software upgrade to fix this remote hacking issue. To tackle this threat, however, the government would need to go after a large number of computer systems.

Finally, *identity theft* has become a growing concern for corporate or governmental leaders. Computer-savvy thieves are able to create fraudulent websites that mimic authentic websites. The unsuspecting consumer may supply an unauthentic website with personal information such as a Social Security number, or bank account and other personal and financial data. Unauthorized use of personal information can cause considerable harm to the consumer. This is likely to have serious implications for corporations because the consumer loses confidence and trust in the e-commerce business to which s/he has supplied personal information. In effect, corporations may lose the consumer's business forever. Identity theft is becoming an epidemic: it is the fastest-spreading crime in the United States. The Department of Justice estimates that 700,000 Americans will be victimized this year by criminals who steal their Social Security numbers and wreak havoc with their bank and credit card accounts.[7] Consumers should shop online only at companies they know and use secure browsers that will encrypt purchase information. They should never reveal personal information not needed for their purchase and should never give out Internet passwords.

HOW GOVERNMENTS AND COMPANIES CAN RESPOND TO AN ATTACK

The likelihood of a cyberterrorist attack on an organization's centralized computer is rapidly growing. Computer crime is expected to increase by an estimated 230 percent. If cyberterrorists were to gain access to the centralized computer system of a major corporation, a national or state water supply, or a major transportation facility, they could bring a country to a halt, reduce production, cause environmental damage, create unsafe working conditions, or cause the loss of intellectual property.

What can a company or organization do to protect itself from cyberterrorists? A company can implement a new tool that helps identify and prosecute perpetrators of computer crime: e-forensics. The Rits Information Security Specialist system has been active in e-forensics, a process that collects technology-generated evidence to form part of a chain of evidence. E-forensics can link and reconstruct an attacker's trail and determine who made the attack, how they penetrated the system, what information they accessed, and where they sent it. Most cases that result from e-forensics are resolved outside of court. E-forensics can also aid in identifying the source of inappropriate e-mails being sent to a company's staff. Under section 9 of the Criminal Justice Theft and Fraud Offences Act, it is a criminal offense to use a computer dishonestly to make a personal gain at the expense of another. The perpetrator may be sent to prison for a ten-year term.

The federal government has been working to combat cyberterrorism. After September 11, the Bush administration created the Department of Homeland Security, which oversees cybersecurity. In February 2003 the administration implemented the National Strategy to Secure Cyberspace. The president signed the cybersecurity strategy a week after the Sapphire worm slowed Web traffic and disrupted bank cash machine services, airline flights, and other critical parts of the Internet infrastructure. The strategic process informs public and private businesses of practical solutions that may reduce the risk of cyberterrorism. The budget to apply the suggestions made by the White House is left to the discretion of each company. The National Strategy to Secure Cyberspace also establishes government leadership in the fight against cyberterrorism by tightening our nation's security in federal information systems. Furthermore, President Bush also signed the first national antispam bill into law in December 2003, outlawing some of the most annoying forms of junk e-mail and prescribing jail time and multimillion-dollar fines for violators.

In addition to these attempts at preserving cybersecurity, the government should provide funding or tax breaks for companies that incorporate programs to fight cyberterrorism. It should also play an active role in sharing information on security issues and in participating in joint public and private security initiatives. Government agencies have neither sought nor set aside adequate funding to implement the goals of the Cyber-Security Research and Development Act.[8] Eighty to 90 percent of the country's infrastructure is under private control. Leaving the cybersecurity budget up to the discretion of a private company creates confusion and false illusions of how the company perceives the threat.

Currently, corporations are not applying the right security against cyberattacks. They have been slow to implement e-security. Many do not realize how serious the cyberterrorist threat is to their business. Cyberspace is still underappreciated as a source of security threats, and the solutions to prevent breaches of security within cyberspace aren't as obvious as the preventive measures taken to safeguard physical security.

There are many ways a corporation can protect itself from cyberterrorism using less-expensive methods. These measures include backing up data, installing antivirus software, using firewalls and detection networks, tracing software, and protection suites.

Backing up data is absolutely essential. It is important to keep hard copies on backup floppy disks, zip drives, rewritable compact discs, and removable hardware. A corporation can also back up data using a secure computer that is not connected to the Internet—a computer that mirrors the Internet-connected computer and stores all information in real time.

Antivirus software offers continuous protection and automatically scans all file inputs, outputs, downloads, and so forth. It offers the user the option to clean or delete infected files. Firewalls or detection networks screen and filter out all communication to a system.

Tracing software is designed to trace exactly where anyone connecting to the company's network is coming from. It gives the user detailed information on the registered owner's name, address, and other information.

A protection suite is custom-tailored software designed specifically for the company and its needs. Off-the-shelf protection software may have loopholes that hackers already know how to configure.

A corporation can also educate all of its employees and require them to make sure that all accounts have passwords, to frequently change passwords, and to use passwords that are unusual and alphanumeric. The corporation should also change network configurations when defects are known, get upgrades and patches, audit systems and check logs to detect intruders, and not access suspicious e-mail from unknown addresses.

Despite talk immediately after September 11 about the threats of cyberterrorism, a survey of 227 information security professionals conducted by security audit company RedSiren Technologies, Inc., a year afterward showed that 30 percent of respondents said their companies didn't have adequate plans for addressing security and cyberterrorism issues. In addition, nearly 40 percent said senior management did not regularly review their companies' security policies and plans.[9] This illustrates that many executives still don't consider security a critical part of their companies' strategic plans, despite the continued increase in the number and severity of attacks on corporate networks. One of the most interesting findings of the survey is that 48 percent of respondents said the 9/11 attacks had no effect whatsoever on their levels of concern about cyberterrorism or the threat it might pose to their organizations. In addition, an equal number said that their companies had not changed their resource allocations for information security in the wake of the attacks.

The biggest barrier that will have to be overcome in preparing countermeasures to cyberterrorism will be the policymakers' and business managers' lack of awareness of the threat. Acknowledging the threat translates into increased dollar signs: The policymakers and business managers might be reluctant to publicly acknowledge the threat, if that means incurring additional expenses. Many corporate managers think cybersecurity is an investment that neither increases corporate revenue nor improves daily customer service. Due in part to the political unrest in the Middle East, companies have been increasing their security monitoring and dedicating more resources toward looking for potential threats. There has been a big shift in the critical thinking of security managers, who now finally see nonemployees as the biggest threat to their businesses, according to *Information Week*'s 2003 Global Information Security Survey. Fifty-eight percent of surveyed companies cited hackers or terrorists as the primary source of attacks, while only 22 percent blamed unauthorized users or employees.[10]

On the government side, during his term, President Bill Clinton sought an additional $2.8 billion for defenses against cyberterrorist attacks, as well as against attacks by chemical and biological weapons. In May 2001, however, the General Accounting Office identified the ineffectiveness of the National Infrastructure Protection Center (NIPC). The shortcomings included staff shortages, ineffective counteragency reporting, and the FBI's reluctance to share sensitive information on potential cyberattacks. Basically, the NIPC echoed alerts that security professionals had already discovered through other channels, such as the CERT Coordination Center. The NIPC has inherent challenges due to the difficulty of identifying potential cyberattacks, including viruses and coordinated attacks, before they occur. Furthermore, the former White House cybersecurity czar Richard Clarke thinks that the government is doing an unacceptable job of helping the private sector lock down the nation's critical infrastructure. He stated that part of the problem was that many people who were supposed to join DHS from other government agencies opted to stay where they were and caused severe damage to the department's efforts to get up and running.[11] In March 2003 Clarke left his position as chairman of the president's Critical Infrastructure Protection Board (PCIPB), which dissolved when the DHS became operational.

GOVERNMENT AGENCIES THAT ADDRESS CYBERTERRORISM

Everyone hopes terrorists will never again strike on American soil. But if they do, having a plan to protect our systems will minimize unnecessary risks. There are some government agencies that plan, measure, and prevent possible terrorists threats: the Department of Homeland Security (DHS), the National Infrastructure Protection Center (NIPC), the Computer Emergency Readiness Team Coordination Center (CERT/CC), the Federal Bureau of Investigation (FBI), and some other incident response teams and security-related organizations. For example:

- *Department of Homeland Security (DHS)*. The creation of the DHS is the most significant transformation of the U.S. government since 1947, when President Harry S. Truman merged the various branches of the U.S. armed forces into the Department of Defense to better coordinate the nation's defense against military threats.
- *National Infrastructure Protection Center (NIPC)*. The NIPC is an interagency center located at the FBI. Created in 1998, the NIPC is

the focal point of the government's efforts to warn of and respond to cyberattacks, particularly those that are directed at our nation's critical infrastructures. These infrastructures include telecommunications and information, energy, banking and finance, transportation, government operations, and emergency services.

- *CERT Coordination Center (CERT/CC).* The CERT/CC is located at the Software Engineering Institute (SEI), a federally funded research and development center at Carnegie Mellon University. It monitors public sources of vulnerability information and regularly receives reports of vulnerabilities.

STRATEGIES FOR GOVERNMENT POLICYMAKERS

Since the September 11 attacks, federal officials have been telling anyone willing to listen that terrorists have the knowledge and equipment to carry out sophisticated information warfare attacks against targets in the United States. The administration has planned to spend $20 billion on security in fiscal years 2004 through 2006 and to put more efforts into improving coordination and response among all information security organizations under the umbrella of the Department of Homeland Security.[12]

On February 14, 2003, the Department of Homeland Security released its final version of the National Strategy to Secure Cyberspace, which calls on private industries to show unprecedented cooperation with government agencies in the name of network security.[13] The strategy recommends that the private sector develop a centralized network operations center to access Internet health information and complement the DHS's centralized capability and the overall national cyberspace security response system. The five priorities of this strategy are to

- Build a national cyberspace security response system.
- Create a national cyberspace security threat and vulnerability reduction program.
- Develop a national cyberspace security awareness and training program.
- Secure government cyberspace.
- Enhance international cyberspace security cooperation.

This plan depends heavily on network operators and on industry groups sharing government information on network attacks, security threats, and widespread vulnerabilities.

On the national front, the FBI established the National Infrastructure Protection Center, which is a public/private venture that aims to prevent and respond to cyberattacks on the nation's critical infrastructures, such as the telecommunications, energy, banking, transportation, and healthcare sectors. To encourage private sector cooperation, government officials have reached out to enlighten people in private industry, providing threat briefings, issuing analyses and threat warnings, and speaking at industry conferences. Furthermore, the attorney general and the Information Technology Association of America announced a set of initiatives as part of a "cybercitizens' partnership" between the government and the information technology industry. One initiative involves providing IT industry representatives to serve in the NIPC to enhance the technical expertise of the organization and understanding of the information and communications infrastructure.

The government expects the private sector to do its part. Congress passed the USA Patriot Act, which required banks to do more to help the government track money launderers who might be funding terrorist organizations.[14] To further the planning against cyberattacks, the members of the Honeynet Project, would maintain several unprotected computers on the Internet as a way to gain intelligence on current attack methodologies for further research. The Bush administration also authorized the National Science Foundation to create cybersecurity research centers, college grants, and fellowships as part of an approach to boost computer security in academic fields.[15] In addition, an annual cyberdefense exercise is part of cadet training at the U.S. Military Academy at West Point, the U.S. Air Force Academy, the U.S. Naval Academy, the U.S. Coast Guard Academy, and the Naval Postgraduate School to compete in a real-world environment.

Furthermore, the government may even try to reform hackers in order to protect the homeland infrastructure. An example of this tactic is its work with the most-wanted Internet hacker, Kevin Mitnick, who once broke into the networks of Motorola, Novell, Nokia, and Sun Microsystems. Recently, Mitnick met with the Commission on National Security to share his illegal hacking techniques to help deal with the menace of international technoterrorists.

STRATEGIES FOR CORPORATE MANAGERS

Most of the victims of cybercrimes are private corporations. Therefore, successful investigation and prosecution of cybercrimes depend on the private sector reporting incidents to law enforcement and cooperating with investigators. An effective operation of securing critical infrastructure would require management's observing several important principles:

- Understand that the control system is a vulnerable point of an attack with potentially serious consequences.
- Recognize that security tools designed for higher corporate-level information security do not adequately address control-layer security threats.
- Build a defense policy that will handle attacks from outside and from within the enterprise.
- Apply a best-practice model in creating a control-level security system that will perform the functions of monitoring, detecting, notifying, protecting, and recovering.

For a decision-maker, it is important to stay proactive in defending the computer networks in any way possible. A security policy should specify the technologies and procedures that will provide protection by such tools as antivirus software, firewalls, intrusion detection, and data backup systems. The policy should include details such as how employees identify themselves and how often they must change passwords. It is also helpful to update operating systems and software regularly, to disable any unnecessary services, and to lock down systems whenever appropriate. The most important is to make management and users aware of why there is a need for such steps to be taken, to make them aware of the threat to their organizations, and to encourage them to do their parts in protecting the organization's infrastructure. This action requires the full support of the chief executive officer of each corporation.

CONCLUSION

Despite many cybersecurity measures adopted by the government over the past years, a lack of focus and leadership within the federal government's security community has made it unlikely that many of the initiatives will ever be implemented successfully, especially those in the recently released National Strategy to Secure Cyberspace. The impact of this strategy may be as minimal as any of the countless policy statements that come from Washington. We may not have a real strategy to secure cyberspace until the government, businesses, and civic leaders work together.

The other obstacles to protecting cyberspace are too few incentives for private corporations to comply with proposed mandates, and a lack of clear funding sources for many of the proposed programs. Ideally, everyone in a company should be responsible for whatever number of Internet-connected computers are needed to take the actions necessary to secure against cyberterrorism. Fortunately, we will have several sophisticated counterterrorism plans before real digital warfare can arrive.

NOTES

1. Hinde S. Cyberterrorism in context. Oxford: Elsevier Ltd.; 2003.

2. Misra S. High-tech terror. Amer City & Country 2003 June.

3. Haugh R. Cyber-terror. Hospital and Health Networks 2003 June:60–4.

4. Souter G. Companies urged to prepare for cyberterrorism. Bus Ins 2003 Aug.

5. Hamm S, Greene J, Edwards C, Keistetter J. Epidemic. BusWeek 2003 Sep 8 (Issue 3848):28.

6. Kirkpatrick D, Tkaczky C. Taking back the Net. Fortune [Europe] 2003 Sep 27;148(6):73.

7. Kutler J. Ahead of the game. Inst Inv 2003 Oct 4;37(8):15.

8. Lesher S. Lawmakers see cyberterrorism vulnerability. Lexis Nexis Academic, Capitol Hill Publishing Corp.; 2003 May 28.

9. Fisher D. Survey: planning for cyberterrorism lags. e-Week 2002 Sep 16.

10. Hulme G. Global watch: attacks come from just about anywhere. InfoWeek 2003 Sep.

11. Fisher D. Clarke takes government to task over security. e-Week 2003 July.

12. Fisher D. How real is the threat? e-Week 2002 Aug.

13. Gonsalves C. Feds unveil cyber-security plan. e-Week 2003 Feb 14.

14. Colkin E. Banking and financial services. InfoWeek 2002 Sep:171.

15. Chabrow E. Cyber security research a go. InfoWeek 2002 Nov:35.

4 Is the Securitization of Terrorism Risk Realistic?

Sylvie Bouriaux

The U.S. insurance industry has long faced the specter of large, unexpected losses from natural catastrophes such as hurricanes and earthquakes. The September 11, 2001, terrorist attacks clearly demonstrated a new form of catastrophic risk of human origin. The damages in property and life are now well known, as estimates of insured losses deriving from these events range from $40 billion to $54 billion. The 9/11 terrorist attacks renewed the capacity problem that the insurance industry has faced in the underwriting of catastrophic risk. This chapter explores the feasibility of capital market alternatives to conventional insurance, and analyzes whether the capital market could provide extra capacity to absorb terrorism risk.

The capacity issue was first raised in the aftermath of 1992's devastating Hurricane Andrew in the southeastern United States. It was then partly forgotten or ignored as the market for insurance and reinsurance catastrophic coverage softened in the second half of the 1990s. Due to the severity of losses, the World Trade Center attacks rekindled concern about the industry's capacity, and particularly, about the possibility of a new kind of catastrophic-loss event. The capacity issue is especially relevant for reinsurers. The Risk Management Solutions Company estimates that, on average, less than 35 percent of the overall gross insured losses in Hurricane Andrew and the Northridge, California, earthquake disasters were paid by reinsurers.[1] For 9/11, however, a 2002 report from the Insurance Information Institute trade association estimates that 67 percent of the insured losses were covered by the reinsurance industry. Moreover, it is important to point out that the terrorist losses were not limited to "traditional" property exposures or business interruption, as is typical of natural events. According to the institute report, 46 percent of the total claims related to 9/11 were casualty, liability, and life insurance exposures.

Given the potential severity of the terrorist risk capacity problem, the U.S. Congress adopted the Terrorism Insurance Act in November 2002. The Act calls for insurance companies in 2003 to retain an amount equal to 7 percent of the premiums they collected the previous year. The percent deductible rose to 10 percent in 2004 and to 15 percent in 2005. In the event of a terrorist attack, the federal government would cover 90 percent above the deductible with insurance companies financing the other 10 percent. The Terrorism Insurance Act has a three-year sunset provision and, in the absence of a major terrorist act, may not be reconducted.

This chapter evaluates the feasibility of capital market investors to absorb the property loss risk of terrorism. First, it will discuss why the customer risk-pooling mechanism may not be appropriate in the case of terrorism. Then, drawing on the past experience of insurance-linked securities and derivatives developed in the 1990s, it will assess the pros and cons of a possible securitization of insurance risk.

NONAPPLICABILITY OF CONVENTIONAL INSURANCE MECHANISMS TO TERRORISM RISK

In their traditional role, insurance companies shift the risk of each individual to a pool of similarly exposed individuals. Customer pools enable the sharing of the cost of losses among all members of the group. Insurance companies are willing to pool risks when their customers' future losses may reasonably be estimated, and when risk is uncorrelated among the members of the pool. Under the *law of large numbers*, the larger the data set measuring the extent of past losses and the larger the group of policyholders, the more accurate the statistical estimate of future losses. Therefore, employing the law of large numbers gives insurance companies confidence that they have collected enough to cover potential losses.

Unlike many conventional risks, however, terrorism risk does not lend itself to the customer pooling mechanism. There are three key reasons:

1. *No historical database is available to predict terrorism losses.* Although there has been a handful of human-made disasters in the United States that could qualify as terrorists acts (arsons, the Los Angeles riots, the

Oklahoma City bombing), there is no underlying body of data for terrorism-induced property losses. As a result, insurance companies cannot utilize the law of large numbers to formulate good estimates of potential losses. Instead, companies are forced to make subjective inferences of losses based upon *ad hoc* criteria. These forecasts have little predictive capability. In fact, insurance companies have reduced their offerings of terrorism coverage because they are unable to reliably predict the occurrence of terrorist events. One can argue that natural disasters are also generally unpredictable, yet insurance companies did not cease to offer catastrophe insurance.[2]

2. *Terrorism risk is hard to quantify.* In the case of natural disasters, it is possible to simulate catastrophic events based on their own characteristics and to assess the financial impact they would have on a particular community. The problem with terrorism risk is that the inputs needed to simulate the financial and business consequences of a terrorist attack are unknown. There are no wind factor or fault line characteristics attached to a terrorist event, and predicting the next tools used by terrorists to launch a new attack is extremely difficult. Nevertheless, recent studies have attempted to address the modeling and quantification of terrorism risk. Terrorism risk differs in kind from natural catastrophe risk because of the human element.[3] In his opinion, human intent (by terrorists) and human intelligence (by counterterrorists) can be modeled using game theory and search theory. Woo,[4] while acknowledging the difficulty in predicting a terrorist event, suggests that tools like complexity theory can help identify the business and financial consequences of terrorism acts. Although these studies open new doors in the prediction and quantification of terrorism risk, the complexity and sophistication of the tools proposed might nevertheless deter insurance companies from undertaking terrorism coverage.

3. *The pooling of customer risk assumes homogeneous risk exposures.* Such assumption may not hold in terrorism risk. For instance, terrorists may be keener on hitting a landmark skyscraper in New York City than a small retail shopping center in an Arizona town. Having violated a major tenet of the law of large numbers, the accuracy of loss estimates is significantly diminished. Moreover, it is unfair to set equal premiums for members of a group whose risk exposures are heterogeneous.

Since customer risk pooling cannot safely estimate the potential losses of terrorist attacks, insurance companies must maintain a significant amount of surplus beyond the premiums collected. This could prove difficult for many companies. Mutual companies, which are less able to raise external funds, may end up charging extra premiums to their customers. This could raise the cost of terrorism insurance to prohibitive levels for the public. Even stock companies could have trouble raising capital, as existing or potential stockholders may reject investing in companies that undertake such unconventional risks. Therefore, terrorism risk requires new risk-underwriting alternatives.

CAN CAPITAL MARKETS SECURITIZE TERRORISM RISK? PROS AND CONS

The Rationale for Securitization of Insurance Risk

The 1990s saw the emergence of the securitization of insurance risk. While insurance-linked securities and derivative instruments have so far mostly targeted the risk of natural disasters, it is fair to ask whether such instruments could be adequate risk-transfer tools for terrorism risk.

The need for extensive reserves behind terrorism coverage suggests the need for risk transfer, as opposed to risk pooling. In *risk transfer*, risk bearing is removed from entities exposed to risk and transferred to others not exposed to it, but nevertheless willing to accept it and provide the reserves necessary to absorb it. Those who accept the risk, then, would not be the pool of policyholders, but instead would be external professional risk-takers. This risk transfer function is appropriate to the capital market, which has a long history in risk management.

In theory, capital markets are good candidates to undertake terrorism risk coverage. Capital markets have long been underwriters of risk. Investors place funds to earn a "risk premium," or a payment for assuming risk. While financial and business risks differ from property risks, the risk underwriting process is the same. Just as with business and financial risk, capital market investors are enticed into insurance risk by the expectation of profit; that is, a risk premium for their services. Investors manage this risk not by pooling, but instead by diversifying their holdings of risky assets in order to reduce the overall risk of their portfolios.

The willingness of capital market investors to assume terrorism risk can have important benefits:

- *Additional capacity.* If capital markets could augment the insurance industry by providing terrorism coverage, the extra capacity provided would lessen the pressure on premiums.
- *Lower production costs.* Capital markets may introduce efficiencies in the underwriting, monitoring, and settling of terrorism insurance. If so, premium costs of terrorism insurance could be lower, as the risk-analysis function is separated from the risk-bearing function. Terrorism risk exposures could be pooled by originating entities in the capital

market. These entities could, in turn, create and issue new insurance-linked securities against the pool. The originating financial entity undertakes the risk-analysis function required in evaluating the potential terrorism risk exposure, and the investor in the securities issued by the pool becomes the bearer of the risk. This principle has already been effectively applied in mortgage securitization. Financial institutions efficiently provide the risk analysis when they originate mortgage loans as the initial lenders. Then they sell these instruments to outside investors, who bear risk but cannot evaluate it as efficiently as the lenders can.

- *Risk diversification.* Investors may further diversify the overall risk in their portfolio of assets by combining insurance risk with financial risk. For instance, some studies have shown that capital markets participants create more efficient portfolios by allocating a small percentage of their assets in insurance-linked securities. Generally, the returns on securities that have payoffs triggered by natural-disaster losses display a low correlation with stock and bond returns.[5] Whether or not this diversification element would work in the case of terrorism is not clear. The U.S. stock market fell as a result of the 9/11 terrorist attack while bond markets remained fairly stable.

The Reality

Capital market products with payoffs tied to insurance risk first appeared in December 1992 when the Chicago Board of Trade (CBOT) introduced the first exchange-traded derivatives instruments with payoffs linked to industry-insured losses. Soon thereafter, insurance securitization developed, mostly in the form of catastrophe (CAT) bonds. Below is a description of the characteristics of these two instruments:

- *Exchange-traded insurance derivatives.* The CBOT catastrophe insurance futures contracts were designed to allow insurance or reinsurance companies to hedge insured losses resulting from catastrophic disasters, such as earthquakes and hurricanes. The losses relevant to these contracts were not specific to individual insurance companies, but rather, included in an index of losses sustained by all insurance companies. Therefore, these instruments can be best defined as hedge tools for generalized catastrophe risk. In 1995 the CBOT restructured the futures contracts as cash options, enabling the contracts to mimic traditional layers of reinsurance. Insurance companies could, in effect, purchase synthetic layers of reinsurance from capital market investors. The CBOT options ceased trading in 2000.
- *Insurance-linked securities.* Insurance-linked securities like CAT bonds usually carry a coupon income tied to a variable short-term rate.

Investors who invest in such instruments may forego part or all of the coupon income and may even face a loss of the principal invested, if a catastrophe arises and triggers compensation to the insurer or the reinsurer who originally issued the bond. Insurance risk, then, is transferred to capital market investors who, in exchange for bearing the risk arising from catastrophic disasters, receive a higher nominal coupon return on these investments than they would from investing in traditional corporate bonds. When the payoff is triggered by the insured losses of an insurance company's actual portfolio of business, insurance-linked securities are called *indemnity-based* or *company-specific* instruments. When the payoff is triggered by the performance of a broad, industry-based index, insurance-linked securities are called *index-based* or *non-indemnity-based* instruments.

The theoretical benefits of insurance-linked securities and derivatives as alternatives or complements to traditional reinsurance have been documented in numerous papers and publications. Yet, to date, these instruments have encountered limited success among issuers and investors. In previous research, the author of this article addressed the common factors that have limited the growth of insurance securitization. Lack of dual coincidence of wants between issuers and investors in the securities, basis risk, low secondary market trading, and an unfavorable regulatory environment are among the culprits.[6,7]

The growth of catastrophe-linked risk transfer mechanisms in the capital markets was also hampered by investors' difficulty in accurately predicting the frequency of natural disasters. One can argue, however, that it is somewhat possible to simulate catastrophic losses caused by natural disasters, based on the events' own characteristics and to assess the financial impact they would have on a particular community. The problem with catastrophic risk caused by man-made disasters is that the inputs needed to simulate the financial and business consequences of a terrorist attack are unknown.

In addition, for capital markets to successfully underwrite terrorism risk, investors must be adequately compensated for investing in insurance-linked securities. Adequate returns are possible when premiums charged for terrorism coverage are high enough to cover the potential insurance losses and still provide an adequate payment to investors. Nevertheless, the premiums cannot be so high as to make insurance synthetically provided by the capital markets prohibitively expensive. Bouriaux and Scott[8] presented simple simulations of the risk-reward trade-off faced by investors who might consider underwriting terrorism risk. The premise of the simulations was that investors should receive a rate of return on insurance risk that must at least equal the rate of return of any efficient portfolio composed of both Treasury bills and risky securities. The authors calculated equilibrium rates of return (conceptually similar, in the insurance jargon, to rates online) based on hypothetical lognormal probability distributions for terrorism losses. The results of the simulations could not support the statement that investors in the capital markets would charge significantly cheaper premiums than those charged by insurance companies for terrorism risk. As a result, while capital markets may provide additional terrorist coverage capacity to private corporations and/or insurance companies, the coverage is likely to come at a high cost.

Terrorism coverage is also a longer perspective business, compared to catastrophe coverage, which makes terrorism risk even harder to securitize than catastrophe risk. Insurance market participants generally assume that most claims resulting from a catastrophic event will be paid within twelve months following the event. Catastrophe-linked securities offered in the capital markets have been designed to compensate the issuer of the security within that time frame. On the other hand, terrorist attacks result in a high amount of liability and workers' compensation claims, which may take years to develop.

Finally, previous experience shows that institutional investors have been reluctant to invest in catastrophe-linked securities because of adverse selection and moral hazard issues. One way to mitigate similar problems with respect to terrorism coverage is for insurance companies to transfer all of their terrorism risk to a pool that would issue securities with a payoff linked to the pool's overall loss. Some countries, such as the United Kingdom and France, have already created terrorism insurance pools, but with government backing only. The role of capital markets as a partial guarantor of losses incurred by a pool along with the federal government needs to be investigated further.

Public/Private Initiatives to Finance Terrorism Risk

Congress's decision to pass the Terrorism Insurance Act on November 25, 2002, underscores the extensive social costs associated with inadequate private insurance coverage. It also acknowledges that terrorist acts not only impact properties and people directly involved, but also the larger economy. In this context, government aid is not just a subsidy for insurance companies and their customers; it also benefits society and the economy as a whole, so that the use of public dollars to support terrorist insurance may be justified.

However, the Terrorism Insurance Act has a three-year sunset provision. If no widespread terrorist event occurs in the next two years, the future of a federal solution will be in doubt. Politicians are known to react to immediate crises, but not to hypothetical future situations. The time to investigate public/private initiatives to finance terrorism risk is before another attack happens.

Among new ideas developed is the auction of excess-of-loss reinsurance contracts. A similar initiative was considered in 1996 and 1997 for natural disasters.[9] The idea was for the federal government to set a reserve price above which it would sell excess-of-loss reinsurance contracts. The reserve price would be indexed to aggregate industry capital and auctioned in the public markets. Unfortunately, the initiative fizzled away in part because of the Treasury Department's opposition to it.

Another concept calls for the government to purchase contingent corporate "catastrophe" bonds issued by the insurance industry. While this idea has merits, the contingent offering could be expanded to private investors.

Finally, one could envision an alternative solution in which insurance and reinsurance companies could transfer all their commercial terrorism policies to a pool (either state or national) that would issue securities to private investors. This idea can be summarized as follows: the securities issued would have a payoff linked to the pool's loss experience (possibly measured in loss ratio terms) up to a maximum amount (say $40 billion worth of losses). The federal government would become the guarantor of last resort above this threshold.

The securities would have to be issued in small denominations to attract not only large institutional investors but also retail investors. Bouriaux and Russell[7] have argued that insurance-linked securities issued in small denominations and possibly traded on an established exchange (for instance, the American Stock Exchange) may attract individual investors. Terrorism-linked securities could also be marketed to small investors as "charity" or "war" investments and might become popular as alternatives to donations because they would have an upside yield potential if no terrorism event occurred. Nontaxability of income received from owning such securities could also boost their attractiveness to investors.

CONCLUSION

This analysis concludes that it is possible for capital markets to securitize terrorism risk, provided that the return paid to investors on any form of insurance-linked securities is high enough and in line with other investments of similar risk. Securitization of terrorism risk may be more difficult to achieve than securitization of other lines of insurance business, due to the longer tail aspect of the risk and due to the current reluctance of investors to develop a liquid secondary market in insurance securities.

As a result, it may be more appropriate to envision joint solutions from the private and public sectors in which insurance and reinsurance companies could transfer all their commercial terrorism policies to a pool (either state or national) that would issue securities to private investors. In this framework, the securities issued would have a payoff linked to the pool's loss experience up to a maximum amount. The federal government would become the guarantor of last resort above this threshold.

NOTES

1. Risk Management Solutions, Inc. Managing risk in the aftermath of the World Trade Center catastrophe. Risk Management Solutions, Inc.; 2001.

2. Note that, after the occurrences of Hurricane Andrew in 1992 and the Northridge earthquake in 1994, some states had to intervene to provide additional catastrophe coverage to the general public. California created the California Earthquake Authority (CEA), and Florida forced insurance companies to create an insurance pool backed by a state guarantee.

3. Major JA. Advanced techniques for modeling terrorism risk. J Risk Fin 2002;4(1):7–14.

4. Woo G. Quantitative terrorism risk assessment. J Risk Fin 2002;4(1): 15–24.

5. Unless, of course, the catastrophe brings the economy down. For instance, in Japan, the large economic losses resulting from the 1994 Kobe earthquake caused a steep decline in the Nikkei Index.

6. Bouriaux S. Basis risk, credit risk and collateralization issues for insurance-linked derivatives and securities. J Ins Reg 2001;20(1):94–120.

7. Bouriaux S, Russell DT. Loss ratio on insurance equity securities: a new step in insurance securitization. J Risk Fin 2002;3(4):73–82.

8. Bouriaux S, Scott WL. Alternative solutions to terrorism risk coverage [working paper]. Katie Insurance School; 2002.

9. Lewis CM, Murdock KC. The role of government contracts in discretionary reinsurance markets for natural disasters. J Risk and Ins 1996;63(4): 567–97.

5 Terrorism: The Response and Interplay of Insurance and Business

James Barrese, William L. Ferguson, and Nicos A. Scordis

All too little understood, the uniqueness of the strategy lies in this: that it achieves its goal not through its acts but through the response to its acts. In any other such strategy, the violence is the beginning and its consequences are the end of it. For terrorism, however, the consequences of the violence are themselves merely the first step and form a stepping-stone toward objectives that are more remote. Whereas military and revolutionary actions aim at a physical result, terrorist actions aim at a psychological result.... But even that psychological result is not the final goal. Terrorism is violence used in order to create fear; but it is aimed at creating fear in order that the fear, in turn, will lead somebody else—not the terrorist—to embark on some quite different program of action that will accomplish whatever it is the terrorist really desires.

—Professor David Fromkin, Boston University[1]

The notion of terrorism as a form of warfare is consistent with the common saying that "one man's terrorist is another man's freedom fighter."[2,3] The word *terrorism* has been traced to revolutionary France and the Reign of Terror (1793 through 1794), yet a formal and universally acceptable definition of terrorism today continues to be elusive. With current efforts to exclude "terrorism" from insurance coverage, having an agreed definition of terrorism is highly desirable for both insurers and policyholders, as well as for more effective and efficient functioning of the insurance transfer mechanism in the general economy.

Unfortunately, there is no consensus on a definition of terrorism, even among U.S. law enforcement and intelligence communities. For example, the Federal Bureau of Investigation (FBI) defines terrorism as "the unlawful use of force or violence against persons or property to intimidate or coerce a Government, the civilian population, or any segment thereof, in furtherance of political or social objectives."[4] The Central Intelligence Agency (CIA) defines terrorism as "premeditated, politically motivated violence perpetrated against noncombatant targets by subnational groups or clandestine agents, usually intended to influence an audience."[5]

In the wake of the September 11, 2001 terrorist attacks discussed later, the Insurance Services Office (ISO), a major U.S. insurance industry-sponsored trade association, quickly developed an optional new war *and terrorism* exclusion (emphasis added) to replace existing standard war exclusion clauses for member commercial insurance policies to take effect with contract renewals beginning in January 2002.[6] Terrorism had historically been viewed under U.S., English and other international law as separate and distinct from war, which involves sovereign or at least *de facto* governments.[7] This addition of "terrorism" to time- and court-tested standardized contract language regarding war was quickly approved for use in most U.S. states and territorial jurisdictions. In general, the initial ISO terrorism endorsement, dated January 2002, defined the term *terrorism* quite broadly, subject to various loss thresholds not discussed here, as follows:

> [T]errorism means activities against persons, organizations or property of any nature:
>
> 1. That involve the following or preparation for the following:
>   a. Use or threat of force or violence; or
>   b. Commission or threat of a dangerous act; or
>   c. Commission or threat of an act that interferes with or disrupts an electronic, communication, information, or mechanical system; and
>
> 2. When one or both of the following applies:
>   a. The effect is to intimidate or coerce a government or the civilian population or any segment thereof, or to disrupt any segment of the economy; or
>   b. It appears that the intent is to intimidate or coerce a government, or to further political, ideological, religious, social, or economic objectives or to express (or express opposition to) a philosophy or ideology.

This ISO definition of terrorism, although virtually replaced by wording dictated to precisely match the provisions of the federal Terrorism

Risk Insurance Act (TRIA) passed in late 2002, was significant in that it represented the first truly "mass market" attempt to apply a workable definition of terrorism, which would indicate when such an exclusion would operate in the contracts of insurance that are marketed to millions of individuals and commercial entities every day. This definition, and related exclusions, may still apply in certain limited situations not prohibited under TRIA as discussed later; for example, to losses not "certified" as an act of terrorism or below certain threshold loss levels.

EVOLVING TERRORISM

The Council on Foreign Relations identifies "at least six different sorts of terrorism: nationalist, religious, state-sponsored, left wing, right wing, and anarchist."[8] Nationalist terrorism is difficult to define because many groups accused of being terrorists claim they are freedom fighters, hence the well-known saying. Religious terrorists seek to use violence to further what they see as divinely commanded purposes. State-sponsored terrorist groups are used by radical states as foreign policy tools. Left wing terrorists desire the replacement of capitalist with communist or socialist regimes. Right wing terrorist groups, such as neo-Nazi groups, desire the replacement of liberal democratic with fascist states. Anarchist terrorism was a global phenomenon from the 1870s through the 1920s.

The use of tactics that are characterized as terrorism occurs because these tactics are typically low-cost activities designed to instill psychological intimidation. Physical force is involved, but it is less often true that the terrorist believes a goal can be accomplished through the force alone.

The use of terrorism as a tactic has a long history. Historical references cited by Alexander and Alexander[9] include: "attacks mounted by the Jewish religious extremists, known as Zealot Sicarii, against the Romans in occupied Judea as well as the martyrdom missions of the Muslim Hashashin (assassins), targeting the Crusaders in the Middle East. The former were active for seventy years in the first century and latter between the eleventh and thirteenth centuries." Despite centuries of terrorist tactics, commentators focus on the late 1960s as the modern watershed for international terrorism. Developments in technology, communications, and travel contributed to growth in the number of terrorist groups. It is difficult to say which came first, but these changes, coupled with the rise of Palestinian terrorism following the Arab defeat in the Six-Day War of 1967, are coincident with an increase in the level and scope of international terrorism.

The tools and tactics of modern terrorist groups include arson, bombings, kidnappings, hijackings, facility attacks, destruction of property, slaughter of innocent people, and assassinations. Groups studying terrorist activities and tactics believe the activities employed by terrorists soon will include biological, chemical, and nuclear attacks. Discussions about the destructive impact of these attacks mention as possibilities millions of casualties, major disruptions of government and businesses, and widespread public panic.

A frequently cited example of this growing possibility is the Aum Shinrikyo incident. In 1995 this Japanese cult released sarin gas in the Tokyo subway system. In addition to causing twelve deaths and over 5,000 injuries, investigators also discovered that Aum Shinrikyo were seeking more lethal weapons at the time its leaders were arrested, and that the group had attempted to release anthrax from atop several Tokyo buildings the year before.

The attacks of September 11, 2001, were the most devastating terrorist attacks to date, yet they required very little in terms of expense, technology, or weaponry. Instead, the attacks involved sophisticated logistical analysis and execution. Nineteen terrorists boarded four planes, each loaded with fuel for a transcontinental flight, in a kamikaze operation against at least two known targets: the World Trade Center (WTC) in New York City and the Pentagon in Washington, DC. Armed with simple knives and box cutters, the men hijacked the planes and used them as guided missiles. Three of the planes hit their targets. The timeline for the flights is well known:

1. At 7:59 a.m. American Airlines Flight 11 took off from Logan Airport in Boston; at 8:46 a.m. the flight struck the North Tower of the WTC complex.
2. At 8:14 a.m. United Airlines Flight 175 also took off from Logan Airport, and at 9:03 a.m. hit the South Tower of the WTC.
3. At 8:20 a.m. American Airlines Flight 77 departed Dulles International Airport in suburban Washington ten minutes after its scheduled departure; and at 9:38 a.m. struck the Pentagon.
4. At 8:42 a.m., forty-one minutes after its scheduled 8:01 a.m. departure time due to a runway delay in Newark, United Airlines Flight 93 took off and ultimately crashed into a field in Pennsylvania at 10:05 a.m.

All four crashes were the result of a coordinated terrorist attack.

As a result of these four crashes, the World Trade Center complex collapsed, the Pentagon was damaged, over 3,300 people died, thousands were injured, billions of dollars of immediate damage occurred, and the daily lives of millions have been, and are likely to continue to be, disrupted for years. In New York, the area south of Canal Street came to a virtual standstill in the days following the collapse; for some in the area, their lives and business activities were disrupted for months. More than two years after the event, the lives of many remain disrupted. Millions of square feet of office space were destroyed, and the city and state of New York evacuated those who lived or worked within a large area surrounding the WTC location, some for many months. Subway service was not restored for several years after the event, with the first commuter line going back into service only in late fall 2003. Business relocations have altered the lives of many thousands and affected the financial condition of thousands of businesses that were to provide services to a business community and employees who were located in the millions of square feet of destroyed office space in the WTC area. The monetary and social costs of the attacks—physical, emotional, and financial—remain to be calculated.[10]

The immediate effect of the attacks was devastating but, as with most things, the impact may reasonably be expected to dissipate with time. Some suggest, however, that the effect on the risk consciousness of the public will be long-lasting, not because of the effect of the attacks on the public psyche but because of the effect of the responses to the attacks. The immediate surge in risk awareness following 9/11 was followed by a declining trend in the succeeding months. Risk consciousness may never recede to pre-9/11 levels in part because a portion of the immediate response was the creation of institutions designed to ensure the continuity of a higher level of risk awareness. Enactment of the Homeland Security Act of 2002 alone guarantees at least a modicum of a continued higher level of risk consciousness in the future. Evidence of this heightened awareness is found in a Pinkerton survey of Fortune 1000 companies (table 5.1) designed to determine the current perceived relative importance of a set of twenty-three potential security threats. The top five perceived threats are listed with the relative importance score obtained (a one-to-five scale was used, with five defined as "most important"). The survey was sent to 1,266 security directors and other executives, and 212 returned completed surveys.

Category confusion may affect the rankings; but still, two years after 9/11, terrorism remained among the top perceived business security threats.[11] An example of category confusion is seen in the separate listing of computer crime: a part of computer vulnerability is the threat of cyberterrorism. Following the WTC and Pentagon terrorism attacks,

Table 5.1
Pinkerton Survey of Fortune 1000 Companies

2003 Rank	Security Threat	Average Importance Score
1	Workplace violence	4.02
2	Business interruption/continuity planning	4.00
3	Computer crime: internet/intranet security	3.87
4	Terrorism (global & domestic)	3.78
5	Employee selection/screening concerns	3.68

the FBI's InfraGard Website, www.infragard.net (established in January 2001 to aid in the fight on cyberterrorism) cautioned companies, including data centers, of possible terrorist attacks.

Alexander and Alexander[9] provide a partial list of cyberterrorism possibilities: altering formulae for medication at pharmaceutical plants, "crashing" telephone systems, misrouting passenger trains, changing pressure in gas pipelines to cause valve failure, disrupting operations of air traffic control, triggering oil refinery explosions and fires, scrambling the software used by emergency services, shutting down power grids, and simultaneously detonating numerous computer-operated bombs around the world.

An additional event occurred in 2001 that heightened awareness to biological hazards: anthrax-laced letters were received across the United States. It is now recognized that, for example, an aerosolized release of 100 kilograms of anthrax spores in an enclosed setting is projected to be able to cause over 100,000 deaths.

Part of the higher level of risk awareness is an almost daily acclimatization to hazards that seemed, a short time ago, to be the meat of fiction. In addition to traditional attacks, and to attacks like those of 9/11 that used conventional methods but involved sophisticated logistics and planning, attacks using weapons that result in mass deaths are considered realistic possibilities. Chemical attacks have already occurred, and a nuclear terrorism attack may be considered inevitable. Nuclear terrorism could include the use of a crude explosive device designed to spew radioactive material (i.e., a "dirty bomb"), a truck-bomb attack against an operating nuclear facility, or a jetliner crashing into a facility stockpiling nuclear waste. The cost and availability of both material and knowledge are such that a dirty bomb is well within the reach of a number of subnational or splinter groups.

The frequency and severity of terrorism are expected to increase during the twenty-first century. David Kay, former United Nations weapons inspector, cites four reasons for this expectation. First, terrorism has proved very successful in attracting publicity, disrupting the activities of government and business, and causing significant death and destruction. Second, arms, explosives, supplies, financing, and communications are readily available to terrorists. Third, an international support network of groups and states exists that greatly facilitates the undertaking of terrorist activities. Fourth, certain conditions, such as religious extremism or perceptions that the "cause" is lost, could provide terrorists with an incentive to escalate their attacks dramatically by resorting to weapons of mass destruction (WMD).[1]

Kay also quotes a Deutch-Spector Commission report that ranks terrorist use of WMD as first among the most serious threats facing the United States.[1] Kay observes that media attention to terror weapon possibilities increases the likelihood of the use of weapons of mass destruction: "only a blind, deaf and dumb terrorist group could have survived the last five years and not been exposed to the possibility of the use of WMD while the more discerning terrorists would have found some tactically brilliant possibilities already laid out on the public record.... This all too quick look at the guideposts to analytical surprise suggests ... that there is sound reason for believing that attempts at mass casualty terrorism deserve to be taken seriously."

GOVERNMENT RESPONSE TO 9/11

Within days of the 9/11 attacks, the U.S. Congress passed, and President Bush signed, a $40 billion emergency funding measure to respond to the enormous damage caused by the tragedy. Over the next year, at least two other significant government actions guaranteed that the impact of 9/11 would continue: the passage of the Homeland Security Act of 2002 (Public Law 107:296) and the Terrorism Risk Insurance Act of 2002 (TRIA, Public Law 107:297). As noted previously, overall risk consciousness of the public may have become more acute following the events of September 11, but it is the creation of institutions and laws subsequent to those events that is likely to maintain a higher level of risk awareness.

The Homeland Security Act of 2002

The Homeland Security Act of 2002 provides the basis for the creation of the Homeland Security Department in one of the largest-ever

Organization of the Department of Homeland Security

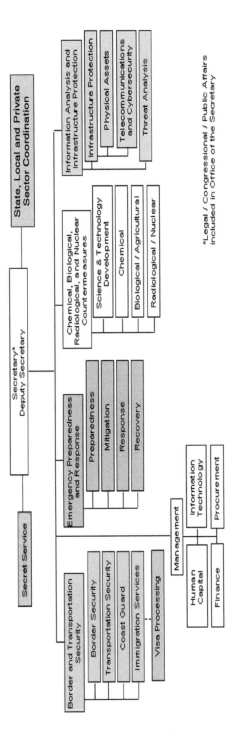

Figure 5.1

The chart shows the organizational components of the newly established Department of Homeland Security. The extent of the altered government organization will create a need for significant restructuring of corporate-governmental relationships, concomitantly requiring businesses to adjust expenses.

reorganizations of U.S. federal agencies, involving some 170,000 federal employees, approximately twenty-two federal agencies, and a proposed budget of $37.7 billion for fiscal year 2003.[12] This reorganization merges federal agencies with widely varying histories and missions, ranging from the U.S. Coast Guard to the Secret Service, into one federal department with a Cabinet-level Secretary heading the office.[13] The mission of the new department, which will not include either the CIA or the FBI, is to help prevent, protect against, and respond to acts of terrorism on American soil. The four main divisions of this department (each headed by an undersecretary) are: (1) information analysis and infrastructure protection; (2) chemical, biological, radiological, and nuclear countermeasures; (3) border and transportation security; and (4) emergency preparedness and response.

Figure 5.1 displays the organizational components of the Department of Homeland Security. The extent of the changes in government organization created a need for significant restructuring of corporate-governmental relationships, concomitantly requiring businesses to adjust expenses.

The Insurance Industry and the Terrorism Risk Insurance Act of 2002 (TRIA)

Insurance involves a contract between a "primary insurance company" and the insured (the holder of the risk in the absence of an insurance contract). Reinsurance is a contractual relationship between insurance companies that allows companies to further share and spread losses. The primary insurer has a legal responsibility to honor and pay the claims for losses of the insured, whereas the reinsurer does not. The contract involving the reinsurer is with the primary insurance company only, not with the insured. Furthermore, the contract between the primary insurer and the insured is subject to many regulatory constraints and guidelines, while the relationship between the primary insurer and reinsurer is considered to be a contract between sophisticated parties such that neither the price nor conditions of reinsurance coverage are subject to direct regulation. The latter point is especially significant given that many reinsurance relationships also cross international boundaries, as geographic dispersion is a very effective method of spreading the burden of risk, and foreign reinsurers may have very unique risk selection, pricing and/or coverage expectations (e.g., terrorism exclusion).

As a result of the 9/11 attacks, insurers (and, in turn, reinsurers) saw an immediate surge in claims across a number of lines of business,

including: life, property, casualty, workers compensation, business interruption, and disability insurance. These claims caused the property-
casualty industry as a whole to record its first-ever aggregate loss. A
period of significant price increases has followed, driven at least in part
by reinsurance pricing and concerns over reinsurance coverage availability. According to Conning & Company, a major industry analyst,
premiums for property and casualty are increasing every year.

Subsequent to the 9/11 attacks, some insurers increased rates by 50
to 100 percent for particular shippers and owners of large commercial
property. Workers compensation rate increases exceeding 20 percent
were reported in 2002. Airlines saw some of the largest rate hikes, with
some premiums up over 400 percent. Fortunately for the airlines, stabilization legislation enacted in the days immediately following 9/11
allowed the federal government to pay any rise in commercial insurance
as well as assume responsibility for third-party liability insurance for
terrorism for half a year. The Council of Insurance Agents and Brokers
announced that rates for insurance policies covering property damage
could be expected to rise by at least 30 to 50 percent. For these reasons,
it was no surprise that five weeks after 9/11, the Bush administration
proposed that the federal government would phase in, over a three-year
period, a plan to take on the most immediate financial risk of another
terrorist attack by paying up to 90 percent of insurance claims resulting
from a future incident. The proposal was based on the approach the
United States historically took toward insuring nuclear power plants:

Year 1: Insurers pay 20 percent of first $20 billion in claims, with the
government paying the remaining 80 percent of first $20 billion in in-
sured claims. The government would also pay 90 percent of claims in
excess of $20 billion, up to a maximum of $100 billion.
Year 2: Insurers pay the first $10 billion in claims and then they split the
second $10 billion with the government, fifty-fifty. Again, the govern-
ment would also pay 90 percent of claims in excess of $20 billion, up to
a maximum of $100 billion.
Year 3: Insurers pay the first $20 billion in claims and then they split the
cost of the next $20 billion with the government, fifty-fifty. The govern-
ment would pay 90 percent of claims in excess of $40 billion, up to a
maximum of $100 billion.

There were few differences between the original Bush proposal and the
final legislation, the Terrorism Risk Insurance Act of 2002. Part of the
reason for the speedy passage of the act was the considerable potential
impact of the issue on financial markets. Reinsurance companies and

pricing had become driving forces that led to the TRIA, which took effect on November 26, 2002.

Unlike insurance contracts, which are renewable throughout the year, most reinsurance contracts are renewable at the beginning of January or July (about 90 percent of all commercial policies renew in January). Following the 9/11 attacks, reinsurance coverage renewable in January 2002 excluded coverage for terrorism. In the short run, this left domestic primary insurers with a much larger potential exposure than they desired and, as their policies became renewable, primary insurers also attempted to exclude coverage or charge prohibitive prices (e.g., using, among others, the ISO language discussed at the beginning of this chapter). Hillman observes that "a number of factors affect both the speed and extent to which primary insurers can insulate themselves from terrorism. First, in contrast to reinsurance, changes in the coverage provided by direct insurers require regulatory approval in most states.... This regulatory hurdle caused ISO, acting on behalf of P/C insurers, to file a request in every state for permission to exclude terrorism from all commercial insurance coverage. As of February 22, 2002, 45 states and the District of Columbia and Puerto Rico had approved the ISO exclusion."[14]

Below are two examples drawn from Hillman of the effect of the increasing loss of terrorism coverage, coupled with a greater awareness of the potential effect of terrorism. These examples demonstrate why the government felt a need to act with speed to pass the TRIA.

> The owners of a major Midwestern mall reported that when their all-risk insurance policy on the property expired at the end of 2001, they purchased a terrorism-excluded insurance policy because they could not find one that would cover the risk of terrorism. The mall's mortgage lender objected to the policy's terrorism exclusion and argued that it violated the "all-risk" insurance requirement stipulated in the loan documents. Consequently, the lender notified the owners that it had purchased a stand-alone $100 million terrorism insurance policy to protect the mall from this risk. Furthermore, the lender demanded repayment by the mall of the $750,000 premium. The mall owners protested the lender's action, arguing that they could not be required to purchase insurance that was not available to them or other owners of similar properties. (pp. 159–160)[14]

Similarly, another lender described the adverse business relationships created as the bank responded to the technical default of mortgages when full terrorism insurance was not in force.

From the bank's perspective, it is being asked to absorb risk that it had not previously priced into the mortgages and is therefore putting pressure on its mortgage holders to obtain terrorism coverage. At the same time, the bank recognizes that the unavailability or increased cost of terrorism coverage will also negatively impact the mortgage holders' ability to service the loans. Consequently, the bank's likely course of action will be to review each loan on a case-by-case basis. (pp. 159–160)[14]

The lack of coverage slowed the market for the securitization of loans, such as mortgage-backed assets, as investors feared the increased vulnerability of the underlying assets. TRIA addressed the problems outlined above by requiring property-liability insurers doing business in the United States to offer commercial coverage for incidents of what might be termed "international" terrorism and by establishing a rein-surance program that would reimburse insurers for a large percentage of any loss paid under the Act.

TRIA defines an act of terrorism as an act that is "certified" as such by the Secretary of the Treasury, the Secretary of State, and the Attorney General of the United States. The act in question must have the following characteristics: First, it must be a violent act or an act that is dangerous to human life, property, or infrastructure. Second, it must have resulted in damage within the United States, or to an air carrier as defined in the U.S. code, or to a U.S. flag vessel or other vessel based principally in the United States and insured under U.S. regulation, or on the premises of any U.S. mission (e.g., embassy or consulate). Third, it must have been committed by someone acting on behalf of a foreign person or foreign interest, as part of an effort to coerce the civilian population of the United States or to influence the policy or affect the conduct of the U.S. government by coercion. Fourth, it must produce property and casualty insurance losses in excess of $5 million. Acts that otherwise meet these criteria but that occur in the course of a declared war cannot be certified as acts of terrorism under the Act, except with respect to workers compensation claims.

TRIA voids all terrorism exclusions on commercial property and casualty policies of participating insurers to the extent that such exclusions eliminate coverage for certified acts of terrorism as covered by the federal program.[15] State regulatory approval of terrorism exclusions is specifically voided by the Act. To be eligible for federal reimbursement of certified terrorism losses, TRIA requires insurers to provide notice to their customers of the premium for coverage being provided under the program and the extent to which losses paid under the program are reimbursed by the federal government. Of course, the insured may decide not to purchase the federally backed coverage.

Reinsurers are not included in the program. Captives and risk retentions groups come under the Act only if they meet the criteria requirements applicable to other insurers: first, they must be licensed or admitted in a state; and second, they must report their direct earned premium information either in an annual statement to the National Association of Insurance Commissioners (NAIC) or to any state.

Each participating insurer will receive reimbursement from the federal government for a percent of paid losses. The percent varies with a time-dependent deductible.[16] The reimbursement also is subject to a cap on aggregate losses.

Impact on Selected Industries

The U.S. economy was arguably at the start of an economic downturn in September 2001, so it is difficult to say precisely how much of the corporate losses of late 2001 are appropriately attributable to terrorism. Business travel fell significantly, and the ongoing security burdens and attendant delay potential greatly increased for those that did travel. For many companies, the weakening economy was the key factor in company performance. Clearly, however, the effect of 9/11 on the economy was not insignificant; for example, 26 percent of chief financial officers (CFOs) responding to an October 2001 Duke University survey said they would postpone investments because of the September 11 attacks, 71 percent said it would not affect planned spending, and the remaining 3 percent said the incidents would spur additional capital spending.

Notwithstanding the CFO survey results, companies were advised to adopt risk management strategies that would alter underlying cost structures, and such altered cost structures undoubtedly are due in part to adverse reactions to the events of 9/11.

Mercer Management Consultants offers advice in at least three areas that would result in higher costs. In the area of inventory management, manufacturers were advised to carry larger stocks of buffer inventory in order to hedge against supply and production-line disruptions. In the area of production input sourcing, manufacturers were advised to be more selective about the location of critical inputs. Finally, regarding transportation, manufacturers and retailers were advised to broaden shipping arrangements.

To further reduce the impact of possible attacks against office buildings, companies were advised to consider multiple electronic means to conduct business: online payments, Websites, participation in electronic business-to-business exchanges, online sourcing and procurement, electronic data exchange, and in the financial world, electronic trading markets.

Before the attacks, the vaunted movement toward telecommuting was a stagnating trend because of inherent difficulties in effectively and efficiently managing a network of dispersed, remote workers. Employees not in frequent face-to-face relationships with their colleagues felt stigmatized. September 11 caused employees and employers to reevaluate potential advantages of telecommuting. Firms benefit from the low-cost dispersion of employees and, in the short run, employees reevaluated their priorities and requested work-at-home options. As a result, several companies providing videoconferencing, teleconferencing, and Internet-based collaboration tools were expected to see a surge in business and the stocks of such firms rose by over 30 percent in the two weeks following the attacks. Unfortunately, as seen in the Pinkerton survey, cyberterrorism and nonpolitical cyber attacks also are seen as serious threats to electronic business that dampen telecommuting benefits.

The American Chemistry Council, the industry association for over 180 chemical companies, aware that its toxic and volatile chemicals could kill thousands during an explosion or fire at a manufacturing plant or storage facility, has encouraged chemical companies to increase their preparedness against attack. Damage to the nation's chemical facilities or water and waste treatment facilities could disrupt the lives and livelihood of millions, in addition to causing large numbers of deaths. Linden[17] notes only about 15 percent of the nation's water facilities service almost 75 percent of the U.S. population, representing a potentially very significant exposure.

Companies with decentralized operational scope—various units spread out among disparate cities or regions—may become a growing trend among firms that seek to reduce the impact of terrorist attack. Some architects and urban planners have argued that in light of possible massive terrorist attacks during this century, it is preferable to avoid building skyscrapers huddled together along endless blocks. Instead, it may be preferable to construct discrete office developments separated by parks and other structures.

There is little doubt that 9/11 has, and will continue to, increase product costs through its impact on the (inter)national transportation system. In addition to business travelers, commercial trucks, licenses and transportation manifests are being examined more closely. Bridges, tunnels and highway toll facilities are under expanded surveillance with consequent delays. In addition to the increased costs required to secure cargo carried in transportation systems, particularly in shipping and trucking, higher costs also are incurred due to the interdependence of the transportation system with tight commercial production schedules. For example, the manufacturing sector of the economy bears additional costs attributed to production delays when supplies are not delivered as expected, and the retail sector experiences costly reductions in cash flow due to the effect of inventory delivery delays on sales revenue timing. Disruptions to distribution systems immediately following the 9/11 incidents caused a number of companies to re examine just-in-time (JIT) inventory techniques, which involve delivery of parts to the assembly line only as/when they are needed. There may be a short-term positive impact on the economy as some companies increase inventories and build additional storage facilities, but in the longer term the cost of carrying higher inventories will be reflected in product prices.

Computer recordkeeping strategies are another source of increasing costs being incurred or considered in light of the damage inflicted during the September 11 terrorist attacks. Companies are investigating expensive backup sites, data storage software and services, and emergency/contingency planning. Some banks and security firms adopted some, or all, of these measures following the bombings of the World Trade Center in 1993, and the speed with which some of the firms located in the WTC recovered their computer presence was positive news for other firms.

One example of the damage possible without such backup systems is a concern that future terrorists may, for instance, attack the Clearinghouse Interbank Payment Systems (CHIPS) in New York. CHIPS is a computer network that links 59 of the world's largest banks operated by the New York Clearing House. Approximately $292 trillion passed through CHIPS in 2000. If this system were not geographically dispersed, an attack could be devastating throughout the world economy.

The banking industry also was affected by a large number of direct and indirect consequences of 9/11, and many of the factors that influence the economy will be felt through the banking systems financial intermediation function. One example of the impact of 9/11 on banking industry activities is in its role regarding anti money-laundering efforts. A "9/11 Report" prepared by the Senate and House Intelligence Committees on intelligence community activities before and after the terrorist attacks of September 11 discusses the U.S. Treasury's involvement in counterterrorism efforts. The report states that prior to the attacks, no single government agency was responsible for tracking terrorist funds, prioritizing and coordinating government-wide efforts, and seeking international collaboration in that effort. Some tracking of terrorist funds had been undertaken before September 11. These efforts were reported to be unorganized, and actions such as seizures of assets and bank accounts were reluctantly taken. Congress reacted by passing the International Money Laundering Abatement and Anti-Terrorist Financing Act of 2001, which imposes numerous additional reporting requirements for banks and other financial intermediaries.

CONCLUSION

The September 11 incidents had an enormous worldwide impact using low technology and little expense. The U.S. economy experienced $50–80 billion in losses (approximately $40 million in direct insured losses); billions in cleanup costs; billions in lost company revenues; reduced tax revenues; increased military and law enforcement outlays; expenditures to support selected industries (e.g., aviation security); and increased private sector spending for security. For the business community, the impact of 9/11 is seen even in changes in worldwide security measures, causing significant ongoing business-expense increases in almost every country. The real estate company Cushman & Wakefield estimates that about 50 percent of multi-tenant commercial buildings will invest in better security, such as: computerized access control systems, video surveillance systems, bomb-detection devices, and x-ray equipment. In 2001 the average corporate security budget was $667,000, up about 5 percent from 2000, according to *Security Magazine*.

The short-term impact of 9/11 included an increase in the number of bankruptcy filings, the sharpest decline in air passenger demand in over 30 years, and an almost immediate review of corporate insurance premiums.

The magnitude of longer-term costs is less certain. In 2002 the Council on Foreign Relations sponsored a study by an "independent task force," chaired by former Senators Gary Hart and Warren Rudman. The task force report, *America Still Unprepared . . . America Still in Danger*, indicates that state and local first responders remained significantly unprepared for large-scale terrorist attacks. The report points out that police, fire, and medical emergency personnel in states and localities had woefully inadequate access to communication equipment and to necessary intelligence data, training and protective gear in the event they had to handle a public emergency created by a terrorist attack. Further, state and local government assets available for response to such emergencies also were not well coordinated and correction of these problems required considerable new or reallocated revenues.

The cost of reducing risk at offices and businesses through adding security guards, purchasing surveillance equipment, acquiring metal- and bomb-detection equipment, buying detectors of chemical and bio- logical agents, acquiring machines that can irradiate mail, and training security and office employees, among myriad potential necessities, undoubtedly will affect competition and profitability. Industries and companies that fail to respond to terrorist risks may save capital by not purchasing antiterrorism products and services, but they will also run a higher risk of human and financial costs if an incident does occur.

Author Stephen Sloan (in Smith and Thomas, 2001) places the threat of terrorism in context.[1] He observes that, in the short term, govern- ment policy and public attention shift focus from one major group or personality to another, from low-level threat awareness to high-level concerns. The changing nature of terrorism, however, requires govern- mental and corporate policymakers, analysts, and planners to look beyond the present threat environment and address the continuing impact of modern terrorism, and the motivation of terrorist groups as varied as those with deeply held religious beliefs or those who use ter- rorism as part of a mercenary tool to acquire political and economic power. Sloan is not encouraged about the success of current activities, concluding that the focus on current threats, together with seemingly intractable domestic and international political and bureaucratic issues, combine to work against a much-needed long-term strategy to address terrorism and its causes. He expresses concern that the twenty-first cen- tury "will be marked by acts and campaigns of terrorism that might lead not only to mass casualties but destroy an increasingly fragile interde- pendent social order."

NOTES

1. Smith JM, Thomas WC, editors. The terrorism threat and U.S. government response: operational and organizational factors. Institute for National Security Studies, United States Air Force Academy; 2001 Mar. Available from: www.usafa.af.mil/inss/books.htm.

2. Roberts A. The changing faces of terrorism. British Broadcasting Corporation Interactive (BBCi). 2002. Available from: www.bbc.co.uk/history/war/sept_11/changing_faces_01.shtml.

3. The fifth-century BC Chinese military philosopher Sun Tze wrote, in *The Art of War*, about the significance of a surprise attack: "The enemy must

not know where I intend to give battle. For if he does not know where I intend to give battle, he must prepare in a great many places. . . . If he prepares to the front, his rear will be weak, and if to the rear, his front will be fragile. If he prepares to the left, his right will be vulnerable and if to the right, there will be few on his left. And when he prepares everywhere he will be weak everywhere."

4. Federal Bureau of Investigation, Denver Division. Counterterrorism: FBI Policy and Guidelines. Available from denver.fbi.gov/inteterr.htm

5. www.odci.gov/terrorism/faqs.html. Extension of 22 USC'2656(f); 2002 Apr 12.

6. As a trade association ISO, among other activities, is a collector and supplier to the industry of legal, statistical and analytical information.

7. See, among others, the case of *Pan American World Airways vs. Aetna Casualty & Surety et al.*, 505 F2d 989 (1974), where the appellate court affirmed a lower court ruling that the commercial hull insurers had failed in their burden to prove the terrorist acts at issue constituted "war" or "warlike operation," and thus barred the insurers from imposing the applicable contract war exclusion in the September 6, 1970 hijacking to Beirut, and destruction in Cairo, of Pan Am Flight 083 from Brussels to New York by members of the Popular Front for the Liberation of Palestine (PFLP). The court also noted that in the two hours immediately preceding the hijacking of Pan Am 083, the PFLP had also successfully hijacked TWA Flight 741 from Frankfurt, SwissAir Flight 100 from Zurich, and had been thwarted in the hijacking of El Al Flight 219 only by security personnel in flight. After releasing all hostage passengers, the two other hijacked aircraft (plus yet a third plane that was hijacked September 9), were detonated on the ground by the PFLP at Dawson's Field (Zerqa), just north of Amman, Jordan on September 12. Pan Am 083 initially was destined for Dawson's Field, but its hijackers had diverted to Beirut, and later Cairo, only after being convinced that a Boeing 747 could not land there.

8. Chossudovsky (2001) suggests that rules of economic behavior dictated, generally, by wealthy nations represent a form of "economic terrorism," but this view is not highly regarded.

9. Alexander DC, Alexander Y. Terrorism and business: The impact of September 11, 2001. Ardsley, NY: Transnational Publishers; 2002.

10. New York City Comptroller Alan G. Hevesi estimated in early October 2001 that the attacks caused $34 billion in property damage, including 13 million square feet of Class A office space. At least 22 buildings were destroyed or severely damaged in the catastrophe. Hevesi projected cleanup and rescue at $14 billion, and other continuing costs in fiscal 2002 and 2003 at a minimum of $31 billion.

11. Industry differences do exist; terrorism is ranked as the most serious threat perceived by the utility industry, an increase over the prior year.

12. Fiscal year 2002 federal appropriations for homeland security, including supplementary sums, were $29.3 billion.

13. President Bush appointed Tom Ridge, ex-governor of Pennsylvania, to be the first secretary of the Department of Homeland Security. New York Times 2002 Nov 26.

14. Hillman RJ. Terrorism Insurance: rising uninsured exposure to attacks heightens potential economic vulnerabilities, in Diana Miller, editor. Terrorism: Are we ready? New York: Nova Science Publishing; 2002.

15. Among the acts that might not easily or readily be "certified" are losses below the $5 million threshold, or any act of "domestic" terrorism (e.g., akin to the Oklahoma City bombing by Timothy McVeigh), creating many potentially complex situations for insurers, risk managers, and insureds alike. Therefore, two versions of the pre-TRIA January 2002 edition ISO terrorism endorsement outlined earlier are still in use, depending upon applicable state law. Why two? About half the states have laws requiring that every property insurance policy must provide coverage at least equivalent to that provided under a standard fire policy (SFP), and some of those states also impose this requirement on commercial inland marine (CIM) policies. Thus, the two pre-TRIA versions may still apply (one for SFP states and one for non-SFP states), preserving coverage for direct loss by fire. However, IRMI (2003) points out this situation may have the unintended effect of inequitably forcing an insurer to pay for a fire loss due to terrorism when in fact their insured had specifically elected not to purchase terrorism coverage. In response, a few states have modified their laws, and ISO has responded such that there are now some eighteen post-TRIA terrorism SFP/non-SFP/CIM endorsement combinations also in existence to better balance the needs of insurers and insureds under TRIA. In sum, insureds still bear the burden of carefully reviewing their potential exposures to terrorism.

16. The deductible rises from one percent of the previous year's direct earned premium in year one of the program to seven, ten, and fifteen percent in the next years. In addition, TRIA contains a cap on paid losses, an aggregate cap of $100 billion.

17. Linden EV, editor. Focus on terrorism. New York: Nova Science Publishing; 2002.

6 Negotiations with Terrorists

Antoinette Collarini Schlossberg
and Harvey Schlossberg

There are some events in history that occur in the blink of an eye, but profoundly change the way that civilized governments function and consequently restructure in order to cope. Citizens face the reality that life will never return to its original form. One such event occurred on September 5, 1972, in Munich, Germany. Eight Palestinians disguised as athletes and carrying weapons in their athletic bags shocked the world by breaking into the Olympic Village to take hostages. By the time the incident ended, eleven athletes, five terrorists, and one German police officer were dead. This event demonstrated to the free world two important lessons that modified the way military and police would respond to crisis situations forever. First, a small group of ragtag malcontents with a variety of psychological problems demonstrated that a small number of people with a few weapons could do something that had never been done before: stop the Olympic games long enough to focus world attention on political issues that few people even thought about. Their infamy was directly attributed to the fact that they could hold the world's attention focused on their ranting, raving, and often illogical rhetoric and at the same time render a well-trained police department ineffectual over several days. This incident culminated in significant loss of innocent lives and created a shock wave that is still felt today. Second, they proved that traditional security measures could not keep a determined group of criminals out of an Olympic Village structured like a fortress, and therefore no location or event could be secure from a determined terrorist group.

The group's actions, however, were not spontaneous, as previously thought; they involved long-term planning. Post-incident investigation revealed evidence that placement of conspirators into low-level work positions well in advance of the time they would be needed gave the terrorists control of the facility when they initiated action.

This simple fact led to a realization that many governments have yet come to terms with: How are organizations going to recruit and screen applicants for the many undesirable jobs that undocumented aliens or terrorists are glad to fill? This may be one of the most significant keys to security, since there are many low-level vacancies and significant numbers of terrorists who would be delighted to do the work. So, for example, cleaning, maintenance, moving heavy cargo, and other "undesirable" work has been terrorist organizations' backbone when placing operators, informants, and killers into positions of striking at the heart of commerce and transportation.

In many incidents over the years, terrorists have gone through airport security and found weapons for a subsequent skyjacking that had been secreted on the airplane while it was being serviced at the terminal by accomplices working on maintenance crews. Two important lessons were learned: first, no amount of security can keep committed criminals from accomplishing their aims. This became clear when sixty American Airlines employees were arrested in August 1999 in Miami for drug smuggling, following a two-and-a-half year undercover operation by the U.S. government that netted ramp agents, food service workers, and cargo handlers. It is abundantly clear that if drug smugglers can do this, so can terrorists. Second, while the force of arms may be victorious in the final analysis, reliance on sophisticated electronic security methods is not an effective deterrent. An example of this was a case involving federal agents at Kennedy Airport on December 1, 2003. They arrested a similar cast of players for drug smuggling. The group included dozens of baggage and cargo handlers. After more than five years of stream-lined airport security, smuggling remains a flourishing airport crime. It is conceivable that terrorists can readily use the same tactics to infiltrate airport operations.

The New York City Police Department was one of the first to realize that what occurred in Munich in 1972 could very easily occur in New York City. In the early 1970s, there were many events—political, theatrical, and sporting—that attracted large numbers of people to New York City. In addition, turmoil on the everyday menu at the United Nations, with demonstrations on both sides of every issue, presented the average discontented, psychopathic personality with ample opportunities to attain world recognition. From the cold-blooded assassination of a celebrity to the explosion of a bomb in an airport locker, one could rise from obscurity to possibly the next world conqueror. These aggressive, psychopathic, paranoid personalities continually bombarded the police department with vague and sometimes specific threats. Because of this threat the New York City Police Department realized that traditional law enforcement techniques, including units trained in special weapons and tactics, were insufficient to deal with terrorists similar to those in Munich. While terrorists could be outgunned, the amount of damage they would leave behind was unacceptable to the civilized world.

This view of terrorism was reinforced in Moscow on October 27, 2002, when fifty Chechen terrorists held over 800 people in a theater. It became clear that the terrorists planned to kill the hostages one at a time, with the aim of getting the Russian government to stop interfering with Chechen politics and to attract world attention to their cause. When the Chechens executed three hostages, the Russian government decided that a tactical forceful approach was needed. In typical fashion, weapons are always supported with ancillary devices such as gas or smoke. In this particular case, a fast-acting gas that could disable the terrorists and hostages was used, since it was not possible to distinguish among the players. The result was that 117 hostages died, the fifty terrorists died, and 195 went to intensive medical care.

The injuries and loss of life were unacceptable to the civilian population and even surprised the authorities who authorized the forceful solution. Yet from a police standpoint, the Russians had no choice but to use force because they could not stand by and watch the systematic killing of hostages. One of the basic truths learned was that when force is used, regardless of the weapons involved, the actions are both unpredictable and irreversible.

The attacks of September 11, 2001, that led to the destruction of the World Trade Center and the deaths of over 3,000 people were the major event whose significance resonated throughout the entire free world and certainly changed the way people in the United States pursued their lives. It became crystal clear that no place was safe from terrorist onslaught. The skies, the waterways, and the roadways were no longer just paths to vacation and business events, but were also gauntlets to be traversed without being killed or captured and held hostage with the risks of rescue as great as those presented by the terrorists.

Since 9/11, it has become clear that the terrorists have entrenched themselves in various countries and have a true international flavor, with recruiters and operatives placed throughout the world, including sleeper cells in the United States that are poised to strike when given the signal to do so. The terrorists' international character, their possible acquisition of weapons of mass destruction, and their extensive use of suicide bombers have put the entire world on a defensive alert that actually resulted in people willing to give up many of the freedoms that were seen as birthrights and taken for granted.

The ability to travel and conduct life safely has been compromised by the government's development of measures to identify, track, and monitor the population while restricting many freedoms. For the terrorist, this is a victory greater than killing large numbers of people, and it has surpassed any prior historical fame once attributed to terrorist activity. That is, while they have not gained sovereignty or real estate, they have obtained recognition as an international force to be reckoned with. No longer can the free world treat terrorist acts as individual, criminal, isolated events. Rather, it must look at them as well-organized military maneuvers by an ambiguous enemy. At one time, a terrorist action could be tolerated with its results being sanitized and ignored.

THE "CONTAIN AND NEGOTIATE" APPROACH

After the 1972 Munich incident, the New York City Police Department decided that no amount of tactical training or armed intervention would have led to a successful outcome in Munich. Instead, a new combined police and psychological approach was developed to deal with terrorist events. This approach recognized that the result of each terrorist action could not be viewed as an independent event but rather an extended event that was ongoing; and that while it might seem isolated, it was a battle plan that the terrorists had in place and were prepared to carry on for years regardless of political attempts to solve issues. For example, attempts of the United States and other nations to bring peace to the Middle East are sabotaged by radical terrorist groups rather than each step viewed as a possible step toward the establishment of stable, cooperative Middle Eastern states. It becomes clear that repairing damaged buildings and killing terrorists does not prevent another occurrence of terrorist violence.

The New York City Police Department developed a team approach involving a system called "contain and negotiate." The system includes well-trained and -equipped tactical weapons units with sufficient power that, if a situation became combative, the team would have the manpower and force of arms to win; however, in the initial phase, this unit is used to isolate and restrict the terrorists' movements. This is the "contain" part.

The "negotiate" part of the system uses negotiators who are trained in psychological techniques of crisis intervention. This system is based on the concept that most of the issues raised by the terrorist are not immediately solvable; but that by using the psychological principle of airing or communicating his grievances, the terrorist can be induced into problem solving. This problem solving leads him or her to realize that killing will not produce anything but dead bodies, and that delaying gratification and respecting life can lead to continued dialogue. The authorities are more willing to listen, and the public is more likely to cooperate, when killing does not take place. In this way, restraining violence and cooperation are rewarded, and violent responses are punished. This system acknowledges that in each terrorist incident, the terrorist goals are often not to accomplish political change, but rather to gain power and recognition by gathering world attention by manipulating media and creating perceived helplessness of civilian populations.

It is interesting to note that in January 1973 on a freezing, rainy afternoon, the New York City Police Department had its first opportunity to test the "contain and negotiate" system with a group of four Hanafi Muslims who entered a sporting goods store to hold it up for money to finance their revolution against the "capitalist, imperialist" government and to gather weapons for their fight. Even after the gunmen killed one police officer and wounded another, the approach to "contain and negotiate" went into operation for the first time and successfully concluded the situation. The importance of this situation was that even terrorists who had killed and sworn never to surrender yielded to negotiations and were satisfied with the media attention they had achieved.

Suicide attacks since September 11, 2001, have brought into question some of the effectiveness of this approach; however, it is still a sound approach and deals with terrorist activities without having to take away individual freedoms. The current use of suicide bombers is not a terrorist push to victory but rather the terrorists' recognition of a last-ditch effort to intimidate and perhaps gain their goal by extortion and public reaction to the loss of freedoms.

We have seen this in much of the American public's reaction to the homeland security measures. For the most part, the homeland security changes have not made the world safer, but have made the average citizen feel a loss of independence and privacy. It is quite clear that when people's freedoms are threatened in a democracy, a process of displacement results in which the public blames not the terrorist for the threat, but the authorities for their intervention. The government is seen in general as weak and ineffective, and the people in a democracy demand change. For this reason, it would be better to return to "contain and negotiate" rather than revoke individual rights and freedoms.

One of the basic tenets of this approach is that if an individual is intent on dying, is suicidal, the "contain and negotiate" process will isolate him and limit the extent of his killing. The capture of Saddam Hussein on December 13, 2003, without a single shot fired sent a message to terrorists worldwide. The most important aspect of this was that Saddam Hussein did not fight "to the death" or blow himself up as he had suggested to his followers, but rather took a chance on dealing with the established authorities. This message, then, minimizes the value of all the young men and women who have destroyed themselves for the cause of finding glory in suicide. Another important outcome will probably be that once the value of suicide is diminished, terrorists will return to skyjacking and hostage holding.

The approach used in "contain and negotiate" is based on two principles. The first is that when terrorists stage an aggressive act, they do it to get attention and recognition for a cause that would otherwise be ignored. It reflects their status as individuals who are unable to achieve their goals through legitimate channels or actions. The targets of the violent act are actually seen by the terrorist as the power figures and indisputably in control. This is not too different from a child having a tantrum when unable to attain what s/he wants, and when the parent is seen as able to provide but unwilling to do so. The child cannot provide for him or herself but needs the parent to do it. The terrorist performs a violent act or takes hostages to force the perceived power to provide what is wanted. On a symbolic level, if the terrorist asks to be provided with something, then the one s/he asks has the power to give it and therefore is recognized as the power. This model makes the parent or established authority powerful, perhaps more than realistically justified, and the child or terrorist is ineffective and unable to problem-solve. In the war on terrorism, this is more serious because the destruction the "child" does is certainly more massive and dramatic; but it is dynamically the same. The terrorist in his act defines the true authority as he sees it.

The second principle is that the terrorist must be careful not to bite off more than he can chew. If he provokes the authorities, then ultimate power in a confrontation will belong to the authorities, and he will be the loser. Again, as with the analogy of the child, if the tantrum is too violent, the parent has the strength and the power to stop all further activity up to and including hospitalization and medication.

There is little doubt that the events of 9/11 were not helpful to the terrorists. The damage led to the attack on Afghanistan and al Qaeda's loss of operational bases. In a similar vein, the war in Iraq cost the terrorists financing and support. In addition, they have brought Saudi Arabia and Iran into focus, limiting those countries' willingness to help the terrorists. The result of these circumstances is the use of suicide bombings to attempt to end the ongoing assaults on terrorist havens. Their bombings in the Philippines, Pakistan, and Turkey have actually reduced support for the terrorists so that, as they feel more helpless, they increase their violence and therefore lose support from those who have been their prior allies.

Suicide bombing is a technique that will be short-lived for a number of reasons. The number of people willing to do it will diminish, and there is a realization that there is no glory in self-destruction, especially if it does not accomplish anything. If we examine the use of kamikaze (suicide) pilots by the Japanese in World War II, it is clear that while it was psychologically powerful, it was militarily ineffective and ultimately, in the face of the more terrifying power of the atomic bomb, resulted in Japan's surrender instead of the announced plan "never to surrender."

The reality is that hostage taking of either groups or individuals still remains one of the primary activities of terrorists. Hostage-taking events play out over a protracted time. They are covered by media for sensational impact. The result is a feeling of total helplessness by those who watch the events unfold. One can easily empathize with the abuse and loss of self-respect that accompany the thought that one may die any minute. The reinforced helplessness that is generated is a powerful vision that most people can easily see themselves in. Current events in Afghanistan and Iraq have simply emphasized the "us versus them" mentality on a more global scale. The United States' use of force was so overwhelming and unexpected that the terrorists, frustrated and desperate, have lashed out in an almost illogical worldwide display of violence with no clear goal or aim except to demonstrate that they still have power.

Ultimately, individual terrorist acts will solidify free nations into recognizing that what is being confronted is a third world power directed at gaining world dominance, and therefore it will be confronted as an organized army and not a small group of ideological zealots. Meanwhile, there is no doubt that hostage taking will increase in the short run as a response to the suicidal bombings' waning effectiveness. It is necessary, therefore, for the free world to apply "contain and negotiate" internationally and respond to individual terrorist acts as the doings of people who feel helpless and inadequate. These situations, such as barricading oneself in a particular place, skyjacking an airplane, kidnapping media personnel or tourists, or general hostage-holding by terrorists, are really no different from hostage-taking or similar crimes by local citizens. Therefore, while it seems more frightening because of the increased number of suicidal personalities involved, the basic rules of hostage negotiations nevertheless apply.

FUNDAMENTAL RULES OF NEGOTIATING WITH TERRORISTS

There are two fundamental rules that apply whether dealing with a group of terrorists abroad or a similar group in the United States. The first rule is that the hostage in and of himself has no value to the terrorist except as a tool or a device for the terrorist to get what he wants from authorities. This means that there has almost never been a case in which the hostage could provide those things that the terrorist was looking for. If the hostage could, the terrorist would simply take from the hostage what was wanted and we would have a different kind of crime. Therefore, any force applied to, or injuries sustained by the hostages are for ultimate effect on the authorities because killing the hostage simply gives the terrorist a dead body and does not move him even one step closer to the ultimate goal. In fact, it could cause the authorities to decide that the use of force, even at the risk of hurting the remaining hostages, was a more viable solution.

The second rule, as we have already noted, is that it is just as much in the terrorist's interest as it is in the authorities' interest not to let a situation turn violent. In a violent confrontation, the established authorities will always come out as the victors. The authorities have the ultimate power to bring the situation to a successful conclusion. Recognizing these rules, the object is to isolate or contain the terrorists, so that support and encouragement from outside is unavailable. If the media could be held away from the situation, and the terrorists deprived of any external information, they would develop the feelings of being abandoned, ineffectual, and unable to proceed because there would be no feedback on the success of their mission. Then they might be satisfied with an opportunity to make a media statement in return for releasing hostages. No matter how frightening and hopeless a situation looks, to the terrorists who are conducting the operation, the hostage situation represents logical, purposeful, and goal-directed problem solving. To them, it is not random violence, but carefully orchestrated behavior. They believe that they will achieve their goals.

Terrorist acts cannot be considered in isolation. Rather, we must look at the personalities of the terrorists. Generally, all terrorists have overwhelming feelings of being isolated and not part of the establishment. It is for this reason they became terrorists. In psychological terms, this means that the common denominator for them is a feeling of inadequacy. Resorting to bombings, murder, and hostage taking certainly represents an inability to achieve one's goals through legitimate channels. So, although some may glamorize terrorists as freedom fighters and ideologists or political heroes, in a relative definition, they represent society's fringe and do not feel part of the social system.

Most experts concur that there are three basic terrorist personality types. The first is usually described as the leader, who is seen as ideologically motivated. The leader is dedicated to a cause and has little consideration for reality. Obstacles only exist as hypothetical constructs and therefore are easily removed without regard for the method. Leaders are fairly well protected from direct assault by established governments because they are usually in hiding or exile.

The second type is the psychopathic or sociopathic activist recruited from the ranks of prisons and mental institutions. He feels no guilt and can easily commit murder and robbery. He needs immediate gratification and has little empathy for others. He is totally oblivious to the needs or concerns of others. Ultimately, he is likely to act in his own self-interest and is more amenable to the negotiation process. The activist individual also represents a threat to the group's goals because with each successful mission, he envies the leader more, and on some level he would like to replace that person. This is the individual who is most likely to be in charge of a field operation or situation and most likely to be dealt with by the authorities.

The third type of personality is the adventurer or naive idealist. These are tangential members of the group. They do not have staying power or long-term membership, and the leaders see them as expendable. This personality group frequently makes up the field soldiers. Often, they include students, and in the early 1970s they included many women. Interestingly, terrorist groups recognize that women could be as effective as men; and in many instances more so, since they could travel in and out of public places with less scrutiny than males. As a side note, many current terrorist leaders are women who have worked their way up through the ranks. The instability of this third personality type is one factor that led to long containments during negotiations, since no one individual really wants to lose relative status within his or her own group. Each is resistant to surrender until there is a group consensus, and no one individual bears the responsibility for weakening first. In a sense, their emotions ping-pong off each other in a mix of bravado and fear. The basic issue facing the terrorist is, symbolically, what does it feel like to be identified as the most inadequate in the group of inadequate personalities? After all, surrendering to the authorities has some kind of negative consequences for the terrorist, so that in the eyes of the community there is a loss of status.

Once the terrorist is contained and isolated with most ties to the outside world eliminated, it will soon become apparent that whatever the original goals of the mission were, the only real factor that has any consequence is how the situation ends. Does the terrorist kill all the hostages and die in a hail of bullets, never knowing whether anyone will be aware of what s/he has done or what its effect will be on the world? The alternative is to work out a settlement, hope for release by the authorities, and bask in the accomplishment among fellow group members.

The actual negotiations with terrorists are extremely difficult because the authorities cannot offer political sovereignty, return of a homeland, or an atomic bomb, nor can they permit the murder of hostages.

THE ROLE OF THE NEGOTIATOR

The role of the negotiator is complex. Since the terrorist is contained and unable to communicate outside of his immediate environment, the negotiator becomes his or her communicator. Symbolically, the negotiator becomes a substitute for the hostages. Prior to the introduction of the negotiator, the terrorist must threaten and/or abuse the hostages to get attention. The negotiator, by offering assistance, makes it no longer necessary for the terrorist to do this. S/he is able to switch attention from the hostages to the negotiator. Sometimes this process is sufficient to give hostages opportunities to escape unnoticed. The negotiator then helps the terrorist formulate demands in a more familiar and sensible fashion. During this process, an important element automatically comes into play: time. Time becomes the principal weapon of the negotiator and the authorities in dealing with the terrorist. There are many natural environmental and physiological needs that come into play as functions of time. For example, once the terrorist is isolated, issues of food, water, heat, sanitary facilities, and the like become important not only for the hostages but also for the terrorist. These are weapons that are supplied by nature and simply need time to develop. Another function of time is the formation of the Stockholm Syndrome.

The Stockholm Syndrome is the formation of a relationship between the terrorist and his or her victims. It forms as a result of survival need: since the terrorist has life-and-death power over the hostage, the hostage wants to incorporate the characteristics of the terrorist so that s/he can be just like the terrorist, and therefore be liked and valued by the terrorist. In many ways, this is similar to the way a child picks up the characteristics, behaviors, and beliefs of a parent through the process of identification. In general, we tend to like people who are like us and dislike people who are different. The more the hostage can be like the terrorist, the more the terrorist will like him or her. The payment for the hostage is that if s/he is liked, s/he will not be killed and will have power like the terrorist. This phenomenon was identified in psychology as identification with the aggressor, meaning that one wants to have the power of the stronger figure.

The Stockholm Syndrome begins to form approximately ten minutes after capture. It increases in strength with time. Usually it is able to sustain itself for approximately six months. Unfortunately, it is also possible to have a negative Stockholm Syndrome. There is no way of knowing in which direction the relationship will go. Fortunately, logic dictates that if no one is killed, the longer the terrorist and hostage are together, the less likely the terrorist will be to kill. It is interesting that, in contrast to logic, the less the terrorist knows about the hostage prior to the current situation, the greater the likelihood of a positive relationship; conversely, the more that is known about the hostage prior to the incident, the greater the likelihood of a negative relationship. Thus, a family member held hostage is more likely to be killed than a total stranger, even though it would be logical that since the hostage is known, it would be more difficult for the terrorist to kill him or her because of hostile feelings that already exist. The point is, if the terrorist had good feelings prior to this incident, then the hostage would not be a victim.

Through the use of projection, the terrorist can attribute to the hostage any characteristics s/he wishes that person to have. Projection, as in a slide show, works better on a blank screen. In the negotiation process, the negotiator is actually utilizing time while discussing what the terrorist wants.

Another role of the negotiator is to act as a crisis-intervention therapist. This role recognizes that a hostage confrontation is not an everyday event, and therefore represents a highly charged situation and a crisis in the person's life. The negotiator creates an identity as a significant other in the situation. A significant other has to meet two criteria, which the negotiator does meet. First, the negotiator must offer to help the terrorist. In reality, if the containment is successfully performed, the terrorist has nobody else to speak to. Then the negotiator must meet the second criterion by letting the terrorist understand that s/he can, in fact, help. This is accomplished automatically by the negotiator's being an official representative of the establishment. By encouraging the terrorist to outline demands, the process of ventilation occurs. "Ventilation" means verbalizing thoughts in a logical fashion and having to repeat them constantly; this often results in the terrorist seeing his or her thoughts for the first time. In that process, the terrorist may recognize that the thoughts are illogical or not as important as previously thought. The end result is a feeling of relaxation and resolution, even though nothing may have really changed. In a less-than-perfect verbal interchange, a substitute or more feasible objective may develop.

The typical negotiating team consists of a minimum of three people: a primary negotiator, a secondary negotiator, and a tertiary negotiator or coach. The role of the primary negotiator is to deal exclusively with the terrorist. Dealing with the terrorist as well as the authorities would become too pressured and conflicting. The primary negotiator is the crisis therapist and in many ways is the tool of the terrorist to achieve his goals. The terrorist may not want to talk to the primary negotiator; needing time to formulate responses, s/he may select a coconspirator or a hostage to deal with the negotiator. If this should occur, the primary negotiator will have to deal with the person selected by the terrorist. In the negotiation process, it is important to remember that a dialogue need not be established for negotiating to occur. The offer to negotiate in and of itself is negotiating because it gives the terrorist an alternate solution to the problem, so that killing a hostage is not necessary to prove a point, since negotiations are still feasible.

The secondary negotiator supports the primary one in making decisions and acting as a sounding board, helping to evaluate information for the primary negotiator, interpreting what the terrorist is saying, and acting as a go-between with the authorities. Screening intelligence information and providing the primary negotiator with ideas and appropriate intelligence are important functions of the secondary negotiator.

The tertiary negotiator or coach records events, including demands, threats, requests, and other information, in chronological fashion. In some instances, more people are on the team; however, the minimum requirement is three individuals. Adding others would simply give those others ancillary roles, such as gathering and sifting through intelligence, helping to set up communication networks, or providing media liaison functions.

All negotiations are usually conducted by telephone communications that are isolated from the public system. This is done to avoid interference by supporters of the terrorists or well-intentioned individuals with their own agendas and solutions. In the early days, face-to-face negotiations were conducted. This type proved to be too dangerous for the negotiators and often too threatening to the terrorists. They failed to consider people's psychological boundaries and required space for interaction. In addition, telecommunication removed the cues of body language and possible paranoid interpretation of eye contact. A telephone, unlike face-to-face contact, can provide psychological feelings of privacy and intimacy. This is demonstrated when we observe people walking down the street or sitting in a restaurant having the most intimate of conversations on the telephone. On a more serious level, known criminals whose telephone lines are tapped will often carry on conversations that lead to their arrests even though they know that their telephones are tapped.

The basic system of "contain and negotiate" has remained constant since 1972. The only major change has been a change in the primary negotiator role. Typically in the negotiating process, while there have been female terrorists the person chosen by the terrorist to negotiate was a male. In the early 1970s it was felt that most males and females in crisis situations usually preferred a male helper so that, regardless of sex, a person who needed a lawyer, physician, or auto mechanic preferred a male helper.

With the advent of the women's liberation movement, more women entered police work. In spite of the pressure to maintain all-male negotiators, it soon became apparent that many women had interest in doing negotiations. The concept of the female negotiator was pioneered mostly in California, since California police agencies were the quickest to open their ranks to women. Many police departments sought women who received training through an initiative by the California Law Enforcement Association in cooperation with San Jose State University. As a result of the training, many female police officers found themselves in the role of primary negotiator. Their performance proved to be fantastically successful. It is interesting to note that in the 1972 Munich Olympic hostage situation, the terrorists actually requested that the Munich Police Department provide them with a female negotiator.

That attempt failed because the woman was used in a face-to-face confrontation, and because of paranoia, the terrorists suspected a police plot to attack them. Since that time, the use of telecommunications for negotiating has resulted in a very effective development of a male/female negotiating team. The system is designed so the negotiations begin with a male primary negotiator establishing authoritarian parameters. After a couple of hours, a female negotiator replaces the male primary negotiator and becomes the primary negotiator. It seems that the sound of the female voice has a calming effect. Verbally, the dialogue is very similar; therefore, the impact of this team must be one that is created psychologically, regardless of the reality.

CONCLUSION

While terrorism has changed drastically in its use of suicide bombers, it is clear that unless at some point the terrorist is willing to talk about viable solutions to political and social problems, nothing will be accomplished except an increased body count on both sides. In the long run, the terrorists must return to the use of media to send fear into the population and to demonstrate the validity of their demands. In order to accomplish this, terrorists must return to the more basic terrorist tools, namely hostage taking, kidnapping, and extortion. The established authorities must maintain the ability to deal with these acts by training and equipping tactical and negotiating teams that can be mobilized and transported to where they are needed.

7 Managing the Business Effects of Terrorist Acts: Does Strategic Planning Play a Role?

John Angelidis and Nabil A. Ibrahim

The terrorist acts of September 11, 2001, marked the dawning of a new era of challenges for the business community. It was the first time that terrorism hit the heart of the most important financial center of the strongest power in the world. The results were devastating in human, economic, and psychological terms. Recent events have clearly demonstrated that virtually no one—including humanitarian groups—is immune from terrorist acts. Although in many parts of the world, some organizations have responded successfully to the new challenges,[1] the vast majority continues to be highly vulnerable to such attacks.[2]

In recent years we have witnessed the remarkable wealth creation that can be accomplished through the free movement of goods, services, labor, and information. This openness of borders can also make it possible for terrorists to operate freely or with fewer impediments. Thus, acts of terrorism have been greatly facilitated by the promises of globalization.[3] Consequently, an unprecedented level of cooperation has been set in motion among governments, businesses, and international organizations.

Despite these efforts, terrorists can still hit business interests all over the world, as the bombing of HSCB Bank in Turkey and other traumatic events have demonstrated. Not surprisingly, then, managers have been forced to confront the task of developing plans to meet the newest major threat of the twenty-first century. Yet a great number of firms and organizations still do not have any plans for how to deal with terrorist acts.[4]

A literature search has found that, although there is a plethora of articles describing how industries and companies coped after 9/11,[1,5] very few have focused on the need to address the business effects of terrorist acts within the context of strategic management. For example, Peter Kennedy, Charles Perrottet, and Charles Thomas provide examples of how scenario planning can be utilized as a strategic tool to manage the impact of a catastrophic event.[6] A different approach is proposed by Jan Torrissi-Mokwa, who describes a "people strategic plan" to deal with terrorism.[7] Finally, Jim Underwood argues that corporate counterterrorism should focus on five tiers, beginning with the global environment and ending with the corporate premises.[8] Although these articles have emphasized strategic issues, they do not discuss specific steps to address this important issue. This chapter attempts to partially fill this void by explaining how companies can respond to the terrorist business threats of the new millennium.

PLANNING FOR A SUCCESSFUL RESPONSE

The strategic management paradigm can provide an anticipatory, systematic approach for developing plans to address the impact of terrorism on business. This approach is based on a stepwise process that includes five parts.

Identification of Significant Terrorist Actions

The process begins with the establishment of a crisis management team that will identify significant terrorist actions that can harm a business. The team should thoroughly scan the environment to identify potential terrorist threats such as explosives, kidnappings, poisonings, data/information contamination, and sabotage. Also, the team should carefully scrutinize international, regional, national, and local media; examine appropriate publications and literature; and take into account any other intelligence sources as they relate to their business organization.

As shown in table 7.1, it is probable that businesspeople will be able to identify some, but not all, types of terrorist actions that can harm their businesses. A diligent search of various sources can uncover other dangers. The airline industry, for example, recognized these dangers and developed plans to deal with hijackings and catastrophic accidents. Also, the oil exploration industry had to develop plans and policies regarding the frequent kidnappings of its employees in various parts of the world. It is

Table 7.1
Types of Factors That Can Cause Harm to a Business

	Known	*Unknown*
Realized		
Unrealized		

important to point out that some potential terrorist actions against certain businesses, such as the nuclear power industry, have not materialized.

Businesspeople are challenged to prepare their businesses not only for known threats but also for unknown ones.[9] To cope with this eventuality, they may want to reduce their risk by setting aside financial resources, purchasing insurance policies, developing cooperative arrangements with other organizations, setting emergency facilities outside the existing ones, and developing corporate crisis management teams, and so forth.[5,10]

Determination of the Likelihood of Terrorist Act Occurrence

The second step of this process involves determining the likelihood of occurrence of each of the terrorist acts identified in the previous step. This is essential because it allows managers to weed out terrorist acts that are unlikely to occur and focus on the imminent ones. The likelihood of occurrence of each terrorist act can be measured on a scale from 1 to 5 (1 = low likelihood of occurrence, 3 = medium likelihood of occurrence, 5 = high likelihood of occurrence).

Identification of Potential Terrorist Targets

This step of the process requires the identification of where the terrorists might strike. Businesspeople must take a systematic view of identifying any possible terrorist targets. One tool that can be utilized is Michael Porter's Value Chain concept.[11] Managers should determine *where* value is created in their organization. They should start with their suppliers, and then look inside their organization by examining their inbound logistics, operations, distribution, and outbound logistics, sales, and the provision of services after the sale. They should consider their human resources, management, information systems, research and development, distribution channels, and customers. Finally, their analysis should expand to include the communities within which the business operates.

Table 7.2
Quantitative Method for Determining the Relative Strength of Impact of a Terrorist Act

Organizational Factors Affected	Weight Indicating the Relative Importance of Each Factor (0–1)	Relative Strength of Impact (1–5)	Weighted Strength of Impact: (Weight × Relative Strength)
Profitability			
Revenues			
Costs			
Quality/product performance			
Reputation			
Capacity			
Financial resources			
Total			

Estimating the Relative Impact of a Potential Terrorist Act

The fourth step is to estimate the impact of the terrorist act on one's organization. There are two components of impact assessment. The first is determining the strength of the impact. Managers have to determine whether a specific terrorist act has a strong, medium, or weak impact on their organization. To make this determination, they must consider the impact of the terrorist act on an array of important organizational factors such as profitability, revenues, costs, quality/product performance, company reputation, manufacturing capacity, and human resources. These can be measured on a scale from 1 to 5 (1 = low impact, 3 = medium impact, 5 = high impact). Because these factors do not have the same significance for the organization, a weighting system is recommended to reflect differences in significance. Table 7.2 provides a format for determining the relative strength of impact of a terrorist act.

This determination is important because it indicates where management should focus most of its attention in planning how to deal with a terrorist act; that is, the type and amount of resources the organization should allocate.

The second component of assessment is the duration of the impact. Businesspeople have to determine whether the results of a specific terrorist act will last for a short, medium, or long time. This analysis will exert an influence on how fast, how strong, and for how long an organization should act in the case of a specific terrorist threat.

Assessing the Relative Threat of Each Potential Terrorist Act to the Business

The fifth step assesses the relative threat that each terrorist act poses to the business. We define the relevant threat as a function of the strength of the impact of the terrorist act (how great the damage will be) and its likelihood of occurrence. This assessment will be used to determine the amount of resources an organization will spend to deal with each threat.

The most helpful method of assessing the relative threat of each terrorist act is a quantitative one. All the required information comes from the previous analyses. More specifically, managers need information about the following:

- Significant terrorist acts that can cause harm
- The potential likelihood of these acts' occurrence
- Potential targets
- Weighted relative strength of impact

Table 7.3 provides a format for determining the relative threat of each potential terrorist threat. To illustrate the use of this table, two

Table 7.3
Quantitative Method for Determining the Relative Threat of Each Potential Terrorist Act

Target	Likelihood of Terrorist Act A (a)	Relative Strength of Impact of Terrorist Act A (b)	Relative Threat of Terrorist Act A (a) × (b)	Likelihood of Terrorist Act B (a)	Relative Strength of Impact of Terrorist Act B (b)	Relative Threat of Terrorist Act B (a) × (b)
Supplier A	3.0	3.2	9.6			
Supplier B				2.0	2.5	5.0
Factory I	3.0	2.5	7.5			
Warehouse L				2.0	1.1	2.2
Shipping	3.0	1.2	3.6			
Product contamination	3.0	4.7	14.1			
Customer G				2.0	3.2	6.4
Database	3.0	2.3	6.9	2.0	2.5	5.0
Information technology	3.0	2.7	8.1	2.0	2.4	4.8
Distribution channels	3.0	1.9	5.7			
Inventory						
Total			55.5			23.4

potential terrorist acts are considered: acts A and B. By examining each of the total scores, we conclude that act A (total score: 55.5) poses a greater threat for one's business than Act B (total score: 23.4).

DETERMINING THE AVAILABILITY OF RESOURCES TO DEAL WITH TERRORISM

The crisis management team should determine how many and what type of resources the organization is willing to put at its disposal before it develops any strategies on how to deal with specific terrorist actions. Determining the final amount of resources might require a lot of interaction between top management and the crisis management team. Top management might want to find out how imminent and how serious is the potential of a terrorist act before they decide when, how, and how many resources to allocate for terrorist protection. This, in turn, will affect the type of counterterrorism strategy the company will develop.

DEVELOPING A BUSINESS COUNTERTERRORISM STRATEGY

At this step, the management team has a clear understanding of what terrorist acts most threaten the business organization (analysis of step 4), and how many resources are available to deal with this problem (analysis of step 5). In developing a business counterterrorism strategy, managers have to answer the following three questions:

1. **What can our business do to protect itself?** This question places all the responsibility for counterterrorism on the firm. The business has an absolute control of what needs to be done, how it is going to be done, when it is going to happen, and who is going to do it. On the other hand, the firm alone has to provide all the required resources for the implementation of this strategy. The firm may or may not have all the required expertise in every area of counterterrorism.
2. **What can our business, in conjunction with others, do to protect itself?** The answer to this question forces management to find stakeholders who share similar concerns. The creation of cooperative arrangements allows the firm to combine its responsibility for counterterrorism with that of its stakeholders. A firm's stakeholders could be competitors acting together to protect the safety of the industry. Another type of stakeholder could be other companies operating in the same geographic area acting together to safeguard their facilities. In such cases, the company might be losing some control over the counterterrorism

strategy, since other entities participate in it, and their interests and opinions have to be taken into consideration. Issues of coordination may arise. Different organizational cultures may hinder the implementation of the counterterrorism strategy. On the other hand, the firm might have to contribute fewer resources than if it chose a "go-it-alone" approach. Another benefit is that many partners may bring together a greater variety of expertise.

3. **What can others do to protect our business?** In this case, management tries to identify entities willing to develop and carry out counterterrorism strategies. One possibility is for the company to hire an outside entity to develop and implement the firm's counterterrorism strategy. Another possibility is to find another entity that provides the resources and develops and carries out a counterterrorism strategy covering the firm's security. Today, many governments have undertaken this task within their overall economic and security responsibilities.

CONCLUSION

The new millennium brought new challenges to the business community. Among these is terrorism. This chapter utilized the strategic management paradigm to propose a seven-step process that companies might use in developing counterterrorism strategies to protect themselves.

Counterterrorism strategies include preventive, reactive, and combination strategies. Preventive strategies focus on how to prevent a terrorist act from taking place. Reactive strategies emphasize how the organization should respond when a terrorist act has taken place. Combination strategies use a combination of proactive and reactive strategies.

Finally, it is important to note that, by their nature, counterterrorism strategies for business are dynamic and continuous. They are dynamic because the factors that were considered when the strategy was developed are always changing. They are continuous because managers have to continuously monitor and make the appropriate strategy changes as the conditions change.

NOTES

1. Fearn-Banks K, Symmes RJ, Murphy M, Amir-Hosseini S, Eder DN, Rogers H, et al. A snapshot of how organizations responded to tragedy. Pub Rel Tactics 2002 Sep;9(9):30–2.

2. Anonymous. The 2003 HBR list: breakthrough ideas for tomorrow's business agenda. Harvard Bus Rev 2003 Apr;81(4):92.

3. Bremer LP, Morse G. Doing business in a dangerous world. Harvard Bus Rev 2002 Apr;80(4):22–3.

4. Anonymous. Crisis? What crisis? Pub Rel Strategist 2003 Winter;9(1):4; Anonymous. Most hospital ERs not prepared for bioterrorism; patient violence biggest threat to ER staff. Health Care Strategic Man 2003 Jan;21(1):7.

5. Strazewski L. Business travel coverage now a risk management concern. Rough Notes 2003 July;146(7):124; Kirchoffner D. Throw out the old handbook in favor of today's crisis drills. PR News 2003 Jan 27;59(4):1.

6. Kennedy P, Perrottet C, Thomas C. Scenario planning after 9/11: managing the impact of a catastrophic event. Strat & Leadership 2003;31(1):4–14.

7. Torrissi-Mokwa J. Are your first things second? How a people strategic plan improves focus and results. J Tax Practice Man 2003 Mar/Apr;2(2):9.

8. Underwood J. Corporate counterterrorism, intelligence, and strategy. Competitive Intel Mag 2002 Nov/Dec;5(6):15.

9. Sanchez C, Goldberg SR. How to handle the threat of a catastrophe. J Corp Acc & Fin 2003 Sep/Oct;14(6):35.

10. Fannin R. Danger abroad. Ch Exec 2003 Jan/Feb;185:30–6.

11. Porter ME. Competitive advantage: creating and sustaining superior performance. New York: The Free Press; 1985.

8   Bioterrorism: Is the Nation's Healthcare System Prepared?

Laura K. Acton and Gerald R. Ledlow

Bioterrorism has been defined as "the intentional release of a virus, bacteria, or toxin upon a population for the purpose of causing illness or death."[1] The United States has had very little experience with bioterrorism. According to Tucker,[2] the Federal Bureau of Investigation (FBI) typically investigated only about a dozen cases per year prior to the late 1990s. These cases involved the acquisition of chemical or biological materials. In 1997, however, the FBI opened seventy-four investigations involving these materials, and in 1998 opened 181. Eighty percent of these cases in 1997 and 1998 were hoaxes; some, however, were unsuccessful attacks. In spite of this increased incidence of cases involving chemical or biological weapons, many experts believe that the risk of an attack of bioterrorism is very low.[2,3] Former FBI director Louis Freeh and former Secretary of Defense William Cohen have testified that "the use of biological weapons must be viewed as a low-likelihood, but high-impact event."[4]

This relatively low risk has not deterred the government and many others in the public health sector from speculating on how to prepare for and manage such an attack. Much of the literature focuses on the biological agents believed to be of highest risk. Educating the public on the transmission, detection, and treatment of the diseases caused by these agents is a very important aspect of a preparedness plan. However, a comprehensive plan must encompass much more. A strong public health infrastructure, advanced communication system, rapid response to an outbreak, and disaster preparedness at the local level, are key to effectively managing an outbreak of disease as a result of biological warfare.[5-7] Our ability to recognize and react promptly and appropriately to a highly infectious and invisible agent without panic, and with a high degree of organization, is of the utmost importance.[1]

HISTORY OF BIOTERRORISM

The use of biological weapons goes back as far as the sixth century B.C. The first recorded incident involved the use of rye ergot, a fungus that infects wild grasses. The Assyrians used it to contaminate enemy wells.[1] Reports of bioterrorism continued throughout history. In the fourteenth century, barbarians catapulted plague-infected bodies over the walls of fortified cities to spread the deadly infection among their enemies.[5] In 1763 at Fort Pitt, Pennsylvania, the English gave smallpox-infested blankets to Indians who were loyal to the French.[5] During World War I, Germany used biological weapons to infect livestock in a number of countries, particularly targeting horses and mules destined for the U.S. Cavalry.[4] During World War II, the Japanese conducted experiments with *Bacillus anthracis*, the bacteria that causes the disease anthrax, on prisoners of war.[1] More recent incidents include the release of sarin gas in a Tokyo subway in 1995[2] and the deliberate contamination of restaurant salad bars with *Salmonella typhimurium* in Oregon in 1984.[8]

The United States researched biological weapons up until 1969; President Nixon then ordered the cessation of all biological weapons programs in the United States. Many other nations followed Nixon's lead to stop their programs. In 1972 several nations enacted an international agreement called the Biological and Toxin Weapons Convention; the convention prohibited the production and retention of stockpiles of biological weapons.[4] Despite these measures, the threat of bioterrorism remains. In 1991 United Nations weapons inspectors discovered warheads with anthrax spores and the toxin that causes botulism stockpiled in Iraq.[1] There is also concern that Russia has continued its biological weapons program, and that the technologies developed by the former Soviet Union have become available to other nations as well as terrorist organizations.[4]

ISSUES RELATED TO BIOTERRORISM PREPAREDNESS

A bioterrorist attack could range from the dissemination of aerosolized anthrax spores to food product contamination. Unlike explosions, these attacks are covert. An act by a lone terrorist could result in a major disease outbreak that is spread in successive waves throughout the population before anyone is even aware that it has happened. The covert nature and low incidence of such acts bring forth several problems that are unique to bioterrorist attacks and that must be overcome in preparing for the possibility of the use of biological weapons.

The first problem is the lag time between exposure and the onset of symptoms, regardless of the agent used. This poses a problem because the disease could be dispersed throughout the population before officials were even aware that an attack had occurred. As a result of the dispersion, especially in a large community, the population exposed could access the healthcare system in many different ways, such as physicians' offices, hospital emergency rooms, and walk-in clinics. This would also make the attack difficult to diagnose and cause further delays in treatment.[9]

Another issue is that the early symptoms of most biological agents look clinically identical and are similar to those of common ailments, such as influenza and upper respiratory infections. This makes a biological attack almost impossible to diagnose at an early stage. Because of the virulence of many of these agents, significant morbidity and mortality may occur before there is an accurate diagnosis.[9]

Another issue has to do with finances. Darmiento[10] reported that a national trade group report to Congress estimated that it would cost hospitals $11.3 billion nationwide to adequately prepare for an attack by a weapon of mass destruction. This price tag included such things as testing labs, personal protective gear for healthcare workers, additional medical supplies, and more training. The current economic situation in healthcare contributes significantly to the issues surrounding preparedness for a potential emergency related to biological weapons. Hospital budgets are already "cut to the bone," according to McLaughlin.[11] Disaster planning is often a low priority as a result. Rosen[9] stated that "it is hard to raise money to defend against a problem that has such a low incidence."

Rosen[9] also felt that even if an identified agent had a specific treatment or vaccine, there would be difficulty delivering it to the affected area. Supplies may be limited, there may be issues with distance and travel, or citizens might refuse treatment.

The low incidence of such attacks also raises concern about maintained preparedness in spite of written disaster plans.[9] The Joint Commission on Accreditation of Healthcare Organizations (JCAHO) announced that it would take a closer look at compliance to its standard of emergency management in 2003 as a result of this concern. JCAHO requires hospitals to have emergency management plans that are coordinated with the response of the community.[12] Emergency management plans should include disaster drills to maintain preparedness.

Panic and political instability may also arise from a bioterrorist attack.[5] Panic proliferating throughout a population as a result of a biological attack could influence public officials to overreact by revoking civil liberties. This could result in political unrest.[13]

CURRENT LEVEL OF PREPAREDNESS IN THE UNITED STATES

Preparedness for bioterrorism has become the topic of much debate.[14] In October 1999 a General Accounting Office (GAO) report documented significant gaps in the United States' systems for protecting against biological attacks. Investigators found shortages of vaccines and medications, stockrooms full of expired drugs, and careless security measures where crucial drugs were stored.[5] In March 2001 another report by the GAO reported that "20 percent of the nation's pharmaceutical and medical supplies held by the Federal Office of Emergency Preparedness for a bioterrorist attack were stored in a vault whose temperature was 95 degrees and that had no air conditioning. The medicines' potency could be assured only if kept cooler than 86 degrees."

The Centers for Disease Control and Prevention (CDC) in Atlanta reported in January 2001 that the nation's public health infrastructure was "not adequate to detect and respond to a bioterrorist event."[5]

A recent survey of thirty hospitals in four states and Washington, DC, found that hospitals were not equipped to handle a widespread biological disaster. This survey reported that only one out of thirty hospitals had stockpiled medications for a bioterrorism attack, and twenty-six out of the thirty were equipped to handle only ten to fifty casualties at once.[15] In another study done by Wetter, Daniell, and Treser,[8] hospital emergency departments were found to be generally unprepared to treat victims of bioterrorism in an organized fashion. Levels of preparedness were relatively low with regard to awareness, plans, training, physical resources, and medication inventories.

Reports such as these are certainly disconcerting. The good news is that the federal and local governments have not been sitting back and doing nothing. The medical community and the public sector are "stepping up to the plate" to combat bioterrorism.

GOVERNMENT POLICY TO IMPROVE
THE STATE OF PREPAREDNESS

The U.S. government is taking the need to prepare for a bioterrorist attack very seriously. In 1995 the Presidential Decision Directive 39 triggered actions among many national agencies. Congress enacted the Defense against Weapons of Mass Destruction Act in 1996. This act required the development of a domestic preparedness program.[8]

The Clinton administration also developed a bioterrorism initiative that was administered jointly by the CDC and the National Institutes of Public Health. This initiative was aimed at speeding development of protective technologies such as portable DNA diagnostic devices. The CDC has been designated the lead agency for the government initiatives committed to upgrading preparedness and national defenses against bioterrorist weapons.[16]

The federal government has committed significant funds to fighting bioterrorism. In late 2001, President Bush's emergency relief budget request included $1.5 million for the Department of Health and Human Services (HHS) to further strengthen our ability to respond to potential bioterrorist attacks. These funds would support the CDC, the U.S. Food and Drug Administration (FDA), other HHS agencies, and state and local offices. Key targets for these funds include the following:

1. Expanding the National Pharmaceutical Stockpile, including enough antibiotics to protect at least 12 million people from anthrax exposure.
2. Expanding the number of smallpox vaccines enough to protect the entire nation's population.
3. Speeding the development of new bioterrorism tools such as vaccines, drug therapies, and diagnostic tests.
4. Increasing state and local readiness, especially at hospitals and health facilities.
5. Expanding the response capabilities of the HHS to bioterrorism incidents.
6. Improving food safety through more inspections of imported food products and investments in new technology and scientific equipment for the FDA to detect select agents.

This $1.5 million was in addition to the HHS fiscal year 2002 budget request of $345 million for bioterrorism preparedness.[17]

National, regional, and statewide epidemiological[18] systems to quickly identify, track, and control resource allocation are necessary and must be fully integrated within the multitiered medical laboratory system, the CDC (to include the Health Alert Network),[19] and public and community health systems.[20] The CDC received $178 million in fiscal year 1999 with substantial increases every year since to prepare for surveillance for such events as bioterrorism and to establish this network of laboratories (the LRN). In addition, the CDC received $52 million to establish a pharmaceutical stockpile of drugs, vaccines, prophylactic medicines, and antidotes for events such as a bioterrorist response.[21] The key for communities across the nation to have access to the CDC stockpile (or push-packs of pharmaceuticals and supplies) is to develop and file an approved distribution plan for those medical push-packs with the CDC. The integration of the LRN into the National Electronic Disease Surveillance System (NEDSS), a system that would replace more than seventy different disease-reporting systems operated by the CDC into a single system,[19] should be a high priority. Improvement in the capability and communication systems of clinical laboratories is critical in supporting surveillance efforts.[22] It is imperative that the local healthcare facility's microbiology laboratory integrate into the Laboratory Response Network (LRN), where protocols are utilized to either rule out bacterial agents or refer such specimens to the next laboratory level within the network.[22,23] If biological pathogens are impacting a community, then infectious diseases are the second leading cause of death and the leading cause of disability-adjusted life years worldwide.[24] Implementing the appropriate systems to counter the pathogen protects the population, the workforce, and business.

The LRN is a national network of laboratories in the United States assembled to respond to the growing biological threats. The CDC and the Association of Public Health Laboratories, based on a disease surveillance system, have created a four-level system:

1. Level A labs assess risks of aerosols and rule out and forward organisms.
2. Level B labs work with biological agents at biosafety level (BSL) 2 and confirm and transport biological pathogens.
3. Level C is a BSL 3 lab that does molecular assays and has a reference capacity.
4. Level 4 is the highest-level lab at BSL 4 and is a federal asset at the CDC and U.S. Army Medical Research Institute.[23]

The LRN is important not only for identification of biological agents, but also in determining the appropriate treatment options and guiding the public health response to an outbreak situation based on expert-driven protocols and procedures. These protocols were developed in conjunction with the CDC, public health agencies, the FBI, and the Department of Defense.[22,23] Essential to the early identification system, a laboratory's response (and indeed the entire LRN) should be prompt identification of biological agents; notification of local, state, and federal officials; notification of appropriate law enforcement officials; and healthcare provider support to care for potentially large numbers of patients.[21] It is imperative to incorporate all laboratories into the LRN as soon as possible to exponentially increase our nation's ability to conduct timely public health surveillance in deterrence of bioterrorism.

Human surveillance systems should be complemented by animal systems. Veterinary sciences can and should complement human specimen laboratory efforts. "Although veterinarians have been mentioned as an integral part of the biological [pathogen] ... preparedness planning, the importance of improving surveillance among livestock, pets and wild animal populations have [sic] not been emphasized."[25] Animal reporting systems currently exist and in many instances of disease, reporting is required,[26] and should be integrated into the early detection and identification system of the LRN and the NEDSS.

STRATEGIC PLANNING IN THE FIGHT AGAINST BIOTERRORISM

In "Biological and Chemical Terrorism: Strategic Plan for Preparedness and Response," the CDC[16] identifies five key focus areas:

- Preparedness and prevention
- Detection and surveillance
- Diagnosis and characterization of biological and chemical agents
- Response
- Communication

Each of these areas integrates training and research. The preparedness efforts focus on agents that are felt to have the greatest impacts on U.S. health and security. The top six bioterrorism candidates identified by the CDC are anthrax, smallpox, pneumonic plague, tularemia, botulism, and viral hemorrhagic fevers.[27]

The U.S. Department of Health and Human Services (HHS)[6] also identified five areas for its antibioterrorism initiative. Those five areas include:

- Improving the nation's public health surveillance network to quickly detect and identify the biological agent that has been released.
- Strengthening the capacities for medical response, especially at the local level.
- Expanding the stockpile of pharmaceuticals for use if needed.
- Expanding research on the disease agents that might be released, rapid methods for identifying biological agents, and improved treatments and vaccines.
- Preventing bioterrorism by regulating the shipment of hazardous biological agents or toxins.

When comparing the key elements identified by both the CDC and HHS, similarities become evident. Communication (including surveillance), preparedness, response, and research are common themes. The implementation of these key components in the fight against bioterrorism is a very complex process that must involve numerous partners and activities. State and local governments, along with the medical community and the public sector, are becoming very involved in the fight. How is the implementation of each of these common key components being accomplished?

IMPLEMENTING THE STRATEGIC PLAN

Communication

Enhancing communications between the medical and public health communities is essential in fighting bioterrorism. This includes not only surveillance strategies but also how information regarding disease is disseminated and outbreaks are being reported throughout the world.

There have been concerns about the public health system and the current procedures for reporting outbreaks. The December 2001 *Healthcare Purchasing News* reported that the "nation's public health system relies far too heavily on paper records which slow the reporting of potential outbreaks of diseases or bioterrorism attacks."[28] This concern stems from the fact that many physicians, laboratories, and public health agencies are not connected to the Internet.[29] A report from the National HealthKey Collaborative, a consortium of healthcare groups working to develop standardized e-health security policies and solutions, suggests that reporting speed for outbreaks of disease would improve "if more physicians, hospitals, and laboratories could communicate via the Internet."[28] This would significantly improve communications in the medical and public health sectors.

The CDC has proposed a plan to work with state and local health agencies to develop a "state of the art" communication system. Beginning in 2004 this system will support disease surveillance, rapid notification and information exchange regarding disease outbreaks, dissemination of diagnostic results and emergency health information, and coordination of emergency response activities. Terrorism-related training for emergency responders, emergency department personnel, hospital staff, and laboratory personnel will also be available via this network.[16]

As mentioned before, the CDC has a program in place called the Health Alert Network. This program's purpose is to equip and train local public health agencies, provide access to surveillance data and CDC response protocols, and to assist local agencies in developing and applying performance standards for addressing bioterrorism and other threats. The Health Alert Network has funds allocated in thirty-seven states and three urban public health agencies. To date, these funds, 85 percent of which must be used locally, have been used to link local health departments to state public health agencies, purchase decontamination equipment, and develop training materials for the public health workforce on bioterrorism and emergency response.[11]

Clinical laboratories in both the private and public sectors are key to identifying biological agents and preventing their spread. There is an effort underway to establish a national laboratory system, which would enhance communications among federal, state, and local public laboratories, as well as laboratories in hospitals and physician's offices. This system would allow laboratories to rapidly share information electronically.[29]

The Association of Medical Publications has also launched a public service campaign to communicate information about the diagnosis and treatment of diseases caused by biological warfare agents. This campaign includes advertisements targeting physicians and other healthcare professionals, directing them to an Internet website containing in-depth information on bioterrorism-related diseases. This campaign intends to raise the awareness of healthcare professionals. The pro-bono advertisements state, "Medical professionals are America's first line of defense against bioterrorism."[30] Communications of this sort are essential in the fight against bioterrorism. An aware medical community is also a prepared medical community.

Preparedness

The preparedness of physicians and other healthcare providers, especially at the local level, is another key component in the fight against bioterrorism. Preparedness for a biological attack depends on the ability of the nation's healthcare systems to identify and respond quickly and appropriately. Atlas[4] noted that in order to limit the spread of disease and minimize the number of casualties, healthcare workers and first responders must know what to do.

Healthcare workers, especially physicians, must be alert to illness patterns and diagnostic clues that may indicate the use of a biological weapon.[31] Preparedness depends on knowing what to look for. The American Academy of Family Physicians has outlined seven signs of a potential bioterrorist attack. These include the following:[4]

- A rapidly increasing disease incidence in a normally healthy population
- An epidemic curve that rises and falls during a short period of time
- An unusual increase in people seeking care, especially those with fever, respiratory, or gastrointestinal complaints
- An endemic disease that rapidly emerges at an uncharacteristic time or in an unusual pattern
- An increased incidence of illness among people who frequently go outdoors, compared to those who typically remain indoors
- Clusters of patients arriving from a single locale
- Large numbers of rapidly fatal cases

Another resource is *Primer on 10 Classical Biological Agents*, developed by the U.S. Army Medical Research Institute of Infectious Disease to increase the likelihood that medical personnel will properly recognize the symptoms of diseases caused by biological warfare agents.[16]

In addition to providing information on the recognition of biological agents, response protocols to those agents are essential. The CDC is providing public health guidelines, support, and technical assistance to local and state public health agencies as they develop plans and response protocols.[32] These guidelines developed by the CDC for responding to anthrax, smallpox, and other biological agents are available on the Internet and are being utilized by healthcare organizations and local public health officials across the country as they develop emergency preparedness plans.

An excellent example of how the CDC has assisted with preparedness is seen at Covenant HealthCare. Covenant HealthCare in Saginaw,

Michigan, quickly developed "Weapons of Mass Destruction (Biological/Chemical Readiness Plan)" in the wake of the terrorist attacks of September 11, 2001. This plan was a joint effort of the hospital's safety committee and infection control committee. It is housed on the hospital's intranet computer system and has Internet links to the CDC's published guidelines, the Michigan Department of Community Health, and the Michigan Infectious Disease Society's *Guidelines for Health Care Providers, Hospitals, and Emergency Departments Responding to Concerns about Exposure to Anthrax.* Covenant HealthCare's plan is comprehensive, including protocols for first response, triage, patient management, detailed disease management, internal and external emergency contacts, and how information will be communicated to the public. This is a fifty-eight-page policy with references to the CDC throughout.[33]

Parma Community General Hospital in Parma, Ohio, is another example of how the federal government has assisted in the development of disaster plans involving bioterrorism. The director of security for this 337-bed hospital developed and tested a plan for responding to a terrorist attack involving biological weapons after attending the Weapons of Mass Destruction Responder Awareness and Planning seminar presented by the U.S. Army and several federal agencies. Parma Community General Hospital's plan includes training staff, decontamination and isolation areas, safety equipment, waste disposal, legal considerations, and the development of response teams. The hospital staff received training from local fire department HAZMAT specialists.[5]

The utilization of local fire and police officials for training physicians and hospital staff is an excellent avenue for preparing for a bioterrorist event. These professionals have had specific training for public safety emergencies.[19]

The HHS has also established the Metropolitan Medical Response System (MMRS) in many locations across the country. This system brings together such diverse local stakeholders as police and fire officials to develop local response plans. As these plans are developed, they are tested using field exercises and "table top" simulations. The MMRS is sponsored by the federal government but is controlled locally.[19] The groups involved are law enforcement agencies, fire departments, poison control centers, local and state public health officials, local National Guard units, and local hospitals.[11] The plans developed by the MMRS groups define medical requirements and target populations to be immunized, the use of auxiliary personnel, other treatments, and facilities to be utilized in the event of a bioterrorist attack.[34]

Emergency medical services (EMS) providers will also be among the first responders to a covert biological attack. The U.S. Department of Health and Human Services' Office of Emergency Preparedness has contracted with the American College of Emergency Physicians to develop strategies and objectives to prepare EMS personnel, emergency nurses, and emergency physicians to respond to weapons of mass destruction incidents. This is an integrative effort to provide seamless care from out of the hospital setting to inside the hospital setting.[15]

Bioterrorism-focused educational programs that are targeted for first responders such as emergency physicians, nurses, and EMS personnel are becoming commonplace in the United States. In May 2002 Cross Country University, for example, offered a conference in Washington, DC, called America's Hospitals on Alert. Cross Country University has assembled a coalition of resources to address how to prepare healthcare workers for bioterrorism.[35] Berklan reported that infection control professionals have had increased requests to give presentations on bioterrorism and the nation's preparedness level.[36] Boni and Earls also recommended the incorporation of bioterrorism training into medical and nursing school curricula to increase awareness and knowledge among the next generation of healthcare professionals.[4]

Not only must frontline responders know what to do, but they must also be protected.[37] There is still much debate about vaccinating healthcare workers against smallpox and other infectious diseases prior to an outbreak. The Interim Smallpox Response Plan and Guidelines calls for a contact-based approach for vaccination after a case has been confirmed. According to this plan, the priority for vaccination includes staff involved in the direct medical care, public health evaluation, or transportation of confirmed or suspected smallpox victims.[38] Additional groups could be considered for voluntary vaccinations in the event of a smallpox outbreak. These groups are identified in the Interim Smallpox Response Plan and Guidelines; however, the decision to offer voluntary vaccinations to nonpatient contact groups will be made by the director of the CDC.[39]

Response

The development and stockpiling of vaccines and antimicrobial drugs to protect the public is an essential component of the response to a bioterrorist attack. Currently, the smallpox vaccine in the United States is in very limited supply and may be declining in efficacy due to age.[5] The CDC has contracted with two biotechnology companies to make and stockpile 40 million doses of the smallpox vaccine that is currently being produced.[6]

The HHS initiative for response includes the National Pharmaceutical Stockpile. The role of this program is to maintain a national repository of life-saving pharmaceuticals and medical supplies that will be delivered to the site of a bioterrorism event in order to reduce morbidity and mortality in civilian populations. These materials are intended to be available within twelve hours of an authorization to deploy from national stockpiles.[16]

The CDC and HHS have committed to ensuring that the federal response team is adequate to respond to bioterrorism. They will deploy response teams to investigate unusual etiologic agents and provide onsite consultation regarding medical management and disease control. The CDC is also involved in the National Pharmaceutical Stockpile.[6]

Research

Pharmaceuticals are also the target of research being done in the fight against bioterrorism. The HHS is increasing its support of research related to likely bioterrorism agents. The results of such research are expected to help in the development of diagnostic methods, antibacterial or antiviral therapies, and new vaccines.[4]

Research is also being done in the areas of detection and protection. Early detection capability is essential in the event of suspected cases of biological warfare. The Defense Advanced Research Projects Agency is funding research programs for developing early detection systems and other ways of protecting against biological weapons.[40] The use of biochips or microscale biosensors implanted under the skin is being developed as an early detection system.[39]

CONCLUSION

There is a rapidly growing body of research suggesting that the danger of intentional release of a biological agent to cause illness, death, and political unrest by various terrorists or governments is increasing, as demonstrated by the anthrax case in the United States.[39] Van McCrary[2] reported that a recent literature search revealed over 200 publications on bioterrorism-related issues during recent years. Incidents involving toxic or infectious agents have been on the rise since 1995.[13] There is increasing concern among governments of the world and academic analysts that terrorists will escalate to weapons of mass destruction, including nuclear, biological, or chemical agents.[4] There are several reasons for this increased concern over the dangers of bioterrorism.

One of the factors related to the increasing risk of bioterrorism is the rapid advance in technology made in the past few years. Biological weapons can be easily obtained. Technologies for the production and weaponization of biological agents are also readily available.[4]

Other factors contributing to the increased risk of bioterrorism are the fact that only limited finances and training are needed to establish a biological weapons plan. Biological weapons also have low visibility and are relatively easy to disseminate.[13]

The number of chemical and biological weapons is increasing throughout the world. The U.S. Department of State has identified seven countries as sponsors of terrorism, and all are suspected of having acquired or attempted to acquire chemical or biological weapons. This is in spite of efforts of the United Nations and other organizations to reduce or eliminate the threat of bioterrorism altogether.[4]

The literature on bioterrorism consistently states that the best way to combat biological terrorism is to be prepared to respond immediately to any threat. A comprehensive plan involving a strong public health infrastructure, advanced communication systems, rapid response, and disaster preparedness plans at the local level is key to saving lives and denying terrorists their goal of creating panic and crisis.

There has been considerable speculation surrounding the preparedness of the nation's healthcare system. The general consensus is that we are currently not prepared, but we are moving in the right direction. The government has made a commitment to supporting the key elements necessary for a high level of preparedness. This commitment includes funding, policies, guidelines, and the human resources necessary to win the fight against bioterrorism.

NOTES

1. Hagstad D, Kearney K. Emergency: bioterrorism. Amer J Nurs 2000; 100(12):33–5.

2. Tucker JB. Historical trends related to bioterrorism: an empirical analysis. Emerg Infect Dis [serial online] 1999;5(4). Available from: www.cdc.gov/ncidod/eid/vol5no4/tucker.htm. Accessed February 15, 2002.

3. Lemonick MD. Bioterrorism: The next threat? Time.com. 2001. Available from: www.time.com/time/nation/printout/0,8816,176066,00.html. Accessed February 15, 2002.

4. Atlas RM. Combating the threat of biowarfare and bioterrorism: defending against biological weapons is critical to global security. Bioscience. 1999. Available from: www.findarticles.com/cf_0/m1042/6_49/54823664. Accessed March 3, 2002.

5. Weiss R. Bioterrorism: an even more devastating threat. The Washington Post [online]. 2001. Available from: http://www.washingtonpost.com/ac2/wp-dyn?pagename=article&node=&contentId=A41225-2001Sep16. Accessed February 15, 2002.

6. U.S. Department of Health and Human Services. HHS initiative prepares for possible bioterrorism threat. 2001. Available from: www.hhs.gov/news/press/2001pres/01fsbioterrorism.html. Accessed February 19, 2002.

7. American Society for Microbiology. Bioterrorism: frontline response, evaluating U.S. preparedness. 1999. Available from: www.asmusa.org/pasrc/bioterrorismdef.htm. Accessed February 18, 2002.

8. Wetter DC, Daniell WE, Treser CD. Hospital preparedness for victims of chemical or biological terrorism. Amer J Pub Health 2001;91(5):710–6.

9. Rosen P. Coping with bioterrorism. Brit Med J. 2000;320:71–72. Available from: bmj.com/cgi/content/full/320/7227/71. Accessed February 16, 2002.

10. Darmiento L. Bioterrorism's hefty price tag before officials—Los Angeles County hospital preparedness. 2001. LA Bus J. Available from: www.findarticles.com/cf_0/m5072/46_23/80165401. Accessed March 3, 2002.

11. McLaughlin S. Thinking about the unthinkable. Where to start planning for terrorism incidents. Health Fac Manag 2001 July:26–30.

12. JCAHO surveyors focus on preparedness. Hospital Employee Health 2002;21(1):4.

13. Stern JE. Terrorism. In: Koop CE, Pearson CE, Schwartz MR, editors. Critical issues in global health. San Francisco: Jossey Bass; 2001. p. 272–9.

14. Geiger JH. Terrorism, biological weapons, and bonanzas: assessing the real threat to public health. Amer J Pub Health 2001;91(5):708–9.

15. Cross Country University. 2002. Available from: www.crosscountryuniversity.com/ccu/conf/save.html.

16. Centers for Disease Control and Prevention. Biological and chemical terrorism: strategic plan for preparedness and response. Morb & Mort Weekly Rep 2000;49(RR04):1–14. Available from: www.cdc.gov/mmwr/preview/mmwrhtml/rr4904a1.htm. Accessed February 15, 2002.

17. Sweeney R. $1.5 billion requested to help HHS combat national bioterrorism. American Family Physician. 2001. Available from: www.findarticles.com/cf_0/m3225/11_64/80813341. Accessed February 18, 2002.

18. Sandström G. A Swedish/European view of bioterrorism. Ann NY Acad Sci 2000;916(1):112–6.

19. Fraser MR, Brown DL. Bioterrorism preparedness and local public health agencies: building response capacity. Pub Health Rep 2000;115(4):326–30.

20. Henderson DA. (2000). Bioterrorism. Int J Clin Prac [Supplement 115] 2000;115:32–6.

21. Leach DL, Ryman DG. Biological weapons: preparing for the worst. Med Lab Obser 2000;32(9):26.

22. Jortani SA, Snyder JW, Valdes R Jr. The role of the clinical laboratory in managing chemical or biological terrorism. Clin Chem 2000;46(12):1883–93.

23. Vanner CL, Combs WS, Bertrand T, Bandy U. Identifying bacterial agents of bioterrorism: the pivotal role of the Laboratory Response Network. Med and Health Rh Isl 2001;84(5):178–80.

24. Fauci AS. Infectious diseases: considerations for the 21st century. Clin Infec Dis 2001;32(5):675.

25. Ashford DA, Gomez T, Noah D, Scott D, Franz D. Biological terrorism and veterinary medicine in the United States. J Amer Vet Med Assoc 2000; 217(5):644–7.

26. Fitzpatrick AM, Bender JB. Survey of chief livestock officials regarding bioterrorism preparedness in the United States. J Amer Vet Med Assoc 2000;219(9):1315–7.

27. Physicians central to bioterrorism response. Patient Care. 2001. Available from: www.findarticles.com/cf_0m3233/22_35/80864500. Accessed March 3, 2002.

28. Report: paper records hinder fast reaction to bioterrorism. Healthcare Purchasing News. 2001. Available from: www.findarticle.com/cf_0/m0BPC/12_25/81413193. Accessed March 3, 2002.

29. Szabo J. Is your laboratory prepared for a bioterrorism attack? In the wake of recent anthrax infections, laboratories must play a key role in identifying and preventing the spread of biological and chemical agents. Med Lab Obs 2001. Available from: www.findarticles.com/cf_0/m3230/12_33/81582424. Accessed February 18, 2002.

30. Leading U.S. medical publications join in public service campaign to educate healthcare professionals about bioterrorism; pro bono ads from McCann's Regan Campbell Ward to direct healthcare field to new btresponse. org website. PR Newswire. 2002. Available from: www.findarticles.com/cf_0/m4PRN/2002_Jan_4/81298203. Accessed March 3, 2002.

31. Recognizing bioterrorism-related infections. Contemporary OB/GYN. 2001. Available from: www.findarticles.com/cf_0/m0BGG/12_46/81465388. Accessed March 3, 2002.

32. Covenant HealthCare. Weapons of mass destruction (biological/chemical terrorism readiness plan). Policy number: ECR-014. 2001.

33. Bioterrorism and hospitals: Parma Security's plan to meet the threat. Hosp Secur and Safety Manag 1999;20(8):11–4.

34. Waeckerle JF, Seamans S, Whiteside M, Pons PT, White S, Burstein JL, et al. Executive summary: developing objectives, content, and competencies for the training of emergency medical technicians, emergency physicians, and emergency nurses to care for casualties resulting from nuclear, biological, or chemical (NBC) incidents. Ann Emerg Med 2001;37(6): 587–601.

35. Berklan JM. ICP's preparing for updated bioterrorism readiness plan. Healthcare Purchasing News. 2000. Available from: www.findarticles.com/cf_0m0BPC/10_24/66491793. Accessed March 3, 2002.

36. Boni CE, Earls EA. Hospital preparedness for acts of bioterrorism: an assessment of emergency preparedness plans of hospitals in Rhode Island. Med and Health Rhode Isl 2001;84(6):199.

37. Should you vaccinate HCWs against smallpox? Hosp Empl Health 2002;21(1):3.

38. Centers for Disease Control and Prevention. Executive summary for CDC Interim Smallpox Response Plan and Guidelines. 2002. Available from: www.cdc.gov/DocumentsAPP/smallpox/RPG/index.asp. Accessed February 19, 2002.

39. Van McCrary S. Smallpox and bioterrorism: a growing threat. 1999. Available from: law.uh.edu/healthlawperspectives/Bioethics/990803Smallpox.html. Accessed March 3, 2002.

40. Bashir R, Gomez R, Sarikaya A, Ladisch MR, Sturgis J. Adsorption of Avidin on microfabricated surfaces for protein biochip applications. Biotech and Bioeng 2001;73(4):325–8.

9 Community Preparedness

Diane E. Knudsen

Emergency preparedness (EP) has been a hot topic since the terror attacks of September 11, 2001. Long before 9/11, it became very apparent that the nation needed a major revision to our nation's ability to handle large-scale disaster on the home front. Emergencies have affected many people before and after 9/11. Many types of emergencies are responded to on a daily or weekly basis. These emergencies run the gamut of natural to man-made, to war, to deliberate acts of terror. These emergencies have their own cascade effects on the immediately affected communities as well as surrounding areas. Some emergencies extend beyond the local perimeters and have national and worldwide impact. Bioterrorism was associated with military campaigns, not with civilian populations. It was also perceived as an entity that occurred in someone else's backyard, such as a war-torn country somewhere remote. In recent years we as a global community have had our minds changed for us.

Emergency preparedness means many things to many different people. Within the healthcare arena, this is also true. There are many components or facets to emergency preparedness. There are specialized groups for different types of emergencies, but there are also some commonalities among all emergencies. The major players in emergency preparedness include healthcare workers, mental health caseworkers, first responders, firefighters, police, utilities managers, voluntary agencies (such as the Red Cross), volunteers, emergency medical services (EMS), the National Guard, and morgue services on various levels. There are private and governmental agencies involved with emergency preparedness. There are several areas that appear to require improvement to be more efficient at delivering required services. There is a need to improve communications, standardize training for all healthcare personnel, and to allocate resources and equipment.

We have gone through several changes in a short period since the events of 9/11. If one needs to see a silver lining in a black cloud, necessary attention was given to the area of emergency preparedness virtually overnight in the aftermath of the attacks. While this has been a great shot in the arm to emergency preparedness, it is only the beginning. We need to develop an emergency preparedness system that will work regardless of the need or event occurring.

THE HISTORY OF COMMUNITY PREPAREDNESS

Emergency preparedness appears to be in its infancy. Hopefully, it will grow rapidly to meet the needs of Americans. This is only because of the amount of attention this area has received since 9/11. The development needs to occur at a rapid pace to provide the necessary resources and personnel in the event of an emergency.

The concept of emergency assistance has been here for two centuries. Long before the 1990s, there was much activity and energy devoted to the development of biological warfare. Bioterror is not a new phenomenon. The earliest reported cases occurred in the sixth century BC, when the Assyrians poisoned enemy wells with rye ergot, and Solon used the purgative herb hellebore during the siege of Krissa. In 1346 plague broke out in the Tatar army during the siege of Kaffa in the Crimea. The attackers hurled the infected bodies over the city walls; the plague epidemic that followed forced the defenders to surrender, and some of the infected people who left Kaffa may have started the Black Death pandemic that spread throughout Europe, killing one third of the population.[1] In modern times since as early as World War I, governments have used, and some still try to use, biological warfare against humans and animals to advance their strategic and tactical objectives.[2] The use of chemical and biological weapons was flourishing on both sides of the Atlantic and Pacific Oceans. Governments recognized that these weapons had great impact on enemy armies while incurring little expense. Ricin appeared early as a battlefield weapon, while work continued to further develop biological and chemical weapons.[3]

The Federal Emergency Management Agency's (FEMA) earliest beginnings can be traced to the Congressional Act of 1803. This act, generally considered the first piece of disaster legislation, provided assistance to a New Hampshire town after an extensive fire. In the century that followed, *ad hoc* legislation was passed more than a hundred times in response to hurricanes, earthquakes, floods, and other natural disasters.

FEMA officially became recognized as a federal agency in 1979. Its first director was John Macy. With a vision of "a nation prepared," FEMA's mission is to lead America to prepare for, prevent, respond to, and recover from disasters. In March 2003 FEMA became part of the Department of Homeland Security.[4]

The institution and creation of the Department of Homeland Security has been a major addition to the arsenal of emergency preparedness agencies. The key to success at this point is to bring everything together to make the agencies work together smoothly and efficiently. Although this is easily stated, it is by no means an easy task to accomplish.

The U.S. Congress developed a comprehensive legal framework to prevent illegitimate use of toxins and infectious agents. Congress has defined as a federal crime every conceivable step in the process of developing or acquiring a biological agent for use as a weapon. Congress also vested federal law enforcement agencies with the broad civil and investigative power to intervene before such weapons are used or even developed.[5] The following is a chronological list of legislation developed and ratified by the international community and the United States:

- 1925: The Geneva Protocol, ratified by allied nations, prohibited the use of chemical and bacterial agents in wartime.[6]
- 1972: The Convention of Prohibition, ratified by more than one hundred nations to agree to stop development and stockpiling of biological and toxin weapons.[7]
- 1979: The United States amended the Export Administration Act, which banned the export to prohibited countries of agents that would "directly and substantially assist" development of biological weapons.
- 1989: The United States Biological Control Act, an attempt to curb the transfer of biological agents to other countries.
- 1991: The United States Chemical and Biological Weapons Control Act, which led to the development of economic sanctions and export controls.
- 1996: The United States passed the Anti-Terrorism Act, an attempt to reduce danger by:

  a. Imposing criminal penalties for possession, development, or use of biological agents.

b. Letting the government seize material for use in biological weapons development.

c. Creating regulatory control of the use and transfer of hazardous biological materials.[5]

COMMUNITY EVALUATION

In a paper published in 1992, Saundra K. Schneider stated that there was an existing gap in the aftermath of virtually every disaster between emergent norms that guided the social interactions and the bureaucratic norms that dominated governmental activity. If there is a large gap, the relief activity is viewed as a failure. If the gap is small, the relief activity is viewed as a success.[8] Some of the topics discussed with a field expert repeated some of the issues identified by Schneider more than a decade before. There are many pieces that could be grouped into a few categories.

Some of the major obstacles and challenges being experienced today that hinder the system from operating smoothly and efficiently include resource allocations, training, appropriate equipment, and the disorganization and turf wars that occur between agencies. There are many levels and people at each of these levels who need to be involved and need to know how to obtain necessary information, assistance, and supplies.

The issues can be placed into a few major categories: resource allocation, education, effective and efficient organization management, and removal of interdepartmental barriers. Improvements in any of these areas will result in better overall functioning in the system. Complete success will be attained once all areas are reviewed, improved, and functional. Experts and leaders in emergency preparedness have and are developing systems and subsystems to improve the efficiency and effectiveness of emergency preparedness. They also recognize that there is still a lot of work to be instituted and completed. Communication and collaboration need to improve across all levels of emergency preparedness management. In addition to improving communication and collaboration, the feelings of ownership and competition need to decrease across these same boundaries.

There has been a gap between the needs of the communities and the actual delivery of equipment and supplies to communities that have experienced a major terrorist event. A system to allocate and deliver the necessary tools to the communities needs to be developed so the communities have what they need at the time they need these resources. All levels of emergency preparedness personnel need a standardized education program.

Standardized responsibilities will enable all personnel to clearly identify the responsibilities and roles expected of all emergency response personnel. Each educational program should clearly define the scope of responsibility before, during, and after a major event. There is a need to establish standards of emergency preparedness to enable communities to identify their particular strengths and weaknesses, regardless of their size.

There needs to be focus on the different facets of emergency preparedness at the community level regarding terrorism, weapons of mass destruction, and natural disasters. The facets that should be assessed for the level of emergency preparedness in a community assessment include chemical, biological, nuclear, radiological, and explosive types of terrorism as well as natural disasters.

An established database designed to identify where the community stands regarding the level of preparedness and identification of risk factors specific to that community will assist it in developing a complete, comprehensive emergency preparedness program, which will meet the needs of that community. An established database will also allow each community to compare where it stands against other communities that have similar demographics and risks. In addition to developing its own comprehensive plan, the community has the ability to integrate its plan with other communities, enter mutual aid agreements with surrounding communities and regions, and provide resources that are more comprehensive to all communities involved.

A community evaluation model would be invaluable to the development of an effective, efficient emergency preparedness plan. In addition to providing critical information to the community about the strengths and weaknesses discovered through the community evaluation, the people would also have a basis for developing a plan to decrease and eradicate these weaknesses. At the same time, these same communities could develop an appropriate leadership authority for emergency preparedness protocols. In establishing leadership authority, a community would also establish lines of communication.

An algorithm needs to establish a basic guideline for who and when to call for which service in a timely fashion at the time of an emergency. Having an algorithm in place will help decrease the loss of time for notifying appropriate agencies, because there will be a set of steps to follow. The algorithm may be amended to fit a specific event, but it provides a basic plan of who will, and when to, communicate with necessary agencies during specific emergent events. Protocols would establish customs and regulations of the communication hierarchy, while algorithms would establish a set of steps specific to the type of emergent event.

The planning of an effective, efficient emergency preparedness plan would also prescribe the amount and levels of training required by the community to be adequately prepared if a major event were to occur. Education is an important facet of emergency preparedness because a well-informed community will be better educated regarding steps to take in identifying suspicious behavior or during an actual emergency event. The community evaluation would also be able to assist in developing the protocols for activation, response, chains of command, and communication as part of the emergency preparedness plan.

Starting at the community level would provide crucial information to assist in developing a systematic, organized method of providing the resources to a particular area when the need arose, regardless of that area's size. This area of emergency preparedness has far-reaching effects on the nation as a whole, as well as for those individuals who have been personally affected by an emergent event. Building a community risk assessment database would provide the necessary building blocks required to establish a comprehensive emergency preparedness plan. The community risk assessment would identify areas of weakness and strength in each community. It would also allow communities to locate their particular ranks relative to other communities. Identifying strengths and weaknesses would be instrumental in enabling the community to develop a comprehensive emergency preparedness plan to truly meet that community's particular needs. This is necessary to help it thoroughly identify its strengths and weaknesses, which will assist the researchers in improving upon the system as we know it today. Each community must know what is required of it to be considered prepared for an emergent event. The community is the building block of the nation.

Some terms used interchangeably with emergency preparedness include: *disaster management, disaster planning, emergency management, crisis management*, and *emergency planning*. When the actual definitions are looked at, one can see a common thread among them. They all imply something unforeseen, urgent, and potentially life threatening, which requires immediate intervention. To be able to provide immediate assistance, there must be some type of plan or system available.

Communication is essential to successful outcomes. Without communication, there is little information or vital updates obtained. There is also an increased risk of additional negative events occurring and increased risk of unsuccessful event outcomes. Table 9.1 presents definitions of commonly used concepts.

Each community must know what is required for it to be considered prepared for an emergent event. There is a need to establish standards of emergency preparedness to enable communities to identify their particular strengths and weaknesses, regardless of their size. An established database designed to identify where the community stands in regard to the level of preparedness and identification of risk factors specific to that community will assist it in developing a complete, comprehensive emergency preparedness program, which will meet the needs of that community. An established database will also allow each community to compare where it stands with other communities of similar demographics and risks. A standardized database could also offer communities information for locating resources to assist them in achieving their desired levels of preparedness.

With the help of this database, the researchers would be able to quantify the risks within their region. These would include types of emergencies they may be vulnerable to, the level of qualified personnel present within their community, educational needs to establish and maintain qualified emergency preparedness personnel, type and amount of necessary equipment, resources and personnel available, and contingency plans for different types of major events.

Table 9.1
Definitions of Concepts Used to Describe Emergencies

Concept	Definition
Catastrophe	Sudden, widespread disaster.
Cataclysm	A violent upheaval, especially of a personal or political nature, or sudden and violent physical action producing changes in the earth's surface.
Crisis	A state in which a stage in a sequence of events at which the trend of all future events is determined.
Disaster	Calamity.
Disaster area	A locality or region affected by a major disaster.
Emergency	Sudden or urgent, usually unforeseen occurrence or occasion requiring immediate action.
Experience	Knowledge gained from what one has observed, encountered, or undergone.
Management	Act of person or persons controlling and directing the affairs of an institution, or a person who controls and manipulates resources and expenditures.
Manage	To guide, conduct, regulate, engineer.
Plan (planning)	A method of action or procedure; to arrange or project a plan or scheme for any enterprise.
Preparedness	The state of being prepared, or readiness.

Source: The Random House college dictionary. Rev. ed. New York: Random House, Inc.; 1980.

These major events can be natural, such as earthquakes, floods, hurricanes, forest fires, or blizzards. They can also be man-made, such as building collapses, plane crashes, or gas explosions. These major events could also be intentional acts of violence such as the use of biological weapons, radiological weapons, chemical weapons, or other weapons of mass destruction. Contingency plans for these events would include the liaisons for communication and collaboration to provide efficient and effective response and management of a major event. Depending upon the type of major event, the appropriate contingency plans would be implemented with an appropriate allocation of necessary resources, personnel, and equipment to effectively manage the event. An established list of responsibilities and roles that adheres to a national standard for all levels of healthcare providers and that clearly outlines scopes of responsibilities before, during, and after an event would also be part of the contingency plan particular to each event.

EFFECTIVE EMERGENCY MANAGEMENT

Once an incident has occurred and is recognized, there may be little time to respond to limit the reaction to crisis. There are usually two medical management modes initiated at this point: mass prophylaxis and mass casualty management.[9] Deciding to perform mass prophylaxis requires a complex chain of events to unfold. After the decision is made, it must be communicated to the appropriate resources to facilitate delivery of an adequate supply of medications to meet the needs of the entire population at risk—in a very small window of opportunity. The distribution points must not only be set up quickly, but also announced so the community can readily access the distributions.

During disasters, healthcare professionals are obliged to treat as many victims who have a chance of survival as possible. Disaster medicine deals with large populations. Triage is common to all disasters. Triage is a dynamic process, constantly changing with victim status and resource availability. Triage is the principle of mass casualty care, followed by standards and procedures, and evacuation. The Potential Injury/Illness Creating Event (PICE) disaster nomenclature provides a method of consistency in classifying disasters.[10]

Little consideration has been given to understanding specific stressors likely to affect emergency managers, or those stressors' implications for a manager's thinking and management skills when responding to a disaster. In addition to having to deal with complex, unpredictable, and dynamic response management environments, emergency managers may have to contend with a degree of personal danger, although this will vary, dependent upon the disaster. There are other stressors, including responsibility, the sight of casualties, communications, dealing with the media, and operating a team or integrated emergency management context.[11]

Likewise, when casualty management is initiated, the system can become overwhelmed very quickly. It is especially difficult when mass-casualty victims are known to the healthcare providers, and when first responders are treating or pronouncing victims as deceased. Specific strategies need to be in place to respond to this situation and provide relief to the system. Managers can accomplish this by developing dialogue with surrounding communities; they provide support to an affected community through various methods. These methods may include personnel, equipment, and medical supplies. Depending upon the scope of the incident, the affected community may require more resources than can be offered by the surrounding communities; it may require state or federal intervention.

Good communication is essential for ensuring that appropriate information is available and delivered in a timely manner. Making effective use of information underlines the importance of decision-making and the need for those in leadership roles to adapt their decision styles and utilize different decision-making procedures.[11]

Emergencies usually require interorganizational cooperation if they are to meet the unusual demands of emergency response. By their orientation, however, emergency organizations tend toward formal structures and organizational cultures that make such cooperation difficult. Taken together, it is clear that a substantial number of diverse organizations are likely to be active in the various phases of emergency response. Rivalry is not foreign to emergency services, where response agencies are under great pressure to prove themselves. Resources for emergency response to any type of event are relatively scarce. Achievement of genuine cooperation among emergency responders must not be taken for granted by planners and cannot be overemphasized.[12] State government is responsible for providing leadership that brings together public and private partners to strengthen state capabilities of responding to and recovering from all disasters, including acts of terrorism. To fulfill this responsibility, the state emergency management agency must coordinate its efforts with all levels of government: state, federal, local, executive, legislative, and judicial. It takes total intergovernmental and interagency coordination to prepare the response to and recovery from disasters. The private sector is a significant stakeholder in emergency preparedness initiatives. Two major areas of concern to those in the field of emergency management are the security of critical assets and the assurance that businesses can continue their operations during times of crisis.[13]

Multiagency response and cooperation can be improved through joint planning and exercises that serve to validate plans and enable staff to familiarize themselves with arrangements and assist in training.[14] A key facet to effective emergency decision-making and operational performance is situational awareness.[15] Another key emergency decision process is "distributed decision making,"[16] which acknowledges that effective disaster response requires contributions from people who differ in professions, expertise, functions, roles, and geographic locations.[14]

IMPORTANCE OF PREPAREDNESS, RESPONSE, AND RECOVERY

The key challenge to bioterrorism preparedness is that we cannot predict how, when, or where a terrorist will strike within the United States. Preparedness is crucial and will have to occur at all levels of the public health system. There should be clearly defined performance standards, training to meet or exceed those standards, and self-evaluation through multidisciplinary exercises. Preparedness will require building new partnerships with the medical community, law enforcement and public safety, emergency services, disaster management personnel, and government officials. Hospital preparedness is also critical. The Centers for Disease Control and Prevention will provide public health guidelines, support, and technical assistance to state and local health agencies as they develop coordinated bioterrorism preparedness plans and protocols.[17]

A successful comprehensive, risk-based emergency management program of preparedness, response, and recovery will reduce life and property loss. Having the right people and agencies involved from the beginning, coupled with annual drills and evaluation of the disaster scenario, will go a long way toward establishing confidence and direction when a disaster does occur. Response involves conducting emergency operations to save lives and property by positioning emergency equipment and supplies; evacuating potential victims; providing food, water, shelter, and medical care to those in need; and restoring critical public services. Key members of the response team include representatives from the state office of public health; the departments of social services, transportation, natural resources, corrections or state police; the fire department; waste management; various healthcare provider groups; and community organizations that address special needs. Open communication in a collaborative partnership across departments is the first step in successfully implementing a disaster planning protocol.

The differing levels of preparedness needed to respond depend on a number of demographic characteristics: the health of the community, special needs of community members, and the commitment of those responsible for assuring the safety and health of this population. A disaster management plan must be based on the community's health status, available resources, and the cohesiveness of the community members. The need for self-contained power is absolutely critical. Self-contained portable cellular sites and switching equipment must be designed to operate independently from the regional power grid.[18]

Regardless of whether disaster-resistant or disaster-resilient communities, sustainability, invulnerable development, or any other concept becomes the unifying theme for a worldwide movement to reduce vulnerabilities, it is clear that the disaster problem will require increased attention in the future. Education about triggering agents and vulnerabilities must become top priority. Barriers separating disaster-related actors and institutions from one another must be torn down. Political support, further legislation, the use of carrots and sticks, and the provision of human and material resources for disaster management purposes will be necessities.[19]

The plans must incorporate training and recognition of potential bioterror agents for several types of responders to have an effective plan. The public at large needs to be aware of the types of agents that could affect them. Many times, private citizens may not be aware that they have been infected, and they continue to have contact as usual with others. This usually is the period of time when they are in the most contagious stage of the illness and can cause the most spread of infection. By the time the public realizes they may be infected, they have been exposed to several infecting people. Thus, the epidemic ensues.

Often the private citizen recognizes these events first, however delayed they may be. They usually present to their private healthcare practitioner or local emergency department. It is often by emergency medical services or in the hospital that the healthcare providers acknowledge a trend of complaints and symptoms. The time frame usually depends upon the agent used; some agents have longer incubation periods than others. Terror groups look for opportunities to strike at the weakest links. Table 9.2 provides a summary of several biological agents, the diseases they are responsible for causing, the types of agents they are, the incubation period, the treatment of choice, and early signs and symptoms of the diseases.

Table 9.2
Most Threatening Biological Agents, Based on Development and Ease of Production[20]

Agent	Disease	Class	Incubation Period	Treatment	Early Signs and Symptoms
Bacillus anthracis	Anthrax	Bacteria	1–5 days	Ciprofloxacin, Doxycycline	Fever, malaise, fatigue, cough, discomfort with dyspnea, diaphoresis, stridor, cyanosis
Francisella tularensis	Tularemia	Bacteria	1–10 days	Streptomycin, Doxycycline	Fever, chills, headache, malaise, substernal discomfort, prostration
Coxiella burnetti	Q fever	Bacteria	14–26 days	Tetracycline, Doxycycline	Fever, cough, pleuritic chest pain
Brucella species	Brucellosis	Bacteria	5–21 days	Streptomycin, Tetracycline	Fever, headache, weakness, fatigue, chills, diaphoresis, arthralgias, myalgias
Yersinia pestis (contagious)	Plague	Bacteria	1–3 days	Ciprofloxacin, Doxycycline	High fever, chills, headache, hemoptysis, dyspnea, stridor, cyanosis
Variola (contagious)	Smallpox	Virus	10–12 days	Supportive care	Acute onset with malaise, fever, rigors, vomiting, headache, followed by lesions in 2–3 days
Venezuelan equine encephalitis virus	Venezuelan equine encephalitis	Virus	1–6 days	Supportive care	General malaise, fever, rigors, severe headache, photophobia, myalgias
Staphylococcus enterotoxin (b)	Intoxication (aerosol exposure)	Toxin	1–6 hours	Supportive care	Sudden onset of fever, chills, headache, myalgia, nonproductive cough, possible chest pain and dyspnea, nausea, vomiting and diarrhea (if swallowed)

Source: Slidell, Patrick, and Dashiell. U.S. Army Medical Research Institute of Infectious Diseases. 1998.

THE ROLE OF TRAINING IN COMMUNITY PREPAREDNESS

According to Paton and Flin, training plays a pivotal role in managing stress reactions. The authors considered stressors relating to environmental, organizational, and operational demands. They reviewed the mediating roles of personality and transient physical and psychological states in terms of their influence on stress, judgment, and decision-making. They also discussed strategies for identifying which of these potential risk factors could be controlled or reduced, and they discussed strategies for training emergency managers to deal with the other risk factors.[11]

Fundamental to disaster readiness planning is developing training strategies to compensate for the limited opportunities for acquiring actual disaster-response experience. Regarding communication, decision-making, and integrated emergency management response, the need to develop mental models capable of reconciling knowledge of multiple goals with the collective expertise of those responding is a significant challenge for training. Assessment centers offer participation in multiple exercises and simulations, as well as observation and evaluation of performance against predetermined task-related behaviors by a team of trained assessors.[21] Interagency communications is essential for understanding complex, dynamic, and evolving emergencies, and for providing information for decision-making.[11,22]

Scenario methodology is widely used in investigating hazards and disasters. Although scenarios are often constructed to study past events, and are essential bases of planning for tackling future events, remarkably little has been written about their use in counter-disaster training. It is highly appropriate to teach emergency managers how to use scenarios as a basis for formulating disaster plans, as the scenarios indicate the amount and nature of resources needed to combat the hazards and how the resources must be deployed. The ability to manage emergencies well can be neither acquired fully in the classroom, nor learned entirely by experience. Scenarios are also useful for testing students' abilities to respond effectively to practical problems and hence can be used to screen applicants for courses and to examine them at the end of their training. Thus, the principles of emergency management are taught by practicing them. These methods presuppose a level of experience of the emergency management field that increases from the first to the third of the approaches listed. They are thus suited to different clienteles: the "traditional linear" approach works best with neophyte emergency management students who must learn basic principles, while the third

Table 9.3
Agenda for Local Jurisdictions Endeavoring to Create an Effective Plan and Response Protocol to Counter Biological Terrorism

Planning Issue	Objective(s)	Agencies Needed
Threat/risk assessment	Identify actual threats as well as possible threats. Based on local population density, economics, etc., attempt to validate the planning process.	FBI, state, local law enforcement, public health, emergency management
Hazard analysis	Identify potential worst-case and other scenarios to base planning.	FBI, state, local law enforcement, public health, emergency management
Public safety agencies capabilities	Assess, enhance local capabilities for plans and materials for field biological HAZMAT operations, proper level of personal protection and training, documentation and recording, testing, sample collection and analysis, interagency participation.	Fire department, EMS, HAZMAT team, local law enforcement, public health, emergency management
Health surveillance	Assess local public health surveillance to identify sensitivity to biological agent release. Develop and establish routine surveillance of local indicators (EMS demand, hospital acuity, medical examiner volume).	Emergency management, EMS, public health, hospitals, medical examiner/coroner
Laboratory capabilities	Assess state and local public health labs' capability to analyze biological samples. Enhance capabilities to rapidly identify biological agents locally.	State and local public health agencies, fire department, FBI, emergency management, local law enforcement
EMS capabilities	Assess capacity of local EMS system to manage surge of calls for service. Develop regional mutual aid agreements. Train EMS personnel to recognize biological agent signs and symptoms. Provide personal protection when confronted with a contagious agent.	Regional EMS, agencies emergency management
Mass prophylaxis	Develop a mechanism to distribute medication/antibiotics *en masse* using community-based distribution centers.	Emergency management, public health, EMS, law enforcement, National Guard
Medical systems capabilities	Assess the patient capacity at local hospitals. Identify on-hand and just-in-time stocks of antibiotics (ciprofloxacin, doxycycline, penicillin, tetracycline, streptomycin, gentamycin, and others as determined by public health). Identify regional quantities of ventilators	EMS, hospitals, public health, emergency management, FEMA, U.S. public health services, NDMS

Table 9.3

	(needed for many inhaled infectious agents, e.g., anthrax and tularemia). Develop capabilities to rapidly expand hospital internal and external patient care capabilities. Undertake initiatives to fill identified gaps.	
Medical examiner capabilities	Assess capacity of regional mortuaries. Expand mortuary processing and storage capabilities. Train medical examiner personnel in personal protection.	Local and regional medical examiner/ coroner, U.S. public health service, NDMS
Emergency management capabilities	Assess emergency management agency capability to coordinate the response to a major, region-wide, public health emergency. Assess capacity of local emergency response operation center and its technology. Coordinate the biological terrorism planning program.	Local and state emergency management agencies
Field incident (biological HAZMAT)	Assess and expand local capability to operateat field biological incidents, e.g., suspicious packages, substances.	Fire department, HAZMAT team, EMS, emergency management, FBI, local law enforcement, public health

FBI = Federal Bureau of Investigation; FEMA = Federal Emergency Management Agency; HAZMAT = Hazardous Materials Team; NDMS = National Disaster Medical System; EMS = Emergency Medical Services.
Source: Kuhr S, Hauer JM. The threat of biological terrorism in the new millennium. Amer Behav Scientist 2001;44(6):1032–41.

approach is appropriate in refresher courses given to active emergency management personnel. Field research has shown that the ability of disaster relief coordinates to visualize emergencies spatially, through response maps[23] is critical to their success as managers. This skill can be taught by turning the verbal descriptions in scenarios to sketch maps. The maps drawn by different students can be compared and analyzed in class time. Scenarios are a form of communications model, and as such they fall along a continuum defined by the number of roles and the degree of complexity of simulation.[24] In essence, the scenario method has considerable potential for further development as a means of teaching principles of emergency management, especially as it is easily integrated with other forms of model and simulation used in this field.[25]

The ultimate goal of the disaster management plan is to effectively allocate resources in a timely manner.[18] Table 9.3 gives an agenda for creating an effective community preparedness plan and response protocol.

The increase in natural and human-derived disasters has significantly escalated both the degree of suffering and the costs of restoring existing economic and social systems. The financial impact of disasters has risen dramatically because of the cost of restoring the existing infrastructure and efforts to prevent future occurrences. As a result, increasing pressure has been placed on material managers to do more with less, while also providing the necessary resources to respond efficiently and effectively during an emergency.

Although natural disasters will always occur, a multidisciplinary approach to preparedness, response, and recovery is essential to successfully returning the organization and community to an optimal level of functioning. Developing a disaster plan and evaluating the outcome during non-emergency periods is often the most effective strategy in minimizing the human and financial costs following a disaster.

Recognizing the possibility of positive reactions and growth outcomes in this context necessitates developing alternative models and, in particular, accommodating resilience constructs in research and intervention agendas. The recognition of a relationship between disaster experience and positive growth outcomes introduces a need within disaster management to seek ways in which such outcomes can be facilitated. Calhoun and Tedeschi[26] discuss how growth and distress outcomes need to be mutually exclusive. The authors of this paper extend this model to include mitigation and recovery planning also. Crucial issues here include the identification of resilience and vulnerability variables and defining the mechanisms by which they lead to growth and distress outcomes.[27]

McEntire, Fuller, and Johnston state that scholars are calling for a shift in paradigm to facilitate the understanding and reduction of disaster. They propose the paradigm called comprehensive vulnerability management, which could be defined as holistic and integrated activities directed toward reducing emergencies and disasters by diminishing risk and susceptibility and by building resistance and resilience. The values, decisions, and policies that guide comprehensive vulnerability management are based on careful and continued assessments of liabilities and capabilities from the physical, social, and organizational environments. Comprehensive vulnerability management is a concerted effort to identify and reduce all types of disaster vulnerabilities.[28]

Comprehensive vulnerability management is a more efficient, effective, and appropriate form of disaster response because it increases the capacities of responders by delegating authority to the local level, avoiding overly stringent bureaucratic operating procedures, encouraging self-reliance among the affected population, improving decision-making in crisis situations, and discouraging the creation of dependency through well-intentioned, but sometimes ineffective and counterproductive, relief operations.[28]

In the course of meeting the needs of disaster-affected individuals and communities, relief workers may themselves experience dysfunctional reactions, often for periods extending beyond the terms of their direct involvement.[29-31] The recognition that disaster workers are not immune to experiencing problems has raised questions about the effectiveness of their preparation for the demands of disaster work.[32-34] While this has been recognized, intervention has focused on providing support or counseling rather than preparatory strategies designed to promote adaptation and minimize impact.[25,30]

"Mental models" provide a psychological basis for understanding, response planning, and for predicting outcomes. Many of the facets of these performance schemata become implicit or "taken for granted" aspects of the performance environment. Their importance as determinants of well-being and performance effectiveness may go unrealized until people are faced with operational demands that challenge these assumptions.

A comprehensive inventory of disaster stressors can facilitate the identification of high-risk situations, provide a basis for anticipating the intensity of reactions, and alert the organization to likely support requirements. Inventories of this nature can also provide an input into training needs analysis and the development of training program content, contribute to the design of realistic disaster training simulations, and promote a more flexible and adaptive response capability.[30,35]

Lack of warning increases physical and psychological demands on workers because it reduces mobilization time and opportunities to determine the nature and extent of impact. Family or community associations increase the workers' perceived identification with a disaster, and thus risk status. In addition to knowing the victims, these associations can be prominent stressors among uniformed professionals or members of a close-knit disaster response group. The sense of shared fate associated with high levels of identification with those killed or seriously injured can heighten the impact.

Disaster relief workers faced with substantial physical and time pressures risk developing "counter disaster syndrome,"[36] a state where they feel success only if the relief effort hinges on their personal involvement. The ensuing fatigue and continued exposure to traumatic stimuli can significantly increase risk status. Heightened exposure to the suffering of victims, or colleagues also increases the risk status.

The loss of infrastructure or the large number of agencies associated with the disaster relief effort may create difficulties establishing and maintaining effective coordination and communications systems.[37] Repetition of search and other tasks, and poor communication as well, can fuel frustration and feelings of inadequacy and helplessness. Paton also notes that inadequate planning and the communication and coordination problems that frequently typify the early stages of disaster relief work can generate conflict among agencies and blur roles and responsibilities. Workers can find themselves dealing with interagency conflict, or having to redefine their roles. Engagement in activities other than the express relief role can fuel feelings of inadequacy and helplessness.

Disaster relief workers should be prepared, both technically and psychologically, for disaster relief work. Training should take place in different contexts to generalize understanding; promote predictability, control, and adaptability; and ensure that operational schemata will promote well-being and performance effectiveness under a wide range of circumstances.[38] Cooke, Salas, Cannon-Bowers, and Stout also support the concept of a team mental model, stating that effective multiorganizational and multidisciplinary coordination and performance thus requires a "team mental model" specifically relating to that information pertinent to accomplishing a common goal.[39]

After reviewing the literature, one can see that the need for uniformity and standardization is obvious. There are many people trying to do many good things, but not many seem to connect with each other. Developing a systematic approach to assessing community risk factors can assist the communities in accurately identifying their particular risks and their level of preparedness. Having a uniform approach to identifying risk factors in communities' emergency preparedness would assist in decreasing the amount of redundancy present in today's efforts to prepare for emergencies.

CONCLUSION

As a global community, we need to develop and implement comprehensive plans to assist in the detection of and response to an actual event. These plans must be able to change as the needs change. They must be simple enough for the general population to understand the basic directions of what to look for, whom to contact, and where to go for assistance. The plans must be dynamic and continually updated to stay current with all the changes in technology, biological agents, medications, and treatments. In addition to all of these requirements, these plans must be able to be integrated with surrounding communities, regions, and/or nations. Bioterrorism has the potential to appear at any time, and the surveillance that occurs is able to filter out large quantities of information to determine what is or is not credible, but it is still subject to human intervention.

NOTES

1. Christopher GW, Cieslak TJ, Pavlin JA, Eitzen EM Jr. Biological warfare—a historical perspective. JAMA 1997;278(5):412–7.

2. Iavorone M. Armory: gas warfare [online]. 2000. Available from: www.worldwar1.com/arm006.htm. Accessed September 11, 2003.

3. Sidell FR, Takafuji ET, Franz DR. Medical aspects of chemical and biological warfare (Textbook of military medicine. Part 1, warfare, weaponry and casualty, v. 3.). Medical aspects of chemical and biological warfare. Falls Church, VA: Office of the Surgeon General, U.S. Army; 1997.

4. FEMA history. Available from: www.fema.gov. Accessed August 1, 2003.

5. Ferguson JR. Biological weapons and U.S. law. JAMA 1997;278(5):357–60.

6. Protocol for the prohibition of the use in war asphyxiating, poisonous or other gases, and of bacteriological methods of warfare. 1925 June 25 [online]. Available from: www.lib.byu.edu/~rdh/wwi/hague/hague13.html.

7. Convention on the prohibition of development, production, and stockpiling of bacteriological (biological) and toxin weapons and on their destruction [online]. 1972. Available from: fletcher.tufts.edu/multi/texts/BH596.txt.

8. Schneider SK. Governmental response to disasters: the conflict between bureaucratic procedures and emergent norms. Pub Admin Rev 1992 Mar/Apr; 52(2):135–45.

9. Kuhr S, Hauer JM. The threat of biological terrorism in the new millennium. Amer Behav Scientist 2001;44(6):1032–41.

10. Burkle FM Jr. Mass casualty management of a large-scale bioterrorism event: an epidemiological approach that shapes triage decisions. Emerg Med Clinics of NA 2002;20(2):409–36.

11. Paton D, Flin R. Disaster stress: an emergency management perspective. Disast Prev and Manag 1999;8(4):261–7.

12. Granot H. Emergency inter-organizational relationships. Disast Prev and Manag 1999;8(1):21–4.

13. Gordon EM. Leadership commitment to strong emergency management. J St Gov 2001 Fall;74(4):9–11.

14. Payne CF. Contingency plan exercises. Disast Prev and Manag 1999; 8(2):111–8.

15. Endsley MR. Toward a theory of situation awareness. Hum Factors 1995;7:32–64.

16. Rogalsky J, Samurcay R. Analyzing communication in complex distributed decision making. Ergonomics 1993;36:1329–42.

17. Kahn AS, Morse S, Lillibridge S. Public-health preparedness for biological terrorism in the USA. Lancet 2000;356:1179–82.

18. Bechtel GA, Hansberry AH, Gray-Brown D. Disaster planning and resource allocation in health services. Hosp Materiel Manag Quarterly 2000; 22(2):9–17.

19. McEntire DA. Triggering agents, vulnerabilities and disaster reduction: towards a holistic paradigm. Disast Prev and Manag 2001;10(3):189–96.

20. Sidell FR, Patrick WC III, Dashiell TR. Janes's chem-bio handbook. Arlington, VA: Jane's Information Group; 1998.

21. Ballantyne I, Povah N. Assessment and development centres. Aldershot, UK: Gower Publishing; 1995.

22. Smallman C, Weir D. Communication and cultural distortion during crisis. Disast Prev and Manag 1999;8(1):33–41.

23. Dymon UJ. Mapping the missing link in reducing risk under SARA II. Risk: Health, Safety & Environment 1994;5(4):337–60.

24. Foster HD. Disaster planning: the preservation of life and property. New York: Springer-Verlag; 1980.

25. Alexander D. Scenario methodology for teaching principles of emergency management. Disast Prev and Manag 2000;9(2):89–97.

26. Calhoun L, Tedeschi R. Early post-traumatic interventions: facilitating possibilities for growth. In Volanti JM, Paton D, Dunning C, editors. Post-traumatic stress intervention: challenges, issues, and perspectives. Springfield, IL: Charles C. Thomas; 2000.

27. Paton D, Smith L, Violanti J. Disaster response: risk, vulnerability and resilience. Disast Prev and Manag 2000;9(3):173–80.

28. McEntire DA, Fuller C, Johnston CW, Weber R. A comparison of disaster paradigms: the search for a holistic policy guide. Pub Admin Rev 2002;62(3):267–81.

29. Dixon P, Rehling G, Shiwach R. Peripheral victims of the Herald of Free Enterprise disaster. Br J Med Psych 1993;66:193–202.

30. Paton D. Disasters and helpers: psychological dynamics and implications for counseling. Couns Psych Quarterly 1989;2:302–21.

31. Taylor AJW, Frazer AG. The stress of post-disaster body handling and victim identification. J Hum Stress 1982;8:91–103.

32. Dunning C. Mental health sequelae in disaster workers: prevention and intervention. Intern J Ment Health 1990;19:91–103.

33. Lundin T, Bodegard M. The psychological impact of earthquake on rescue workers. A follow-up study of the Swedish group of rescue workers in Armenia, 1988. J Traum Stress 1993;6:129–39.

34. Paton D. Dealing with traumatic incidents in the workplace. 2nd ed. Queensland, Australia: Gull Publishing; 1994.

35. auf der Heide E. Disaster response. St. Louis, MO: C. V. Mosby; 1989.

36. Raphael B. When disaster strikes. London: Hutchinson; 1986.

37. Paton D. Disaster relief worker: an assessment of training effectiveness. J Traum Stress 1994;7:275–88.

38. Paton D. Training disaster workers: promoting wellbeing and operational effectiveness. Disast Prev and Manag 1996;5(5):11–5.

39. Cooke NJ, Salas E, Cannon-Bowers JA, Stout RJ. Measuring team knowledge. Hum Factors 2000;42:151–73.

10 The Role of the Department of Veterans Affairs in National, Regional, and Local Emergency Management

Jonathan H. Gardner and Dan L. Johnston

When asked about the Department of Veterans Affairs (VA), most people think of the GI Bill, home loans, and educational benefits. Others might think of the VA healthcare system that provides medical care to millions of our nation's veterans. Even fewer people think of the VA's role in medical education and clinical research. However, one of the VA's most important roles involves emergency management of national, regional, and local disasters. For example, did you know that over 1,000 VA staff were deployed to every nationally declared disaster since Hurricane Andrew in 1992, when the Federal Response Plan was first used?

The VA comprises three administrations: the Veterans Health Administration (VHA), the Veterans Benefits Administration (VBA), and the National Cemetery Administration (NCA) (see figure 10.1).

Each of these administrations has a distinct and separate mission to serve veterans. The VHA's mission includes:

1. Providing healthcare to veterans.
2. Providing medical education for future physicians, nurses, and other healthcare-related disciplines.
3. Conducting clinical research.
4. Participating in our nation's emergency response plan. This includes the VHA's responsibilities for

   - VA contingencies.
   - Department of Defense (DoD) contingencies.
   - The National Response Plan (NRP)/Federal Response Plan (FRP).

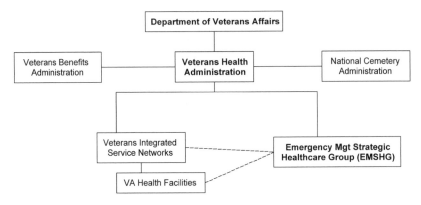

Figure 10.1
Simplified VA organizational chart.

- The National Disaster Medical System (NDMS).
- Radiologic emergencies.
- Continuity of operations/continuity of government (COG).[1]

As the largest integrated healthcare system in the United States, the VHA is uniquely positioned to respond to national disasters. Its medical assets are located in each of the fifty states, Washington, DC, and U.S. territories. These assets and their numbers are described in table 10.1.

In addition to the number of VHA facilities located throughout the nation, the administration employs over 205,000 staff representing the entire clinical and administrative disciplines characteristic of a national healthcare system (table 10.2).

The Emergency Management Strategic Healthcare Group (EMSHG) is the VHA's executive agent for its fourth mission. As stated in EMSHG's brochure, "EMSHG provides Comprehensive Emergency Management

Table 10.1
VHA Facilities

Facilities	Number
VA hospitals*	162
Ambulatory care clinics	>800
Nursing homes	130
Domiciliaries	40
Homecare programs	73
Counseling centers	206

* VHA facilities are organizationally aligned into twenty-one veterans integrated service networks (VISNs).

Table 10.2
VHA Staff Numbers

Staff Position	Number of Staff
Physicians	15,000
Dentists	1,000
Nursing staff	55,000
Pharmacists	4,500
Support staff	130,000
Total:	205,500

services to the Department of Veterans Affairs, coordinates medical backup for the Department of Defense, and assists the public via the National Disaster Medical System and the National Response Plan."[1]

With the large number of VA medical facilities and staff, VHA is in a unique position to respond to national, regional, and local disasters. VHA facilities also have the procurement systems in place to provide the medical supplies that are required during a disaster response. VA resources have been used in every major domestic disaster since Hurricane Andrew demolished south Florida on August 24, 1992. Since then, VA employees have been deployed to every presidentially declared disaster and many high-threat events.

The VA's role in national disasters became clear when the Federal Response Plan (FRP) Emergency Support Function (ESF) #8 designated the VA as a primary support agency to the Department of Health and Human Service's Public Health Service (PHS). Since 1992, VA employees have deployed to disasters such as Hurricane Hugo; the Northridge earthquake in California; the Oklahoma City bombing; Tropical Storm Allison; and the September 11, 2001, terrorist attacks in New York City, the Pentagon, and the crash site in Pennsylvania.[2] Examples of high-threat events to which VA staff have deployed include the NATO fiftieth anniversary celebration in Washington, DC; the 1996 Atlanta Summer Olympic Games; the World Trade Organization conference in November 1999; presidential inaugurations; the State of the Union address in January 2000; the Republican and Democratic National Conventions in August 2000; the United Nations Millennium Meeting in September 2000;[3] the 2002 Salt Lake City Winter Olympic Games;[4] the papal visit; and numerous Super Bowls.

HISTORY OF VA EMERGENCY MANAGEMENT

Initially, the Office of Emergency Management and Preparedness (OEMP) managed the VA's role, the National Disaster Medical System,

VA/DoD contingency planning, and other emergency management-related responsibilities. OEMP was reorganized in the late 1990s, and its name changed to the Emergency Management Strategic Healthcare Group (EMSHG). Its major function and mission have remained largely the same as OEMP's, but following 9/11, EMSHG gained more prominence as the VA became increasingly more involved in national emergency management issues and programs. During the response and recovery of the effects of Hurricane Isabel, the VA looked to EMSHG to provide emergency management leadership and coordination. While EMSHG has received increased focus since 9/11, the VA continues to increase its departmental focus on emergency management through the new Office of Policy, Planning, and Preparedness (P3). Through P3, the VA's emergency management mission aligns more with similar activities of other federal departments.

The Emergency Management Strategic Healthcare Group coordinates the VHA's role in VA contingencies, the VA/DoD Contingency Hospital System, the National Disaster Medical System, the National Response Plan, radiological emergencies, and continuity of government.

THE VHA FOURTH MISSION

VA Contingencies

Like any other hospital or healthcare system, VA facilities must be prepared to respond to a variety of disasters in their communities or at their facilities. In addition to events mentioned above, VA staff have had to respond to natural disasters, such as earthquakes, hurricanes, flooding, ice storms, and snowstorms; and man-made disasters, such as the loss of electrical power for an extended period of time, civil disturbances, and a variety of other emergency situations.

A good example occurred in September 2003, when Hurricane Isabel caused extensive damage along the eastern seaboard. One VA facility was severely impacted, and several others were moderately impacted by this intense storm. The VA evacuated patients from the Hampton, Virginia VA medical center because of the threatening storm and possible flooding. It was a good thing, because the medical center did experience severe flooding and an extended power outage. The patients were transferred to the Richmond Medical Center, as well as other VA medical centers in the state. Several of the Hampton staff accompanied the patients to their assigned facilities. These employees were unable to go home to be with their families and assess damage to their personal property. EMSHG coordinated the deployment of thirty-seven highly specialized VA nurses from around the nation to Richmond, relieving the Hampton nurses of their patient care duties and allowing them to return home.

The VA/DoD Contingency Hospital System

The VA provides primary medical support to the Department of Defense (DoD) medical care system during and following an outbreak of war or national emergency. The VA/DoD Contingency Hospital System plan outlines how the VHA supports that effort.[5]

VA medical centers are assigned one or more of the following missions during a national wartime contingency plan:

a. Primary receiving center (PRC): becoming eligible to receive active duty casualties directly from the DoD patient evacuation system for hospitalization.
b. Secondary support center (SSC): enhancing patient care capacity at PRCs by such actions as accepting stable patients in transfer or sending staff and supplies.
c. Installation support center (ISC): providing healthcare services to active duty staff at an assigned military installation, should existing military services be degraded due to mobilization of staff to wartime duty locations.

During a time of military conflict or national emergency, in addition to continuing the primary mission of veteran care, the major goal of the VA is to provide additional patient care capacity for active duty military casualties in as short a time as possible. The national goal is to make 25 percent of the VA's staffed operating beds available to the DoD within seventy-two hours. With an activation of the VA/DoD contingency plan, active duty military patients are elevated in priority status above all but medical emergencies and service-connected veterans. To date, the VA/DoD contingency plan has not been activated nationally. However, during an activation of the national contingency plan, the primary focus of VA medical facilities will shift to the care of patients in accordance with the following admissions priority:

a. Medical emergencies
b. Service-connected veterans
c. Active duty military casualties/active duty patients
d. All other veterans in accordance with existing priorities

NATIONAL RESPONSE PLAN (NRP)/FEDERAL RESPONSE PLAN (FRP)

The FRP was issued in 1992 by FEMA to describe how the federal government would assist state and local entities in managing major disasters and emergencies declared by the president. The plan was updated in April 1999. The FRP is designed to provide a process and a structure for the systematic and coordinated federal response to a major disaster or emergency declared under the Stafford Act.[6] The plan organizes the types of federal assistance under twelve emergency support functions. The VA supports four of these, including public works and engineering, mass care, resource support, and health and medical services.

Homeland Security Presidential Directive 5 (HSPD-5) led the DHS to develop and administer the National Response Plan (NRP). The DHS released the initial NRP on September 30, 2003. It states, "Accordingly, the purpose of this initial NRP is to harmonize the operational processes, procedures, and protocols detailed in such documents as the *Federal Response Plan, U.S. Government Interagency Domestic Terrorism Concept of Organizations Plan, Federal Radiological Emergency Response Plan, Mass Migration Emergency Plan, and National Oil and Hazardous Substances Pollution Contingency Plan* with the strategic direction provided in HSPD-5 until such plans can be integrated into the full NRP."[7] The initial NRP and FRP will guide the VA's response to national emergencies as directed by the DHS until the full NRP is completed.

NATIONAL DISASTER MEDICAL SYSTEM

The National Disaster Medical System (NDMS) evolved from a long history of responding to national disasters, whether they were man-made or natural catastrophes. The DoD established the Civilian-Military Contingency Hospital System in 1980. The president established the Emergency Mobilization Preparedness Board (EMPB) on December 17, 1981. The EMPB then created the National Disaster Medical System to meet the president's charge to develop a national policy and program to improve emergency preparedness. Initially, the NDMS consisted of representatives from the DoD, Federal Emergency Management Agency (FEMA), HHS/PHS, and the VA. In an interview with the *Journal of Homeland Security*, Dr. Kristi L. Koenig, the VA's chief consultant, stated, "The NDMS is a partnership between four federal agencies: HHS, VA, DoD, and FEMA. HHS is the lead federal agency."[8]

Oversight of NDMS moved under the Department of Homeland Security (DHS) when the Homeland Security Act of 2002 created it. The impact of this change is not fully realized at this time because the DHS is still in the process of completing its organizational structure and assigning responsibilities.

Until the new NDMS policies and procedures are finalized and implemented, many VA medical centers will serve as the NDMS federal coordinating centers (FCC) in their communities. The VA medical center director is designated as the FCC director. Another VA employee is designated as the FCC coordinator. The VA employee's title is EMSHG area emergency manager (AEM). The FCC coordinator, working under the direction of the FCC director, solicits local hospitals to voluntarily agree to make a minimum and a maximum number of beds available to NDMS when there is a need to respond to a mass-casualties disaster. Community hospitals voluntarily commit to this agreement by signing NDMS memoranda of understanding (MOU). The FCC coordinator plans and conducts community NDMS meetings, training, conferences, and exercises, which contribute greatly to a community's preparedness to respond to a variety of disasters.

Meetings

NDMS meetings are multidisciplinary in nature. Led and initiated by the VA, attendees include representatives from community hospitals, fire departments, law enforcement, health departments, the American Red Cross, city communications, city and county emergency management offices, ambulance companies, and other interested parties. They discuss the community's policies and procedures as they apply to the NDMS system. These discussions often address issues that impact any emergency response. As issues are resolved, they not only benefit the NDMS system, but they also improve the community's emergency management system.

For example, Tucson, Arizona identified the need for better communications among the incident site, city communications, and the hospitals. Through a discussion in the NDMS monthly meeting, a plan to assign Radio Amateur Communications Emergency Services volunteer ham radio operators at the scene, at the city emergency operations center, and at each hospital was developed. At least one other community is considering adopting this model to improve its emergency communications.

Training

As a part of a national system, VA medical centers have access to a large number of educational events, materials, and opportunities. EMSHG, in conjunction with the VA employee education system and the DoD, has sponsored several satellite-training programs made available to NDMS participants and the healthcare community in general. Additionally, the FCCs frequently invite organizations participating in the NDMS to attend training provided to VA staff.

Conferences

The FCC in Tucson sponsored two one-day conferences on lessons learned from the Oklahoma City bombing and violence in the workplace. Approximately 200 participants attended each conference. In November 2001, the NDMS FCC co-sponsored, with the Tucson Metropolitan Medical Response System (MMRS) and the state of Arizona Division of Emergency Management (ADEM), a two-day conference on weapons of mass destruction (WMD). The VA's involvement in these conferences, and many others like them held throughout the nation, contribute greatly to the knowledge base of physicians, nurses, paramedics, emergency management technicians (EMTs), emergency planners, and people of other disciplines involved in emergency management.

Exercises

Many FCCs coordinate and conduct annual NDMS exercises with their communities. Not only do these exercises help the local hospitals meet the Joint Commission on the Accreditation of Healthcare Organization's criteria for participating in a community exercise each year, but more importantly, they provide the community an opportunity to identify areas for improvement in their emergency management plans and systems. Many of the same issues that affect the NDMS system are relevant to other emergency situations as well. Therefore, the VA's leadership in the NDMS contributes greatly to a community's overall preparedness to respond to a variety of potential disasters and other emergency events.

An important area where the VA plays a national role is its management and coordination of pharmaceutical stockpiles for national emergencies. The VA has an MOU with the Centers for Disease Control and Prevention to assist with the Strategic National Stockpile, now managed by the DHS. The VA purchases the pharmaceuticals, sets up the system, and stores the drugs as one component of the overall Strategic National Stockpile. Additionally, the VA has an MOU with the applicable NDMS component to maintain and store certain pharmaceutical caches and a special events cache for the national medical response teams. Components of one of these caches were mobilized following the anthrax attacks in October 2001.

Radiologic Emergencies

The VA staffs and maintains the national Medical Emergency Radiological Response Team (MERRT). MERRT is a twenty-five-member team made of VA physicians, radiologists, health physicists, and other appropriate staff. This team is expected to be onsite within twenty-four hours of being contacted. The MERRT is not a first-response team. The MERRT members supplement medical care at a hospital, provide technical advice during a response to a radiological incident, perform decontamination as needed and as appropriate, and conduct radiological monitoring.

Continuity of Operations/Continuity of Government

EMSHG executes assigned actions for the VHA to support continuity of operations and continuity of government plans.

VA RESPONSES TO NATIONAL DISASTERS

As previously stated, the VA has been involved in all major presidentially-declared disasters since Hurricane Andrew. Its deployments include area emergency managers, nurses, radiology technologists, mental health counselors, and chaplains. The deployed VA staff work primarily in non-VA healthcare settings. They have worked in non-VA hospitals, emergency shelters, and first aid stations located in the disaster area.

In addition to deploying clinical, emergency management, and support staff to various national disasters over the past eleven years, the VA was instrumental in providing medical supplies in disaster response and relief efforts. The Miami VA Medical Center was a major source of medical supplies following Hurricane Andrew. The Houston VA Medical Center served as the center of coordination efforts for the Texas medical centers following the major flooding caused by Tropical Storm

Table 10.3
Emergencies or High-Threat Events Supported by the VA from 1999 to 2003

Contingency/Event	Timeframe
Hurricane Floyd	September 15–October 15, 1999
Egypt Airlines 990 crash	November 22–23, 1999
World Trade Organization conference	November 26–December 7, 1999
Hurricane Lenny	December 1–16, 1999
Support to VA national Y2K efforts	December 28, 1999–January 3, 2000
State of the Union address	January 27, 2000
Operation Sail	June 16–20, 2000
Republican National Convention	July 31–August 3, 2000
Democratic National Convention	August 13–17, 2000
UN Millennium Meeting	September 12–17, 2000
Presidential inauguration	January 21, 2001
Tropical Storm Allison	June 10–22, 2001
West Virginia floods	July 11–13, 2001
Terrorist attacks	September 11, 2001 and beyond
2002 Salt Lake City Winter Olympics	February 4–26, 2002
Typhoon Pongsona	December 11–23, 2002
Hurricane Isabel	September 20–October 2, 2003

Allison. Table 10.3 lists the emergencies or high-threat events supported by the VA from 1999 to 2003.

VA REPONSES TO REGIONAL DISASTERS

As cited earlier, the VHA is structured into twenty-one veterans integrated service networks (VISNs). EMSHG has a minimum of one area emergency manager in each of the twenty-one VISNs. The AEMs serve as emergency management consultants or preceptors to the VISN directors and each of the VISNs' VA medical centers. The emergency managers advise VISN and VA medical center management on JCAHO standards relating to emergency management, assist with the implementation of the Disaster Emergency Medical Personnel System (DEMPS), teach the Incident Command System (ICS), coordinate the NDMS programs within their communities, advise management on the VA/ DoD contingency plan, help establish decontamination teams and programs, and assist with other emergency management-related programs and issues.

In addition to support at all levels to non-VA entities during disasters or emergencies, the VA provides support within its own healthcare system. For example, prior to hitting the east coast, Hurricane Isabel was expected to impact the mid-Atlantic shores. Hurricane Isabel's most likely path was North Carolina, Virginia, Maryland, the West Virginia panhandle, and Pennsylvania. The VA medical centers in these states began preparing for Hurricane Isabel. As stated earlier, the Hampton, Virginia VA medical center evacuated the patients to other VA medical centers and deployed staff to care for the patients. EMSHG AEMs were deployed to Richmond to provide onsite coordination of deployed nurses and to support Richmond and Hampton throughout their recovery efforts. The deployment of VA staff was coordinated and funded entirely by the VA.

VA RESPONSE TO LOCAL DISASTERS

A statement frequently made by many speakers at emergency management conferences held throughout the nation is, "Disasters are local." In other words, regardless of all of the national programs, plans, exercises and funds, when a disaster strikes, whether it is a natural disaster, technological accident, or act of terrorism, the response falls first on the local community and its frontline responders. Depending on the location of the incident, it will take a minimum of twelve to twenty-four hours for federal resources and assets to reach the disaster and begin contributing to the overall emergency response. Therefore, the community's first responders have to deal with the entire disaster response in the initial aftermath.

A VA medical center is a part of its community. As such, VA facilities are encouraged to be active parts of their respective communities' emergency management programs. Although the VA's primary mission is to serve our nation's veterans, that does not preclude it from providing humanitarian service to individuals and the community when necessary and when appropriate.

Federal law dictating the availability of VA resources during an emergency depends on the level of response. For example, if the disaster is declared, a national emergency under the Stafford Act and FEMA assigns a specific mission tasking to the disaster, and VA resources are made available, since the VA will be reimbursed for goods and resources by FEMA. However, if the disaster is not of the magnitude that warrants a federal disaster declaration, then a sharing agreement needs to be in place in order for the VA to use its resources for non-veteran care. Often, sharing agreements are not quickly or easily established. Consequently, it is imperative that local, county, and state governments, along with VA facilities, work together to identify needed sharing agreements and negotiate them in advance of potential emergencies. This would save valuable time, effort, and frustration during an actual disaster response.

The VA has authority to "furnish hospital care or medical services to [non-VA beneficiaries] as a humanitarian service in emergency cases."[9] However, many individuals have incorrectly interpreted the humanitarian services to mean "free" services. This interpretation is entirely incorrect. Written guidance from the VA's general counsel states, "VA appropriations, including the existing appropriation ..., generally include a provision stating that no appropriated funds shall be available for hospitalization or examination of any persons unless reimbursement is made to the medical care account at rates set by the Secretary."[10] Therefore, the VA is required to bill for humanitarian services provided to non-veterans. Hence, a sharing agreement is necessary to cover the humanitarian services provided. Humanitarian services apply to the use of medical supplies, medications, and equipment as well as medical care provided directly to non-veteran patients.

In her interview with *Journal of Homeland Security* regarding the VA's role in homeland security, Dr. Koenig says, "We are somewhat unique, however, in that we are the 'federal presence' in virtually every local community in the country. So, in addition to any support role we [VA] play at the federal level, we are 'in and of the community,' and are there to provide assistance to our local partners. Of course, our veteran population is part of that community...." She also states, "Our facilities and personnel are integral components of the communities and are consistently involved in day-to-day planning and preparedness activities. It is only natural that VA is also involved in local and state response and recovery efforts."[8]

Representatives of local VA medical centers, EMSHG AEMs, and emergency preparedness coordinators contribute to the community's emergency preparedness by providing educational forums, conducting exercises, participating on local emergency preparedness committees and councils, and assisting in the planning process for responding to disasters. Frequently, communities will rely on VA resources to assist with disaster responses. For example, following the bombing of the Alfred P. Murrah federal building in Oklahoma City in 1995, the VA medical center provided space, transportation, and fiscal resources to support the response actions. It also provided mental health counselors to assist people with their emotional trauma from the event. VA x-ray technicians assisted the office of the medical examiner with radiologic forensic support.

Another example is the Houston VA Medical Center's role following Tropical Storm Allison. This storm flooded the Houston area and severely impacted the Texas Medical Center, which is a section of

Houston where ten major hospitals are located within blocks of one another. The VA medical center was the only medical center in this area that was not impacted by major flooding. It became the command center for coordinating the response and recovery activities in that area. Additionally, decades of research specimens and documentation were moved to the VA medical center for safekeeping and preservation from the flooding in the impacted medical facilities. VA staff and supplies were used to assist the local hospitals during their devastating and costly disaster.

On another occasion, the EMSHG AEM in Houston was contacted by the local emergency responders and asked to determine how many cyanide antidote kits were available in the community. Although this would appear to be a community responsibility, the AEM was recognized as a valuable source of information for the community's response to a potential emergency.

The Miami VA Medical Center served as a major source of medical supplies for the response to Hurricane Andrew after it destroyed southern Florida. Again, VA staff, supplies, and equipment were made available to assist the local community with its response and recovery efforts.

Following the federal government's implementation of the Domestic Preparedness Program, where weapons of mass destruction (WMD) train-the-trainer courses were taught to communities throughout the nation, the Southern Arizona VA Health Care System conducted educational forums in Tucson that presented the WMD training to the community and VA staff. Many community first responders, nurses, and physicians were able to receive this information that would otherwise not have been available to them until a few years later.

VA medical centers' primary responsibilities are to their patients, volunteers, and staff to prepare for emergencies, including meeting the JCAHO emergency management requirements. To meet these requirements, each VA medical center conducts a minimum of two exercises annually. At least one exercise each year must be conducted with the community. Additionally, the VA facility conducts internal exercises. These exercises not only meet an accreditation requirement, they train the staff on their responsibilities during an emergency. The exercises also help the facility staff identify opportunities for improvement, once the exercises are critiqued.

All VA medical centers located in urban areas are affiliated with one or more medical schools or university schools of nursing, pharmacy, and allied health. As an affiliated teaching hospital, they have access to some of the brightest and most talented physicians, nurses, and other healthcare providers. These individuals, along with the VA medical center staff, are valuable assets to the community's emergency planning and response activities. Other VA resources include medications, supplies, and equipment.

Likewise, VA medical centers located in rural areas play an equally important role in their communities' emergency response programs because the resources available in rural communities are generally more limited than those in urban cities. Often there is only one other hospital in the rural area where a VA medical center is located. The emergency response resources available to the rural VA medical center are as important to that community as the resources in an urban VA medical center are to its community.

The EMSHG, in collaboration with the VHA Center for Engineering and Occupational Safety and Health (CEOSH), developed an emergency management program guidebook to assist the individual VA medical centers in the development of their emergency management programs. The emergency management guidebook describes how to set up the emergency management program and provides templates for a variety of forms that are used in reporting emergency management incidents and after-action reports.

The VA funded two significant emergency management programs designed to prepare every medical center for terrorist events involving weapons of mass destruction. The VA pharmaceutical cache program provides each VA facility the capability of treating 1,000 to 2,000 patients over a seventy-two-hour period of time. According to VA policy, "VA has established a cache of pharmaceutical and related products. This cache contains products to respond to use of chemical, biological, radiological, and explosive weapons of mass destruction. It will be used, if needed, to treat veterans, VA staff, and other individuals seeking treatment at a VA facility."[11]

The second significant emergency management program funded by the VA is the establishment of decontamination teams at medical centers. VA assessed the decontamination needs and capabilities at each medical center and provided decontamination train-the-trainer preparation. At the conclusion of the weeklong training, the four individuals from each facility lead it in establishing a decontamination team at the VA medical center. The VA provides funding and oversight for the purchase of the comprehensive decontamination equipment items. The program began in 2003 and will not be fully implemented until 2005. Once the program is completed, the selected medical centers will be expected to have the equipment, training, and team to decontaminate patients exposed to hazardous material.

SUMMARY

As the largest healthcare system in the nation, the VA has tremendous resources to assist in local, regional, and national disasters. It is first responsible for providing care and services to veterans. However, as members of local communities, VA medical centers plan and prepare to assist with local disaster responses. As a federal partner, the VA is also available to assist with nationally declared disasters under the Stafford Act.

NOTES

1. Emergency Management Strategic Healthcare Group. Available from: www.va.gov/EMSHG. Accessed December 5, 2003.

2. Major exercises, training and deployment. EMSHG annual report. Fiscal year 2001. p. 7.

3. Deployments. EMSHG annual report. Fiscal year 2000. p. 7.

4. Major exercises, training and deployment. EMSHG annual report. Fiscal year 2002. p. 8.

5. VA/DoD contingency. 2003 July 9. Available from: www1.va.gov/EMSHG/page.cfm?pg=61. Accessed December 5, 2003.

6. Robert T. Stafford Disaster Relief and Emergency Assistance Act. 42 U.S.C. §§ 5121, *et seq.*

7. Initial National Response Plan. Paragraph III, concept B, p. 2.

8. The role of veterans affairs in homeland security. J Homeland Sec 2003 Oct 08. Available from: www.homelandsecurity.org/journal/interviews/displayInterview.asp.

9. 38 U.S.C. § 1784.

10. Guidance on entering into mutual aid agreements. 2003 July 23.

11. Koenig KL. Federal emergency preparedness programs: role of the Department of Veterans Affairs. PowerPoint presentation at the Health Resources and Services Administration (HRSA) Conference. 2003 Nov 7.

11 Preparedness Matters: United Way Community Crisis Response Planning

Michigan Association of United Ways

The terrorist attacks of September 11, 2001, have been eternally frozen in the memories of those who witnessed them firsthand or watched the countless video replays in the days that followed. The events of the day elicited a range of emotions—fear, sorrow, anger—and shattered the notion of American invulnerability. However, at the moment of greatest national peril, countless heroes emerged in New York City, Washington, DC, and in the skies over western Pennsylvania. Hundreds of firefighters and police officers courageously sacrificed their lives rescuing survivors at the World Trade Center; seemingly ordinary passengers aboard United flight 93 gave their own lives to thwart the hijackers' efforts to cause further terror and destruction in the nation's capital; and millions of Americans lined up to donate blood, supplies, and money to assist in the rescue efforts. It was a day that revealed the worst and best of human intentions, and forever changed the way Americans viewed the world and themselves.

The attacks also fundamentally changed our approach to national security and public safety. They caused policymakers and emergency response professionals to examine established crisis response models. Would terrorists attempt another coordinated attack, using airplanes as weapons of mass destruction? Could terrorists employ biological or chemical weapons that would almost certainly spread beyond city limits or traditional jurisdictions? Were local emergency personnel and first responders equipped to effectively manage such a crisis? While many of these issues remain unresolved, the need for greater community crisis response and recovery tools is not in question.

UNITED WAY COMMUNITY READINESS INITIATIVE

The events of September 11 reaffirmed the United Way's role and challenged its strategies as it confronted an enlarged field of responsibility. No longer to be activated only by the natural and humanitarian disasters it had so successfully addressed in the past, United Way was now confronted by a potentially larger threat: terrorism. But as the day's events in New York, Washington, and Pennsylvania demonstrated, United Way's past and ongoing initiatives in crisis management, its sponsorship of the nationwide 2-1-1 system, and, of course, its traditional role as a resource broker demonstrated that it could meet the challenges of terrorism.

Founded in 1887, the United Way has a long history of helping communities cope with challenges in times of crisis by partnering with human service agencies, business, and government to raise resources and address local needs. Though not an immediate disaster response agency such as the American Red Cross or the Salvation Army, which work hand-in-hand with the Federal Emergency Management Agency (FEMA) to assist response and relief efforts, the United Way's vast network of almost 1,400 community-based organizations bring together disparate community agencies to provide assistance months or even years after an initial event. The United Way has traditionally filled a void often overlooked in the immediate recovery effort, such as restoring community services, organizing and mobilizing volunteers, providing information to the public about appropriate response resources, and assisting human service providers with resources required for continued and often expanded delivery of their services.

Many local United Ways trace their origins back to the "war chests" formed during the first and second world wars. These war chests were created as an efficient and effective means of financing war relief efforts and helping communities cope with the wars' effects on families and communities. Several large-scale disaster events during the 1980s spurred the United Way system to focus national attention on how the system could improve its support of communities following a crisis event. Subsequently, in the mid-1990s, United Way of America launched an aggressive educational campaign for its state and local organizations in order to establish firm crisis management programs encompassing an "all hazards" approach. In essence, the United Way system would not limit itself to only one type of crisis such as natural disasters, but would include the full scope of threats and risks faced by communities and individuals alike—including threats to, and breaches of, homeland security.

The events of September 11, 2001, served as a reminder of the importance of long-term dedication to the human side of crisis recovery. Prior to the attacks, response was primarily delivered on a local or regional basis. But with large-scale disasters in three states and the nationally traumatizing nature of the incident, the entire United Way system was counted on to help in the most devastated areas—New York City, Washington, DC, and Somerset County, Pennsylvania—while also providing services to local constituents. Given the national scope and media coverage of the attacks, some of which were broadcast live on network television, the United Way mobilized with its community partners to provide emotional support to those Americans deeply troubled by the events far from their own communities, including providing opportunities for people to help. In addition, because all private air traffic was grounded for the first time in American history, thousands of passengers were stranded at major airports. United Ways in the metropolitan Atlanta area, for example, provided food, shelter, and other assistance to confused and shaken passengers.

As people absorbed the enormity of the attacks, they focused on trying to help in some way. In addition to giving blood and volunteering in recovery efforts, people wanted to give financially to the victims, survivors, and families of those lost that day. The United Way of America activated its crisis response plan and national crisis relief fund to organize and sustain immediate assistance in the impacted areas, as well as the significant work in communities nationwide. As with most disasters, the amount of money needed for the September 11 recovery was unknown in the earliest stage. About all that was known was that the scope of needs was immense, and a long-term coordinated recovery effort would need to be developed and implemented.

UWA's Crisis Response Team scrambled to provide consistent communication as best as possible during the chaos of September 11 and the following days and weeks. Utilizing the organization's own sophisticated intranet as well as available e-mail and phone capabilities, UWA provided guidance while strategizing with executive directors and others across the nation on how to best respond. On an almost moment-by-moment basis, information changed so rapidly that the team appointed a UWA communications manager to monitor and track issues that could become challenges for local United Ways across the country. UWA had to constantly distribute messages that synthesized information and put it into accessible forms; e-mail was used more than ever because it was timely, quick, and direct. Through these predetermined and established communication systems, United Way knew that it was reaching those who needed this important information.

As flight 93, en route from Newark to San Francisco with forty-four passengers and crew, reversed course over Ohio and began flying southeast over Pennsylvania, the executive director of the United Way of Laurel Highlands in Cambria County, Pennsylvania, was shocked to hear of the attacks on New York City and the Pentagon. Minutes earlier, Nikki Yorchak received the first of several crisis response notifications from the national organization—United Way of America (UWA)—located only a few miles from the Pentagon in Alexandria, Virginia. After reading the Internet advisory, Yorchak had no reason to believe that her small United Way was about to be engulfed in the shocking events transpiring in New York City and Washington, DC. Yorchak, who for more than fifteen years had been executive director of the local United Way, was saddened like everyone that morning but originally saw the tragedy as happening elsewhere. She never dreamed that she and her community would soon become one of the horrific television images and that she would be pressed into action helping her community respond to and recover from a piece of the still-unfolding tragedy.

At approximately 10 a.m., after a struggle between passengers and the four hijackers, United flight 93 crashed in an empty field just a mile and a half away from Shanksville-Stonycreek High School. The school building shook on impact as the students' world collided with the horrific events in New York and Washington. "I was scared," sixteen-year-old student Terri Jacobs told reporters. "After that, I wanted to help. I couldn't just sit home and watch this all day on the news."[1]

When Yorchak heard about the crash, her initial response was to review the role United Way played in disasters, and how she and her five-person staff could connect the community with the necessary health and human services, as well as opportunities to participate and grieve in order to begin the healing process. She knew that time was of the essence, and along with other United Way executives, she knew the importance of strategy and organization in crisis response and recovery.

As early as the mid 1990s, UWA launched an aggressive educational campaign for its state and local organizations in establishing firm crisis management programs encompassing an "all hazards" approach. In essence, this focus included the full scope of threats and risks faced by communities and individuals alike. From ferocious hurricanes to devastating wildfires and domestic terrorism in Oklahoma City, United Way has enacted dozens of crisis recovery plans, but none with the scope and breadth of events of September 11, 2001.

In 2002, United Way of America leadership established a "special initiatives" team to explore lessons learned from September 11 and to identify the necessary steps to improve its crisis response and recovery efforts. The team polled state and local United Ways for feedback on crisis recovery efforts. What emerged was a revised and improved crisis response philosophy with a core set of principles, including:

1. Play upon your strengths.

   - Use existing resources and competencies.
   - Turn to others to rely on their strengths and competencies and offer your own to them.
   - United Ways are not necessarily good at sharing resources or leaning on others. The same is true between United Ways and other not-for-profits at the local and national levels.
   - Help others understand the effectiveness of using established outlets versus creating new organizations and efforts.
   - Successful crisis response is not just community-wide, but is also a system-wide operation. Two of our greatest strengths are the depth and breadth of the United Way system.

2. Never underestimate the generosity of the American public.

   - Be prepared to manage the funds.
   - Be clear about donor expectations.
   - Help donors understand the response.
   - Help shape donor activity and involvement.
   - Facilitate opportunities for the public to appropriately participate in the response efforts through donations, volunteering, and dialog.

3. Understand and work within the new influence of the media.

   - They determine who and what is right and who is wrong.
   - They serve as examples for behaving in different situations.
   - There is a need for a community-wide spokesperson or conduit.
   - Provide simple, clear access to response, recovery, and support information through the 2-1-1 system.

4. Be prepared—be ready for crisis response.

   - Have a business continuity and disaster recovery plan.
   - Have immediate cash on hand without extensive bureaucracy.
   - Understand how staff roles would/could change.
   - Inventory available services/strengths of all agencies.

- Establish alternate communication channels and procedures.
- Participate in community crisis response planning.

In response to lessons learned during the 1990s and the September 11 attacks, the United Way established the Community Readiness Initiative. The mission of this initiative is to ensure that United Way organizations and their community partners have the necessary knowledge and infrastructure to prepare for crises and support community recovery following an incident. The events of September 11 and the subsequent long-term recovery efforts confirmed what the United Way system had already recognized: for communities to most effectively and efficiently respond to crisis events and to mitigate the impact of a crisis on the capacity of the human services sector to conduct its regular day-to-day services, response plans—including long-term recovery systems—must be developed and practiced in advance of a crisis situation.

United Way is first and foremost continuing to focus its efforts on community impact. For years, United Way has partnered with human service agencies, corporate and labor leadership, and local and state government to raise funds to meet local needs. These partnerships have matured to include the task of identifying the most critical community needs, finding ways of leveraging local charitable dollars with other resources, and building collaborative relationships that strive to reduce duplication of services and build upon those services that provide the greatest impact. These same systems and relationships are now utilized by United Ways in helping communities prepare for and respond to crises, whether natural disasters or acts of terrorism.

The United Way's crisis response and preparedness reach has expanded across the globe. In August 2003 a terrorist car bomb exploded at the JW Marriott Hotel in Jakarta, Indonesia, killing fourteen and injuring over 150 others. United Way International (UWI) has been working with its member organization in Indonesia, Yayasan Mitra Mandiri (YMM), Marriott International, and other community and global partners to ensure that assistance is provided to victims of that devastating attack.

In December 2003 a massive earthquake devastated the Iranian city of Bam, killing more than 30,000 people and leaving more than 100,000 homeless. UWI immediately established a relief fund to help victims cope and rebuild after the rubble and debris were cleared. With the help of trusted partners, UWI worked to identify and qualify other local, proven, not-for-profit organizations already providing relief and recovery support in the region. It directed initial donations to the General Union of Voluntary Societies in Jordan (GUVS), a UWI member affiliate, and other qualified organizations, to respond to the crisis.

United Way's unique community role is to serve as a convener, bringing the right parties together from business, health and human services, government, faith-based institutions, and other key areas to look at needs, assets, gaps in services, and what resources may be needed. Convening communities around a serious need such as crisis preparedness, whether for war, natural disaster, or any other crisis, is an essential role that the United Way is well positioned to perform in America and around the world.

SPECIFIC CRISIS RESPONSE ROLES
FOR COMMUNITY UNITED WAYS

Never intended to be a first responder in crises, United Way over the years established a well-deserved reputation as a crisis recovery organization. While other groups like the Red Cross and Salvation Army—which both receive United Way funds and are valued community partners—provide essential resources during the first moments of devastation and turmoil, the United Way continues its response many months or even years after the initial trauma. Its experienced managers and volunteers know that in terms of the emotional component of crisis, there is no deadline. Often overlooked in the disaster assistance system in this country are two critical elements: (1) what happens when the organizations that provide health and human services within a community are themselves the victims of the disaster, and (2) responding to the long-term victim and community recovery needs that emerge for months and even years after the initial incident and which require significant allocation of resources.

United Ways across the country have had to face these challenges time and again: services disrupted for months by terrorist attack; a campaign for needed social service dollars halted in a hurricane-wracked region because all energies had to be focused on the tragedy at hand; a daycare center destroyed by floods, preventing parents from returning to regular work schedules; a child who lost a parent and didn't begin to show emotional anguish until the parent wasn't at his next birthday party nine months later. These are all very real examples of the unanswered impacts a crisis can, and often does, have on the delivery of human services long after an event. United Way organizations assess potential needs as part of community readiness and then identify authentic gaps in resources and coordination and attempt to address those needs through a variety of channels.

Helping to Restore Community Services

Social service agencies must remain open so that they may continue to provide services prior to, and immediately following, a crisis. When agencies' facilities are damaged, United Way can provide assistance in either repairing the facilities or locating temporary office space for the agencies. Assistance can be in the form of an emergency grant, or as a "broker" of available workspace. United Way of the Coastal Bend in Corpus Christi, Texas, for example, had arrangements with several local businesses for emergency space that could be used by agencies in a crisis situation. Following Hurricane Andrew in 1992, United Way of Miami-Dade and local government worked with local childcare agencies to clear and secure space at a number of public areas, including shopping center parking lots, to allow the agencies to provide childcare services. These services were deemed essential for emergency response, utility, and government personnel who had young children but were needed on the job.

Serving as a Convener

United Ways can convene local social service organizations—nonprofit, private, faith-based, service club, and government agency—to develop plans that identify the types of assistance and resources that may be needed in different kinds of crises. Counseling/mental health agencies, food banks, childcare organizations, agencies dealing with donated goods (such as Goodwill Industries and Junior Achievement), are examples of organizations that will likely be called upon to provide unique services in times of crisis. Many of these organizations can bring nationwide networks to bear on crisis recovery as well.

Expected needs, such as temporary facilities, emergency identification cards for essential agencies' staff, and providing cell phones can be identified and addressed in the crisis response planning phase. For instance, the aforementioned United Way of the Coastal Bend in Corpus Christi, Texas has an arrangement with a local cell phone provider to make donated cell phones available to essential staff within twenty-four hours of a crisis. Many other United Ways are also involved in issuing picture identification cards approved and recognized by local emergency management teams so that essential social service staff members can be provided prompt and appropriate access to crisis-impacted zones. Secure, approved identification has become an even more crucial preparedness component for United Ways and their community partners, with the greater emphasis on security and law enforcement components associated with homeland security events.

Donations Management

During a time of crisis, United Ways and many of their community partners receive both solicited and unsolicited crisis relief donations in the forms of money, in-kind goods, and volunteer assistance from donors within and outside of the community. In Grand Forks and East Grand Forks, North Dakota, the United Way became an integral part of the recovery process as the two communities began to rebuild after devastating floods in 1993. Working from temporary offices (it would be six months before the UW could return to its flooded downtown location), United Way responded with financial assistance to help nonprofit agencies rebuild and get their programs back up and running. Direct relief came as three United Way relief centers were set up to coordinate the distribution of hundreds of truckloads of donated items that poured into the severely incapacitated community—much of it unsolicited. United Ways work with community partners such as financial institutions, chambers of commerce and corporations, local government, and disaster relief service providers to establish policies and procedures to allow for the efficient collection, solicitation, and timely distribution of these emergency funds, goods, and volunteers. Again, the goal is to make it easy for donors to help. United Way of North Carolina has served as a "bank" for donations for Hurricane Floyd (1999) and Hurricane Isabel (2003) relief efforts. The donations came directly to the United Way of North Carolina through "the Governor's Fund" and were used to help with the unmet needs of local communities as determined by local committees coordinated by community United Way organizations.

Development of Long-Term Recovery Strategies and Systems

United Ways participate in, and establish if necessary, long-term recovery committees (sometimes called unmet needs committees), which are typically partnerships among human service providers, funding organizations, and community leaders. These committees can help identify options to meet the needs of the community, determine service gaps, develop plans for providing resources, and commit their organizations to providing the resources that will help the community during recovery. These committees and their subsequent transitions into the permanent health and human services system provide assistance to victims and the community at large for months and often years after a precipitating crisis event. Following the 1995 terrorist attack that leveled the Murrah federal building in Oklahoma City, post-traumatic stress disorder (PTSD) and other mental health issues became the central focus of the United Way's efforts long after first responders had left. In and around the city, the United Way and its partners continued to focus on the community with grief counseling and other related services through the "resource coordination committee" co-convened by the United Way of metropolitan Oklahoma City. Community United Ways are all unique, with different organizational capacities. Consequently, United Ways utilize their particular strengths in community crisis preparedness/response. Their roles also differ based upon the expectations of local emergency management teams and other community partners. In some communities, the United Way will have a designated workstation inside the local emergency management operations center. Other United Ways not located at the emergency management operations center may be directly linked via phone and/or other forms of communication or participate via a community coalition such as a local VOAD (Voluntary Organizations Active in Disaster).

THE ROLE OF STATE UNITED WAY ORGANIZATIONS

Whatever a United Way's role is in a given community, it is linked with a state United Way organization or association (in most cases) as well as to the national association, United Way of America, and the entire United Way system and its myriad of community, state, and national partners. The current United Way system includes a number of state organizations, associations, and coalitions of local United Ways within each state. These state organizations are developing plans to coordinate United Way crisis response efforts on a statewide level. The state organizations will work closely with the United Way of America Crisis Response Team to assess the needs of any United Way(s) affected by a crisis. The types of assistance that can be provided include communications, coordination of needed resources, and staffing, as necessary. Like community United Ways, state United Way organizations differ in many ways, including organizational capacity. Given these differences, the United Way Council of States—an affinity group for

United Way state-level organizations—adopted "minimum require-ments for a community readiness 'certified' state United Way group" in 2003. Those minimal requirements are as follows:

1. Identify two community readiness specialists to serve as the primary and secondary points of contact for issues related to community readi-ness and crisis response.
2. Develop a United Way state-level community readiness plan. This plan will include a business continuity and crisis recovery plan for the United Way state organization functions as well as outline how the United Way will interface with other responding agencies, organiza-tions, and systems in order to prepare to respond to community crises and assist with the resulting recovery system.
3. Have a plan for contact within twenty-four hours of a crisis event by the designated contact person with a local United Way affected by crises, and follow-up contact with the United Way of American Crisis Response Team.
4. Have a designated United Way staff person who maintains current contact information for all United Way chief professional officers and other key staff and volunteers for immediate contact in the event of a crisis—including cell phone, home phone, and fax numbers; websites; and e-mail addresses.
5. Annually update and distribute the state crisis response contact list (a list of key state, federal, and volunteer emergency response organiza-tional contacts) to all member United Ways.
6. Annually review and update the community readiness plan at a state-wide meeting.
7. Actively engage the state 2-1-1 initiative in the community readiness planning. United Way and 2-1-1 crisis response plans will interface and complement each other.
8. Brief the state emergency management director (and homeland secu-rity director if this person is different) about the United Way com-munity readiness plan. Maintain open communication with the state emergency management and homeland security department(s) follow-ing the initial briefing.
9. Meet and brief the FEMA voluntary agency liaison (VAL) who serves the state. Maintain open communication with the FEMA VAL follow-ing the initial briefing.
10. Identify someone to represent United Way on the State Citizen Corps Council, or participate in another coordinated disaster volunteer man-agement initiative within the state.
11. Join and actively participate in the state VOAD (Voluntary Organiza-tions Active in Disaster). The primary representative for the state VOAD will be a United Way staff person.

The ability to improve lives by mobilizing the caring power of communities at the state and local levels is what has made the United Way system successful. Through standards of excellence, statewide planning, and improved communication, local United Ways have changed people's lives and the conditions of communities. A new initiative to implement 2-1-1 (a nationwide version of 911) services nationwide to better connect citizens with vital information during times of crisis is consistent with this effort, and it promises to strengthen communities in many important ways.

2-1-1: AN ESSENTIAL COMMUNITY PREPAREDNESS RESOURCE

Central to all effective community preparedness is communication. The critical element of being able to inform stakeholders of the scope and breadth of needed action depends on being able to impart information quickly, succinctly, and correctly. Once again, the events of September 11 and the fluidity of information caused by attacks in multiple states, along with wide-scale phone and Internet failures, confirmed important lessons that crisis managers knew from previous catastrophes. Even the most sophisticated communication technologies are useless if affected people are unable to access the information or don't know where to find timely information.

The U.S. General Accounting Office recognized this in a report published in December 2002, which found that while "charitable organizations took immediate steps to get aid to those in need, families and victims generally believed that they had to navigate a maze of service providers and confusion existed about the range of services available to people, particularly those facing job or housing losses."[2]

Although this statement was written to describe challenges faced by victims of the September 11 attacks, similar confusion arises in response and recovery to all community disasters including floods, fires, earthquakes, tornadoes, and other local or national tragedies. Partially for this reason, in 2000 the Federal Communications Commission (FCC) assigned the 2-1-1 telephone number to help avoid that type of confusion.

United Ways can provide ongoing communications to social service agencies during, and immediately following, a crisis, and 2-1-1 systems can be an essential component in establishing a social services information network. United Ways and their 2-1-1 partners prepare and maintain emergency contact information for human service agencies, which include emergency phone numbers as well as alternate phone numbers for essential agencies' key staff. Those staff should have access to emergency numbers of key United Way staff as well. Following a crisis, United Way has ongoing contact with the human services agencies, and 2-1-1 can keep track of what services are being provided, if temporary sites are being used, and the locations of those sites. Information about current services can be shared on an ongoing basis with the emergency management team as well as with the public through an Internet interface. This information will include: what help is available, where to get the help, and appropriate eligibility for services. This information can be shared with the media, which will provide a more comprehensive distribution to the general public.

Following Hurricane Andrew, the United Way of Dade County developed an updated list of human services being provided throughout the affected area, which was published daily in the *Miami Herald*. The United Way also provided information and referral services to thousands of people by expanding their call capacity immediately following the hurricane—using a standard ten-digit number that was unfamiliar to the majority of southern Florida residents—by utilizing their corporate partnerships to establish a temporary call center at the vacant Eastern Airlines Headquarters at the Miami International Airport. Today there is a 2-1-1 system in place and available twenty-four hours a day, 365 days a year in Miami and throughout Florida ready to provide crisis response services complete with surge capacity through mutual aid agreements between all the Florida 2-1-1 centers.

First established by the United Way of metropolitan Atlanta in 1997 with great success, 2-1-1 is an easy-to-remember telephone number used to find or provide help during times of emergency. The number is a key asset for communities preparing for and recovering from community crisis and is a critical information system that is necessary prior to, during, and after such events. Prior to a community crisis, it is vital for a 2-1-1 system to be in place to store information and respond to the crisis at a moment's notice. The 2-1-1 number is available immediately during times of crisis to field questions and direct people to services most appropriate for their needs, and once implemented, it maintains a permanent presence in the community. As a result, people can find the help they need whether the needs arise a week or several years after the crisis event.

Local 2-1-1 systems play several key roles in communities in disaster recovery and response, including:

- Managing and tracking available resources.
- Managing and tracking requests for resources.

- Providing rumor and information control.
- Providing evacuation/traffic/shelter information to the public.
- Providing comfort and assurance.
- Volunteer and donations management.
- Entry points for community case management/victim advocacy.
- Providing information to travelers from out of the area.
- Providing connections to services for long-term recovery.

Though in place in only a small number of communities prior to September 11, 2001, the system proved invaluable, as communications were sporadic and events developed so quickly. Communities that had already implemented 2-1-1 prior to September 11 used their systems to respond to the aftermath of the attacks, fielding calls from people concerned about bioterrorist threats, disseminating accurate information to the public regarding bioterrorism and anthrax, and serving as a centralized communication network for rumor control.

Given its proximity to the World Trade Center in lower Manhattan, the Connecticut 2-1-1 system served as the assistance line for the families of Connecticut residents who were lost in the World Trade Center and answered calls from families looking for victims; frightened children and concerned parents; people looking for ways to help; people who escaped the burning buildings and felt guilty; information on terrorist suspects; and mentally ill persons feeling overwhelmed with disaster, to name only a few. In managing these calls, the certified professionals who staff the 2-1-1 line updated their database with new services related to the disaster, posted information online, and prepared statistical reports. Immediately after the attacks, the governor's office provided citizens with two phone number options to use—1-800-CTHELPS and 2-1-1. Over 90 percent of callers chose to use 2-1-1, a number that was familiar to many residents and easy to remember.

Though the city of Atlanta was not directly attacked, the number of calls to the United Way 2-1-1 line in the week following September 11 increased more than 78 percent from the same period the previous year. Many of these calls were people looking for opportunities to volunteer and donate. UW 2-1-1 professionals also coordinated direct assistance to over 900 people stranded at Hartsfield International Airport. Through partnership with Traveler's Aid and other community partners, these families were provided emergency lodging and food.

The success of 2-1-1 programs is not limited to the terror attacks of two years ago. On May 20, 2003, call specialists received calls from people near Nederland, Texas, where there had been a natural gas pipeline explosion. Residents were particularly concerned at the time of the explosion due to the recent increase in the national terrorist alert level. The 2-1-1 center in Houston was able to field calls from citizens who had questions about the event. Of particular benefit was the voiceover Internet protocol (VoIP) system that Texas 2-1-1 had implemented— the first 2-1-1 VoIP system in the nation. The VoIP system enabled calls to be fielded in both the Houston and Austin call centers, substantially increasing call volume capacity. Callers indicated that they were pleased that 2-1-1 was available, as it saved them from calling 911 for a non-life-threatening emergency.

Prior to the gas explosion, the 2-1-1 system in Texas was able to field calls regarding the space shuttle Columbia tragedy in February. Texas 2-1-1 call specialists across the state (Texas 2-1-1 is currently available to 83 percent of the state) had up-to-date information through the VoIP system, including warnings to callers not to touch the debris and later information about how to notify authorities about the location of debris. Additionally, Texas 2-1-1 was able to provide immediate emotional follow-up to the community through information on grief support and memorial services.

Nor is the success of 2-1-1 programs limited to the United States. In March 2003, the Canadian government identified four cases of severe acute respiratory syndrome (SARS) in Ontario. The World Health Organization (WHO) ultimately confirmed more than 250 cases of SARS and thirty-seven deaths in Canada, the largest number outside of Asia. Though 2-1-1 Toronto was not originally publicized as a phone number to call for information on SARS, it consistently received related calls because many people were not familiar with the numbers that were publicized. An estimated 12 percent of Toronto residents utilized the number, particularly during the initial two-week period when the public was the most concerned.

With the highly contagious nature of SARS, hundreds of people were quarantined, which created many issues that prompted calls to 2-1-1. People in quarantine were not able to go to work and were, in some cases, not being paid. The federal government declared them eligible for unemployment insurance, and 2-1-1 Toronto was able to refer the calls to the appropriate support. Quarantined people also called 2-1-1 because they were unsure about how to get groceries or solicit assistance for elderly relatives they normally cared for, and 2-1-1 Toronto responded with creative solutions such as online grocer access and connecting individuals to elder-care service providers for temporary assistance.

2-1-1 Toronto also launched a significant public education outreach to Toronto populations that spoke Chinese in order to inform them of 2-1-1 assistance. These same populations were then able to call with their SARS-related concerns and receive language-interpretation services. The Chinese communities were able to call 2-1-1 in order to get correct information when they were feeling isolated and stigmatized.

According to the Hotel and Restaurant Employees Union, one third of restaurant workers lost their jobs while equal numbers struggled on reduced pay as the entire hospitality industry was devastated by the significant loss of business. 2-1-1 Toronto referred affected workers to agencies for income and unemployment support. On a related note, 2-1-1 Toronto also formed public–private partnerships with members of the retail and hotel sectors to provide referrals for those who could not pay rent due to SARS-related layoffs.

2-1-1 is more than just an emergency hotline or resource following acts of terror, high-profile disasters, or public health crises. Every minute of every day, people find themselves in need of community support. Many families need information on government and not-for-profit services that address domestic violence; support adequate and stable housing; alleviate hunger; and provide for high-quality day care, after-school activities, summer activities, job training and assistance, elder care, and disaster recovery. Individuals often need support, services, or both when suffering emotional distress, having suicidal thoughts or behavior, contemplating violence, or using drugs or alcohol. With more than 800,000 nonprofit organizations in the United States, individuals and families face a complex and ever-growing maze of human service agencies and programs, spending inordinate amounts of time trying to identify an agency or program that provides a service that may be immediately or urgently required and often abandoning the search from frustration or a lack of quality information. 2-1-1 telephone service facilitates the availability of a single repository where comprehensive data on all community services is collected, maintained, and updated regularly, reducing costs and duplication of efforts. The reliable data provided through 2-1-1 telephone service helps to better assess the needs of our communities and to immediately mobilize resources toward those needs.

Despite these successes by the United Way and its 2-1-1 partners, today only 23 percent of Americans in twenty-one states have access to 2-1-1 services. Recognizing the success of 2-1-1 systems at the state level, and the potential for similar results if implemented nationally, the U.S. Congress authorized 2-1-1 funding as part of the Public Health Security and Bioterrorism Preparedness and Response Act of 2002.

In 2003, Senators Elizabeth Dole (R-NC) and Hillary Clinton (D-NY) joined Representatives Richard Burr (R-NC) and Anna Eshoo (D-CA) in sponsoring the Calling for 2-1-1 Act of 2003, which would authorize $200 million annually to help states implement and sustain 2-1-1.

Senator Dole, a former president of the American Red Cross, supported the national implementation of 2-1-1 long before being elected to the U.S. Senate in 2002. "With the abundance of agencies and help lines, folks often don't know where to turn to get the proper assistance they need," said Senator Dole. "The 2-1-1 line allows families and individuals that are really in need of assistance to find the faith based, community, or government agency to best serve their needs."[3]

As part of its Community Readiness Initiative, the United Way of America has identified implementation of 2-1-1 as a national priority because it is a key asset for communities preparing for and recovering from community crisis and is the first step in the healing and rebuilding process for individuals and families. Nationwide implementation will require a steady source of funding and hundreds of public/private partnerships at the local, regional, and state levels. However, because the need is so great, and the benefits so vital to strengthen communities, full implementation will become a reality with the support of Congress, governors, state legislators, corporate and nonprofit partners, and the public that stands to benefit the most from this important service.

CONCLUSION

September 11, 2001, was quite simply a day that forever changed the world. As vivid images of hijacked planes and collapsing buildings are frozen in our memories forever, there is some solace that the courageous acts of countless numbers of firefighters, police, and crisis managers prevented even more carnage that day. The coordinated hijackings and intentional destruction of the symbols of American economic and military might have brought community readiness and emergency responsiveness to the forefront of domestic public policy.

As community preparedness moves beyond a traditionally local responsibility toward a more national approach, new models of crisis management will emerge. Though local relief organizations and first responders are best equipped to provide assistance during national disasters or possibly further acts of terror, federal lawmakers and local decision-makers should not overlook the local and regional resources that provide the long-term recovery assistance. United Ways continue to advocate for community readiness by pursuing funding for a national

2-1-1 community assistance telephone number currently in effect in twenty-one states and by requesting that the Federal Communications Commission (FCC) maintain the 2-1-1 designation after the statutorily required review of the system in 2005. Finally, by renewing its commitment to collaborate community readiness planning, national organizations such as the United Way of America will continue to help their member organizations and other partners to become an even stronger helping hand to communities across North America and the world.[4]

NOTES

1. Tom Gibb. Sculpture to honor Shanksville residents. Pittsburgh Post-Gazette 2002 Feb 18;Sect. C:13. Available from: www.postgazette.com/regionstate/20020210memorial0210p6.asp. Accessed March 13, 2003.

2. U.S. General Accounting Office. September 11: more effective collaboration could enhance charitable organizations' contributions to disasters. GAO-03-259. 2002 Dec 19. Washington, DC. p. 10.

3. Senator Dole calls for 2-1-1 legislation [press release from Senator Elizabeth Dole's office]. Brian Nick, contact person. Washington, DC. 2003 Sep 16. Available from: www.senate.gov/~dole/index.cfm?FuseAction=PressReleases. Detail& PressRelease_id=236&Month=9&Year=2003. Accessed March 10, 2004.

4. For more information about the United Way, visit www.unitedway.org or www.211.org. Contact information is as follows: Tamara L. Schomber, National Director, Community Readiness, United Way of America, 701 North Fairfax Street, Alexandria, VA 22314, tamara.schomber@uwa.unitedway.org.

12 9/11: A Personal Reflection, My Role, and Responsibilities

Carol L. Holland

I knew the phone would ring.

The university counseling center where I worked had just learned of the first attack on the North Tower of the World Trade Center. Now we can recite the chronology by rote, but that day each news report resonated with shock. The second plane crashed into the South Tower, another dove into the Pentagon, and the last came down in a field near Pittsburgh. The images of that day are forever fixed in my memory. As I stood transfixed and immobilized in front of the television, I knew I would be called.

The growing need for mental health professionals trained to respond to the emotional needs of communities was realized after Hurricane Hugo and the Loma Prieta earthquake in 1989. The American Red Cross (ARC) recognized a need for mental health intervention to manage the high levels of stress experienced by survivors and responders. Many responded, as I did, by being trained as American Red Cross disaster mental health volunteers. A few weeks after the 9/11 attack, I received the call I expected, after which I left for New York City, to assist in the relief efforts. With the support of my employer, Slippery Rock University of Pennsylvania, I boarded a small commuter plane bound for Manhattan. For the next two weeks I worked with the American Red Cross's (ARC) integrated care team to provide emotional support for survivors, family members, rescuers, and other volunteers. Since that time, I have reflected on this experience, my training, my profession's response to terrorism, and my personal and professional sense of community. When I am asked about my ARC experience after

9/11, I respond that it was the most challenging, yet rewarding, experience of my life. I feel a powerful sense of connection to the victims and families and am especially awed by the resilience of the people of New York City and our country, who responded with overwhelming love, respect, and pride.

UNIVERSITY COMMUNITY

My first call from the ARC, on the afternoon of 9/11, requested that I go to the Shanksville, Pennsylvania, crash site to provide mental health support and assistance to first responders. Because of my responsibilities to my university, however, I declined. Anxieties on campus had heightened as phone lines became jammed; students, faculty, and staff could not connect with their loved ones. Within hours, however, the university community responded. The administration decided to have students remain on campus to ensure their safety and ameliorate panic. They kept students informed of events via e-mail and through flyers posted across campus. The counseling center freed up time to accommodate students who walked in, and it dispatched counselors across campus.

Faculty members also played an important part in helping students with their uncertainty, anger, and confusion. By allotting time in classes to discuss the terrorist attack, they gave students the opportunity to express their feelings and fears. Faculty also arranged for panel discussions that included representatives from such appropriate departments as political science, international initiatives, and the counseling center. The media contacted faculty and counselors from campus to share their expertise. This helped educate the surrounding rural community and provided information about normal, expected, and healthy reactions related to secondary trauma, the condition that develops as a result of viewing and listening to firsthand reports from the scene. In the age of real-time reporting, this is a condition that must be addressed.[1]

Students spent hours talking among themselves, trying to understand the senselessness of the attack and consoling one another. The university organized candlelight vigils to provide a formal expression of our collective sadness, to ease loneliness, and to enhance our sense of community. Campus blood drives allowed students to feel less helpless and encouraged healthy grieving and stabilization. Students, faculty, and staff also donated money and nonperishable goods. All of these events helped our university community cope in healthy ways and prevented additional stress. These acts of sharing in the sadness of the experience helped to nurture a sense of resilience, hope, and confidence in our leadership, and provided successes in dealing with all aspects of challenge—physical, psychological, and economic.[2]

THE AMERICAN RED CROSS DISASTER MENTAL HEALTH SERVICES TRAINING

In 1993 we witnessed the fatal standoff in Waco, Texas; in 1995 the bombing of the Alfred P. Murrah federal building in Oklahoma City; and in 1999 the Columbine shootings in Colorado. With so many "human-made disasters" scrutinized from our living room televisions, it became apparent to the mental health professional community and the American Red Cross that a need existed to respond to such tragedies through service and preparedness. The goal of disaster mental health is to provide emergency and preventive mental health services to survivors and responders. Assistance includes education about typical responses, methods of coping, advocacy, crisis intervention, and referral services. The ultimate goal is to decrease the possibility of long-term mental health disorders among survivors and responders. As a licensed psychologist in higher education with experience in crisis intervention, I responded to an article about volunteer opportunities as a Red Cross mental health professional.

My local Red Cross immediately arranged for me to take the preliminary training required by all volunteers. I started by viewing a three-hour, video-based training program, Introduction to Disaster,[3] which defined disasters, their impact on communities, victim responses, and the many roles of Red Cross volunteers. I also completed Mass Care: An Overview,[4] a workshop that introduced the various service opportunities available. Mental health volunteers are only part of the picture. Others set up shelter; prepare food; and provide health care, computer and telecommunications support, public relations expertise, and family financial assistance. All volunteers must also complete a six-hour standard first aid course and CPR certification.[5] Training wraps up with the six-hour Serving the Diverse Community[6] program, which addresses consumer issues.

I also received specialized training from Disaster Mental Health Services,[7] designed to expand the basics outlined above. In an intensive fifteen-hour disaster mental health course, participants focused on the basic concepts of critical mental health intervention and the fundamentals of disaster assignments. Two well-seasoned trainers shared their experiences, provided feedback to role-playing scenarios, and provided instruction on appropriate documentation. After a volunteer's training is completed, the American Red Cross enters his or her name into its national register—to be called upon when needed. While most Red Cross volunteers must make minimum commitments of three weeks, Disaster Mental Health (DMH) workers can volunteer for as little time as ten days.

All Red Cross DMH volunteers must be professionally licensed or credentialed and may include psychiatrists, psychologists, counselors, social workers, and nurses. Licenses are verified, and volunteers must always carry copies. Job descriptions for all ARC positions delineate roles and responsibilities and prerequisite training and experience.

OVERVIEW OF TYPICAL RESPONSES TO DISASTER

Basically, DMH workers assist with any mental health needs that may arise. People in crisis may stare blankly or appear numb and disoriented. The traumatic experience is often overwhelming, so much so that it may be immobilizing. Even mundane tasks become impossible. Farberow[8] outlines the following concerns expressed by those exposed to disaster:

- Basic survival concerns
- Grief over loss of loved ones and/or important possessions
- Separation anxiety and fears for safety of significant others
- Relocation and isolation anxieties
- Need to express thoughts and feelings about having experienced the disaster
- Need to feel that one is part of a community and its rebuilding efforts
- Altruism and the desire to help others cope and rebuild their lives (p. 26)

Age, culture, prior mental health issues, previous experience, and pre-disaster coping skills will determine how people respond. Common responses include:

- Symptoms of acute mild depression and anxiety
- Hyperactivity
- Need to retell or remember details of the event
- Psychosomatic illnesses or exacerbation of preexisting illnesses
- Anger, mood swings, suspicion, irritability, and apathy
- Changes in eating and sleeping patterns (increase or decrease)
- Poor work/school/daily performance
- Withdrawal and social isolation

Onset may be immediate or delayed. Duration varies, but these reactions are considered normal within several weeks of the event. However, if symptoms last longer and/or interfere with daily functioning, then a consultation with a mental health professional is recommended. But when people are provided with social support and reassurance, most prove to be resilient and are able to successfully cope with stressful events.

Resilience

Resilience is "the process of adapting well in the face of adversity, trauma, tragedy, threats, or even significant sources of stress—such as family and relationship problems, serious health problems or workplace and financial stressors. It means 'bouncing back' from difficult experiences." Most people are resilient. Although terrorists attacked the United States on 9/11, individuals and communities immediately began to rebuild their lives. Being resilient does not connote the lack of distress; emotional pain and sadness are common in those who have suffered major trauma. Resilience is, instead, a process, a path that involves significant emotional distress. Resilience is not a character trait but involves behaviors, thoughts, and actions that can be universally learned and developed. The American Psychological Association (APA) brochure, *Road to Resilience*,[9] outlines ten ways individuals can personally enhance this quality:

1. **Make connections**. Healthy relationships with close family members, friends, and others are important. Learn to accept help and support from those who care and will listen. Some people find that being active in civic groups, faith-based organizations, or other groups provides both social support and help reclaiming hope. Assisting others in their times of need can also benefit the helper.
2. **Avoid seeing crises as insurmountable problems**. Highly stressful events happen and cannot be changed—what can be changed are responses to and interpretations of those events. Look beyond the present to the possibility of future improvement.
3. **Accept that change is part of living**. Certain goals may no longer be attainable in the wake of disaster or tragedy. Accepting changed circumstances helps to focus on what can be altered.
4. **Move toward goals**. Develop realistic goals. Do something regularly—even a small thing—that enables movement toward goals. Instead of focusing on tasks that seem unachievable, ask "What is one thing I know I can accomplish today that helps me move in the direction I want and need to go?"

5. **Take decisive actions**. Act on adverse situations as much as possible instead of detaching completely from problems and stresses.
6. **Look for opportunities for self-discovery**. People often experience personal growth as a result of hardship. Many have reported improved relationships, an increased sense of strength—even in the face of vulnerability—improved self-worth, a deeper sense of spirituality, and a keen appreciation for life.
7. **Nurture a positive view of self.** Develop confidence in your ability to solve problems and learn to trust instincts.
8. **Keep things in perspective**. When facing painful events, consider those stressful situations in a broader context and maintain a long-term perspective.
9. **Maintain a hopeful outlook**. An optimistic outlook enables the expectation that good things will return. Visualize desired outcomes instead of focusing on fears.
10. **Take good care of yourself.** Pay attention to personal needs and feelings. Engage in activities that are enjoyable and relaxing. Exercise regularly. Taking care of one's self helps keep the mind and body prepared to deal with stressful situations.

A shared sense of community enhances resilience. Becoming active and engaged in civic or volunteer groups decreases feelings of helplessness and fosters a sense of purpose. Sharing this purpose with others increases feelings of control and can help reclaim hope. Assisting others in their times of need benefits the helper. These are all important components of disaster-relief work.

Crisis Intervention

A crisis occurs when a stressful event overwhelms an individual's ability to cope effectively.[10] A "critical incident," on the other hand, is any stressor event that stimulates the potential for or leads to a crisis.[11] Crisis intervention is defined as the provision of emergency psychological care to victims to assist them in their return to an adaptive level of functioning and to prevent or alleviate the potential negative impact of psychological trauma.[12] The basic principles of crisis intervention are immediate intervention, stabilization of the victims or community, facilitation of understanding, a focus on problem solving, and the encouragement of self-reliance. Various types of disaster mental health interventions exist: on or near-scene emotional first aid, crisis intervention (CI), initial defusing, formal critical stress debriefing (CISD), and follow-up CISD.

Disaster mental health protocol relies on several basic helping processes, beginning with emotional first aid. Some contacts, especially those onsite, may be as short as five to fifteen minutes. In that short time, a simple three-part intervention might include getting people to talk, keeping them busy, and an initial attempt to problem-solve.[13] Crisis intervention is the next step, and moves beyond this initial emotional first aid. CI objectives include relieving survivor or responder anxiety, depression, or guilt; preventing further disorganization; and screening for more serious problems that may require treatment. It is critical, therefore, for DMH workers to maintain a calm demeanor, acquire essential information, use active listening and attending skills, permit victims and responders to vent, present information about normal reactions, and provide information that may help reduce fear.[14]

Another possible intervention strategy is diffusion. Defusing allows victims and workers the opportunity to informally vent about disaster-related memories, stresses, and losses in a safe and supportive environment. A more prescribed avenue is debriefing, a formal meeting that is generally held twenty-four to seventy-two hours after a stressful incident. Debriefing helps the victim deal with the emotional residuals of an event. The ARC's disaster mental health debriefing model is a modified version of Mitchell's critical incident stress debriefing (CISD) model.[15] Jeffery Mitchell is cofounder of the International Critical Incident Stress Foundation. He has authored seven books and over 200 articles in the fields of crisis intervention, disaster psychology, and critical incident stress management. He is considered an expert in disaster work. Mitchell's model involves structured interviews between a trained facilitator and emergency responders who witness a critical incident. In order for such meetings to be effective, given the wide range of personal histories, personality styles, and disaster experiences that may be involved, they must be voluntary. Follow-up mechanisms, which may include further debriefings, telephone calls, mailings, or professional referrals, are also critical to the process.

My Experiences in New York City

While my ARC training focused primarily on work in the aftermath of natural disasters, the September 11, 2001, terrorist attacks on American soil were fundamentally a psychological assault.[16] The most psychologically damaging effects follow extreme violence, mass casualties, massive property damage, substantial financial disruption, and malevolent intent[17]—all of which were present in those fateful attacks. When an act is human-engineered, it intensifies the complex dimensions of emotional responses that victims, family members, and responders experience. Responders are at an increased risk as they react to the pain and suffering of others while trying to deal with their own questions and fears.

I arrived in New York City on October 27—just six weeks after the attacks. As required by the ARC, I reported in to Red Cross upon my arrival at JFK Airport and was directed to a hotel that had donated rooms for the use of Red Cross volunteers. I hopped on a shuttle filled with volunteers from across the country; many wore Red Cross buttons, jackets, or hats. These visible symbols identified us as members of a specific community of helpers. We shared information about prospective job assignments and previous experiences, thus providing an informal icebreaker. Such interaction helped in our transition, as we came from distant towns and cities to a community disrupted by tragedy and prepared to work in extremely stressful conditions. The following morning, along with about thirty other volunteers, I boarded a Red Cross bus for the local headquarters in Brooklyn, where I was assigned to work with an integrated care team.

The Red Cross developed integrated care teams to "facilitate the recovery of individuals and families who, because of loss of life, debilitating injury, or illness or profound emotional/financial losses following a disaster event have a decreased ability to obtain or utilize assistance without intensive Red Cross intervention."[18] In New York such teams worked with families or individuals who were dealing with extenuating circumstances such as the loss of more than one family member, widows who were expecting or had given birth to a child since the attacks, and those who had been married only for a short while to a lost spouse. Teams consisted of one family service worker, one health service worker (usually a nurse), and a member of the mental health services. Because circumstances dictated that teams come up to speed quickly, orientations and introductions were brief. My first assignment was to provide follow-up to previous contacts with phone calls to family members and to arrange appointments at their home or at Pier 94 in Manhattan.

Pier 94, which is an exhibition center near New York's Upper West Side, was designated as a Red Cross family assistance center. A huge hall swathed with American flags, it housed numerous local and national assistance agencies including the Red Cross, Salvation Army, and Safe Horizon, New York City's direct assistance agency. Services ran the gamut from therapy dogs to fax services and included legal advice, psychological referrals, healthcare assistance, spiritual counseling, translators, food services for both volunteers and the families of the victims, and financial assistance. Thousands of colorful origami swans that had been delivered from countries around the globe hung on display throughout the building—a monument to worldwide mourning. Every hour the voice of a New York City police officer singing "God Bless America" resonated throughout the hall—each time, work would stop and people would stand and place their hands on their hearts and sing tearfully along.

Though the twelve-hour days we worked were physically and emotionally draining, I commuted the mile and a half each day on foot to provide myself with time to prepare. While we met with family members at Pier 94, team members worked from an undisclosed location. Our offices were cluttered with five-foot tables encircled with four chairs each. Office supplies, a telephone, and mementos and pictures from home covered the surface of each table. We also had computers at our disposal and, in a corner, several large boxes of stuffed animals. By 8 a.m., the phones were active. Conversations ranged from the mundane to the tragic. We might discuss necessary paperwork and subway directions or provide instructions to a grieving family member about acquiring remains. Each team was designated by a letter of the alphabet and responsible for a specific geographic area. I worked on the S team.

After an administrative supervisor assigned families to our teams, we would make an initial contact by phone to determine their most pressing needs and how best to meet them. Needs might include financial assistance, referrals, and recovery information, or such simple items as "comfort kits" and teddy bears. Most importantly, we provided support by listening to our clients. In addition to these "traditional" services, we might also need to help out-of-town family members with transportation, meals, and lodging as they arrived to attend funeral or memorial services or to provide support to injured or ill loved ones. We also provided follow-up with each family to ascertain whether they might have longer-term needs that we could address. We visited clients' homes, hospitals, funeral homes, and other facilities as needed.

PERSONAL STORIES

Jonah and Michelle Smith[*]

I answered the phone to hear a woman asking if she was eligible for financial help from the Red Cross. Her husband of one year had perished in the North Tower. Six weeks later she was ready to accept the reality of his death and address practical concerns. Where, she

[*] Names have been changed to protect privacy.

wondered, could she pick up the urn filled with dust from the World Trade Center site that would symbolize, for now, the body that might never be identified? She gave me her name and told me a bit about her marriage. She seemed to need to tell someone just how much in love she and her husband had been. They had not had children ... but had planned to someday ... she started to cry when she told me this. The verbal admission that she would never have a child with her husband overwhelmed her.

I arranged for the team to meet her at the entrance to Pier 94. "My name," she told me, "is Mrs. Jonah ... no ... Michelle Smith." My anxiety mounted as I walked through the unusually warm October city streets to meet the first family member I was to help. The exterior of Pier 94 loomed in front of us, plastered with photos of lost family members, mementos left by loved ones, pictures drawn for Daddy, and "Have you seen my sister?" posters. The pictures, with their unremarkable backgrounds hinting at the ordinariness of pre-9/11 lives, were eerie. I scanned the pictures as I passed, making a visceral connection with each person. Directly in front of me was Jonah Smith's photo, his name was printed in large black block letters. I felt my stomach drop. A handsome man with smiling bright eyes, he stood beside his beaming wife, Michelle. At this instant the real tragedy of this attack hit me; it was no longer abstract, nor could I be professionally distanced.

I entered the building and immediately recognized Michelle. I walked up to her, introduced myself, and gave her a hug. I told her that I had seen Jonah's picture and how handsome he was. She began to cry and thanked me for acknowledging his good looks, something others were afraid to talk with her about. In the one hour we spent together, she was able to talk about that dreadful day, the day she lost her husband. But today, six weeks later, she was ready to tackle some practical concerns that she had. For example, some concerns included paying bills, donating Jonah's clothes to a community charity, and exploring whether she should move closer to her family. She was learning to live alone again, though this was the hardest thing for her to do. She tended to be more anxious at night and was having trouble sleeping. Attending a support group for family members in her community was very helpful. This was a safe place to share her feelings, and feel less isolated and more a part of a "very special community" where she was completely understood. She had not been back to work since 9/11 but was planning to return the following Monday.

Astrid Freeman[*]

Mr. and Mrs. Freeman lost their thirty-two-year-old, brown-eyed daughter Astrid. Mrs. Freeman was worried about her husband because he had refused to go to Astrid's apartment since the attack. She thought they should go and pack her belongings. He cried constantly; because of their religious beliefs, they could not hold a memorial service until her body was recovered. Mr. Freeman felt suspended much of the time. Could the integrated care team, Mrs. Freeman wondered, be at the apartment when they arrived?

We waited outside the Manhattan apartment until Astrid's parents arrived. While Mr. Freeman was cordial, he avoided direct eye contact and quickly excused himself to his daughter's bedroom. After a few minutes I knocked on the door and asked if I could come in. I was surprised when he agreed; he was clearly skeptical of our presence. As parents of a victim, they were entitled to financial compensation from the Red Cross to cover three months of usual expenditures, a memorial service, and burial. Mr. Freeman told me that all monies received would be donated to a local Jewish organization in Astrid's name. Here was a father who was aching with grief and was just beginning to face the reality of his daughter's life. I asked if he could tell me about Astrid, what kind of person she had been, and what he wanted others to know about her. He showed me the racing bike on which she avidly competed, and he talked about the depth of her faith—even in the face of a world that seemed to dismiss the importance of religion. He showed me pictures and showed me a journal on his website for all those who knew and loved her. I read an entry he had written and others that were composed by friends and family, and I cried. We both cried.

Later, I spoke with Mrs. Freeman. She dealt with her grief in a different way. She had formed a group for family members in her synagogue, and she spent hours each day calling to comfort other parents who had lost children. She wrote a newsletter, attended numerous memorial services, and advocated for public policy on the war with terrorism. She felt hopeful in a proactive, altruistic approach. This approach aided her in feeling more in control at a time when everyone around her felt out of control.

While the Freemans dealt with the loss of their daughter in different ways, both are examples of expected reactions at a difficult time. We all agreed, however, that the religious community, competitive bicycling community, her family, and the world had lost an important member.

[*] Names have been changed to protect privacy.

Miguel Ramierez[*]

While working at Pier 94, an NYPD police officer approached the microphone and began to sing "God Bless America." Hundreds of people stood. Men removed their hats; everyone faced the ten-foot flag, hands on their hearts, and began to sing along. All, that is, but one young Hispanic man. He remained defiantly seated—his ball cap in place. When the song ended, another police officer approached me and asked if I would speak with this angry young man and his mother.

Mrs. Ramierez had worked for Cantor Fitzgerald on the 105th floor of the World Trade Center. Early news reports indicated that no one from that firm survived. Mrs. Ramierez, however, was late for work that day so was not in the building during the attacks. Because of the persistent report that no Cantor Fitzgerald employees had survived, her name appeared on the death list and each time she tried to apply for benefits, she was denied. Six weeks after the attack, her bills were mounting.

Tragically, however, Mrs. Ramierez had worked with her oldest son, Paolo, who did perish in the attacks. Because she was wrongly listed as dead, and because her name differed from that of her son, accessing her benefits had become a nightmare. Her nineteen-year-old son Miguel could only watch helplessly as his grief combined with frustration, confusion, and a growing animosity. He had already lost his beloved brother and felt as if he was slowly losing his mother in the bureaucracy. He was angry. The integrated care team immediately began to talk with Mrs. Ramierez. I sat quietly with Miguel, hoping he could compose himself, but he only became more agitated.

I continued to sit with him and asked him to tell me about his brother, their relationship, and how close his single-parent family had been. Miguel had worked at a well-known restaurant as a pastry chef, but had not reported to work since 9/11. He told me he was afraid to leave his mother alone. He believed he was now "the man of the house." He grieved for his brother and was consumed by anger. He also believed that he and his mother were the victims of discrimination. For almost two hours, he talked and I listened. He told me stories about his childhood, his mother's strength as she raised two boys alone, and their dreams and aspirations.

By the time our conversation had ended, the computer records were finally corrected. The Red Cross immediately issued both a grocery voucher and an emergency check to cover all bills the family had incurred. We gave the family referral information and telephone numbers

[*] Names have been changed to protect privacy.

they could use to contact us. Before they left, Miguel surprised me by wrapping his arms around my neck and thanking me. He told me that I was the first person to take the time to simply listen. We both had tears in our eyes as he pulled away. His mother confided that this was the first time since the attacks that his anger seemed to be relieved. Perhaps now he could sleep.

I gave Miguel a follow-up call and left a message on his machine. He never called back, but I am grateful for what he gave me—an invitation to share his memories and grief.

The personal stories above exemplify some of the typical needs, reactions, and feelings that are experienced by survivors of terrorism. These family members, while grief-stricken, were able to move toward adapting to life after terrorism.

PROFESSIONAL ORGANIZATIONS AND THE AMERICAN RED CROSS

In 1989, after Hurricane Hugo and the Loma Prieta earthquake, the ARC recognized a need for mental health intervention to manage the increased levels of stress experienced by survivors and responders. This realization provided the impetus to offer mental health services that have since evolved into the Red Cross Disaster Mental Health Services (DMHS).[19] In 1990, the Red Cross began the process by surveying 3,800 of its workers. Results indicated that volunteers suffered high levels of stress and felt unsupported—especially in view of long hours worked in what were sometimes very rugged conditions. Self-care information and time available for decompression were scarce. The ARC convened a multispecialty task force, which from its inception underscored the need to develop a multidisciplinary approach to reduce acute post-disaster stress. The task force compiled a rough draft for a training manual that was implemented with a "train the trainers" approach. A systematic exponential plan provided a framework for training other instructors. Pilot training sessions were implemented and revisions to the training as well as the instructional manual evolved. Next, the trainers were given the task of teaching mental health professionals from psychology, psychiatry, nursing, social work, and counseling the basic principles of disaster work.

Training on a national level was possible when, in 1991, a grant was awarded to the American Red Cross to provide instruction to trainers and additional for supervisory personnel. The award provided support for DMHS workshops to Red Cross chapters in all fifty states.

With the multidisciplinary approach to meeting the wide range of mental health needs of disaster victims, the DMHS was able to integrate diverse skills and contributions of many professional communities. This has underscored the importance of minimizing "turfism" and increasing essential collaboration. With a generic multidisciplinary approach, professional specialty conflicts are reduced. All professional affiliations work together because the duties are basic and universal.

Since 1992 the Red Cross established formal agreements with a number of professional organizations including the American Psychological Association, the National Association of Social Workers, the American Association of Marriage and Family Therapists, the American Counseling Association, the National Association of Hispanic Nurses, the National Black Nurses Association, the North American Association of Christians in Social Work, and the American Psychiatric Association. The goal of these agreements was to establish a working relationship for development of cooperative disaster relief efforts. This non-disciplinary approach fosters acceptance and appreciation that elicit the highest levels of humanitarianism, as exemplified by those professional association affiliates who volunteered time and money as well as personal comfort to aid others in time of need. This provides a context to help discipline specific individuals to respond to each other in a human-to-human way to provide humanistic and altruistic care. To date there have been 9,000 professionals trained.

THE AMERICAN PSYCHOLOGICAL ASSOCIATION'S RESPONSE TO TERRORISM

In December 2001, in response to the terrorist attacks of September 11, the APA board of directors adopted the following resolutions stating how the profession and professionals could help with the war on terrorism:

WHEREAS on September 11, 2001, terrorists hijacked four commercial airplanes and attacked the World Trade Center in New York City and the Pentagon in Washington DC, area and crashed the fourth plane in rural Pennsylvania;

WHEREAS those attacks caused the deaths of thousands and great destruction of property;

WHEREAS the physical impact of terrorism is death and destruction; its behavioral effects include disorganization, fear, anger, and a sense of helplessness, loss of confidence, and problems in coping;

WHEREAS, the fear of anthrax contamination has heightened these psychological states;

WHEREAS different segments of our diverse society use different methods of coping with and managing stress, some being more comfortable with individually focused methods like behavioral, affective and cognitive self-management and relaxation techniques, while others are more comfortable receiving support from their extended families, communities, and places of worship;

WHEREAS psychology as a discipline and a profession has much that it contributes through application of psychological knowledge and expertise;

WHEREAS the events of September 11 have led to a dramatic increase in the incidence of hate crimes based on ethnicity, ranging from harassment at work to murder;

THEREFORE, LET IT BE RESOLVED that the American Psychological Association, and organization devoted to health and well-being, calls upon the psychology community to work toward an end to terrorism in all its manifestations;

BE IT FURTHER RESOLVED that the American Psychological Association:

Encourages its members to use their knowledge and expertise to help alleviate the public's high levels of stress, anxiety, fear and insecurity and to mobilize the public's strength and resilience to cope with terrorism and its aftermaths;

Provides relevant information to its members that will enable them to reduce the public's high levels of anxiety, fear, stress and insecurity;

Advocates at the congressional and executive levels for increased use of behavioral research that will produce greater understanding of the roots of terrorism and the methods to defeat it, including earlier identification of terrorists and the prevention of the development of terrorism and its related activities;

Encourages increased research, treatment and prevention of trauma-related and disaster-induced problems among children, adolescents and adults;

Encourages ways to develop stress management, fear management and support programs specifically designed to help citizens deal with the continuing threat of terrorism;

Condemns prejudice leading to harassment, violence and hate crimes.[20]

CONCLUSION

Like the term *holocaust*, which conjures vivid images, the term *terrorism* will always invoke images of the planes crashing into the towers of the World Trade Center, the smoldering remains at the Pentagon, and the phone messages of the heroic passengers on flight 93, which crashed in a Pennsylvania field on September 11, 2001.

This chapter provided a framework for the roles and responsibilities for disaster mental health professionals after the act of terrorism on September 11. In my role as a mental health responder, working collaboratively with the American Red Cross and countless other volunteers, we provided support in the relief efforts. For two weeks I worked with the American Red Cross's integrated care team to provide emotional support to survivors, family members, rescuers, and other volunteers. Together with the American Red Cross, my profession of counseling, other helping disciplines, my employer, and communities within and outside the United States, I experienced firsthand a global helping community. As a result of my personal experience, my role as a Red Cross disaster mental health volunteer, and my responsibilities in my university and volunteer community, I feel a powerful commitment to using my knowledge and skills in restoring peace.

NOTES

1. Miller J. Reflections on 9/11: vulnerability and strength in the "new world order." Smith Coll Stud in Soc Work 2002;73(1)73–84.

2. Prince R. Voices from New York. Contemp Psychoanal; 2002 38(1): 77–99.

3. American Red Cross. Introduction to disaster services. Washington: Author, 1993.

4. American Red Cross. Mass care: an overview. Washington: Author, 1995.

5. American Red Cross. Standard first aid. Washington: Author, 1993.

6. American Red Cross. Serving the diverse community. Washington: Author, 1995.

7. American Red Cross. Disaster mental health services. Washington: Author, 1998.

8. Farberow NL, Frederick CJ. Training manual for human service workers in major disasters. DHHS Publication No. ADM 83-538 (formerly NIMH). Rockville, MD: National Institute of Mental Health, 1978.

9. The road to resilience. American Psychological Association. 2003 Nov 30. Available from: helping.apa.org/resilience/what.html. Accessed August 12, 2004.

10. Auerbach S, Kilmann P. Crisis intervention: a review of outcome research. Psych Bul 1997;84:1189–217.

11. Flannery RB Jr., Everly GS Jr. Crisis intervention: a review. Internat J Emerg Mental Health 2000;2(2):119–25.

12. Everly GS Jr., Mitchell JT. Critical incident stress management (CISM): a new era and standard of care in crisis intervention. 2nd ed. Ellicott City, MD: Chevron; 1999.

13. Weaver JD. Disasters: mental health interventions. Sarasota, FL: Professional Resource Press; 1995. p. 68–70.

14. Weaver, JD. Disasters: mental health interventions. Sarasota, FL: Professional Resource Press; 1995.

15. Mitchell JT. When disaster strikes ... the critical incident stress debriefing process. J Emerg Serv 1983;8:36–9.

16. Levant RF. Psychology responds to terrorism. Prof Psych: Res and Pract 2002;33:507–9.

17. Eidelson RJ, D'Alessio GR, Eidelson JI. The impact of September 11 on psychologists. Prof Psych: Res and Pract 2003;34(2):144–50.

18. American Red Cross. Integrated care teams. Abstract publication no. 588. Washington, DC: Author; 2001.

19. Weaver JD, Dingman RL, Morgan J, Hong B, North, CS. The American Red Cross disaster mental health services: development of a cooperative, single function, multidisciplinary service model. J Behav Health Serv and Res 2000 27;(3):314–21.

20. The road to resilience. American Psychological Association. 2003 Nov 30. Available from: helping.apa.org/resilience/what.html. Accessed August 12, 2004.

13 One Community's Plan for Safer Schools

Rena E. Richtig

After a series of shootings occurred in schools across America in the 1990s, area law enforcement in the mid-Michigan community of Mount Pleasant, led by Director of Public Safety William Yeagley, held discussions and determined the need for an intervention model emphasizing community involvement to make schools a safer place.

A task force funded by a grant from the Saginaw Chippewa Indian Tribe was created to support the endeavor. Over the next eighteen months, conversations, research, and site visits provided materials for the development of a plan. Central Michigan University professor of psychology Walter J. Lesiak served as consultant and directed the task force. I served as one of seventeen selected members of the task force and was part of the team that made site visits, gathered data, and helped formulate a plan.

The result was a ninety-eight-page document that included a detailed plan and recommendations.

The second phase of the process involved taking recommendations to the community, gathering feedback, adjusting the plan as needed, and beginning implementation.

The third phase of the process was the formation of the current School Safety Alliance, whose responsibility included the continuous operation and updating of the plan. This chapter will detail the three phases.

Included here is an overview of the task force's organization and a description of what was accomplished, and changes in the plan's implementation. The summary describes the School Safety Alliance Committee and its current role in the plan.

OVERVIEW OF THE TASK FORCE

Phase One

Located in the central part of lower Michigan, the community surrounding the city of Mount Pleasant has about 28,000 people with an additional 19,000 Central Michigan University students.

The Saginaw Chippewa Indian Tribal Reservation borders the city limits. The reservation boasts one of the country's largest Native American casinos, which draws thousands into the city daily. The city and surrounding countryside are experiencing an increase in population. The area school districts (four public, two parochial, and two charter) are affected by this growth and support the need for an intervention model.

Interested community members began discussing the rash of school violence occurring in the country. They believed that a community-based approach to developing safer schools was necessary. A review of federal legislation showed that several national goals were related to student anger and violence. One example was goal six of Educate America,[1] which focused on creating safe, disciplined, and drug-free schools. Another was a Healthy People 2000 Goal[2] to reduce weapons-related deaths, reduce the carrying of weapons, reduce the frequency of physical conflicts, and increase the number of youth receiving conflict-resolution training in schools.

A task force was created to develop a community intervention model in the event that a school-shooting incident occurred. Preliminary discussions indicated that it could happen in this community, and a plan to anticipate and prepare for such an incident would be worthwhile.

The development of an intervention model involving community agencies would need a key group of citizens to serve on a task force. Interested community members were approached to serve on this task-force; through a selection process that included a review of their interests, personal interviews, and supporting references, seventeen people were chosen.

In 1999, the Saginaw Chippewa Indian Tribe of Michigan funded the task force by awarding an eighteen-month grant for approximately $55,000. Five police agencies collaborated on this effort, and a project consultant was hired to implement the grant's objectives.

The task force began by gathering data. A review of the literature on the topic of school violence showed that much had been written on the topic, but there was agreement that more could be learned by conversations with individuals in communities that had suffered such tragedies.

Task force members representing various disciplines in the community traveled to various sites of school violence incidents. They asked the following questions:

a. When were decisions made by various agencies (school, public safety, police/fire, mental health, etc.) during the incident? In retrospect, what would have been done differently?
b. What changes in policies and procedures have been made or recommended as a result of the incident?
c. What suggestions do individuals involved with school violence incidents have to prevent such incidents in the future?
d. What can be done as part of the healing and coping process when such tragedies occur?

The personal conversations provided details of the impact on the community as a whole and a deeper understanding of the dynamics of the incidents.

The creation of the task force was not met without criticism, however. When the concept was reviewed in the local newspaper, several mental health professionals denounced the idea, claiming that it would be sufficient to adopt an existing model and bring in trainers from the National Emergency Assistance Team (NEAT) to train people in the community.

Although these were seen as important elements to a successful plan, the task force felt that discussions to more fully grasp the depth and breadth of the tragedy in school communities would help create an effective intervention model.

The members of the task force shared responsibilities as the project unfolded; no particular person or committee took on a leadership role. A collaborative norm was encouraged by Director Yeagley, who allowed it to develop, seemingly on its own, through occasional visits, individual conversations and encouragement, and placing realistic expectations on the group.[3] Leadership was not limited to people holding administrative/supervisory positions.[4] Voices were heard and respected, and people across disciplines contributed meaningfully to the process.

The task force representatives from mental health, schools, media, the university, courts, clergy, and law enforcement gathered data and organized visits to areas that recently had experienced school violence. Sites visited included Paducah, Kentucky; Pearl, Mississippi; Jonesboro, Arkansas; Littleton, Colorado; and Port Huron, Michigan. After spending thousands of hours of effort and creating numerous drafts, the group wrote a seven-chapter document titled *Recommendations from the*

Isabella County Community Intervention Task Force on School Violence.[5] The recommendations dealt with the intervention model and conceptual issues surrounding school and education, mental health and human services, law enforcement/tactical media, and the basis for recommendations. Five chapters were devoted to suggestions for those specific disciplines. A final chapter outlined a plan for implementation. Appendices included additional material such as board policy samples, background information of onsite visits, risk factors, and an incident command structure example. The recommendations described below are synthesized from the book.

The recommendations are written in three categories: pre-plan, incident or crisis, and post-incident follow-up. These categories include specific directives and future recommendations for when the initial plan is in place. They are described below.

Law Enforcement/Court System Recommendations

Pre-Plan

The plan placed strong emphasis on law enforcement, juvenile court, and school administration developing stronger relationships with each other and a more active role in school safety during all aspects of the plan. This was supported by research, group discussions, and conversations with law enforcement at the site visits. Specific security issues were listed for addressing by law enforcement and the school community. Further, implementation of a school violence prevention curriculum was recommended.

The community already had effective court-related programs for youth in place, and the recommendation was that they continue or be expanded. Research and site visit discussion also pointed out the importance and necessity of the youth services unit, which they felt should be expanded. Other recommendations included a family resource center and a juvenile risk/needs assessment center.

Incident/Crisis

The recommendations for law enforcement are extensive because school personnel need to be prepared to react to any type of emergency that could occur in or near a school. Site visits determined that most often a plan was either not in place or did not work. A building-specific plan is recommended, utilizing the Incident Command System (ICS) as the foundation. The ICS establishes a common organization structure, terminology, and operating procedures critical to an effective plan in any emergency. If a school crisis occurs, the emergency services team (EST) will be activated. This is a team of fourteen tactical officers and six negotiators. A school would implement its incident command team, better known as the BERT (building emergency response team). These team members follow the directions of the incident commander and carry out the duties for which they have been trained.

Post-Incident Follow-Up

Communication needs to link closely with the media plan, continue, and give updates to the community. The adoption of a zero-tolerance policy for any copycat/contagious incident is also recommended.

School Recommendations

Pre-Plan

Emphasis on further development of strong working relationships with community groups such as law enforcement, firefighters, faith-based groups, media, hospitals, and mental health workers is key to the plan's success. Research indicated that curricula changes were in order,[6] as were ways to look at the overall design and risk management of the school settings[7] and the necessity of preparedness.[8]

The Incident Command System (ICS) would be created in each school setting. Disaster kits, crisis response boxes, a media plan, and communication links would be developed. The plan would also create building emergency response teams. Conflict resolution and bullying prevention plans were indicated as two specific curricula to be considered for implementation in schools. Policies directed to curricula and other issues need to be developed. The plan also requires communication links and a media plan.

Incident/Crisis

The ICS is implemented. The BERT goes into action. Each school has building-specific plans that would then reflect its setting, student body, location, and other unique characteristics.

Post-Incident Follow-Up

The tremendous impact of the media on school personnel was overwhelming, as determined by conversations at every site visit. A solid plan to handle media effectively is critical, especially after the incident. Mental health will have a more active role in ongoing counseling and debriefing of the school community.

Site visits helped the team determine the value of meeting with parents face to face as soon as possible after the incident. Keeping area schools apprised of the situation also arose as an important consideration.

Mental Health Recommendations

Pre-Plan

Once again, the plan lists the importance of developing strong relationships and holding periodic joint meetings of helping professionals to establish and continue groups working together. It further includes mandatory crisis debriefing with law, school, interested community members, and firefighters, utilizing the Jeffrey Mitchell model of crisis response defusing and debriefing.[9]

Incident/Crisis

The County Crisis Response Team (CCRT) coordinator determines the need to contact the Michigan Crisis Response Team and the National Organization of Victim Assistance (NOVA). The CCRT coordinator works with school personnel to determine logistics of debriefings and defusings.

Post-Incident Follow-Up

The CCRT members will conduct defusing at the site, in hospitals, and with first responders going off duty. Within seventy-two hours of the crisis, debriefings should begin and continue as needed with students, school personnel, law enforcement, and firefighters. Debriefings should also include spouses, family, and the community at large, as needed. Continuing support groups will be scheduled in conjunction with school personnel if required.

Media Recommendations

Pre-Plan

Communication devices are important for media and need to be considered in the overall plan. Easy access materials will facilitate stronger media relations and response to inquiries. A media center will be designated and information disseminated by a designated media coordinator.

Written guidelines outlining communication methods that access information during a crisis are a significant consideration, as are training on the effects of media coverage of violent events, training on victims and the media, and crisis training. To address the high turnover rates of reporters, the plan should offer annual workshops for media to inform them of areas of concern when covering crises. Crisis kits developed for media should be in place.

Future Recommendations

Suggestions include a community resource guide, a mock crisis, and a curriculum addressing student preparation for media inquiries and the rights of students.

Incident/Crisis

The media coordinator reports to incident command. Crisis kits are brought to the scene. Reporting hierarchy is from incident command to media coordinator on a thirty-minute interval for status reports, depending on circumstances. Conferences are set up at a specific place designated as a media center. The incident command approves release of any/all information about the media center. The media coordinator prepares key written messages with incident command's approval after every press conference. Information is distributed on paper and uploaded to the community's website when approved.

Post-Incident Follow-Up

The media help incident command coordinate meetings with other community groups, are on call to create and distribute information and/ or write releases for press and websites, and seek additional information overlooked during a crisis, while offering timely news. Further, media will support reporters' need to meet deadlines, offer guidelines to help those being interviewed, provide written guidelines for victims during or preparing for an interview, and place all information in a virtual newsroom as needed.

Faith-Based Recommendations

Pre-Plan

Communication and relationships once again played a role in the development of this group's plan. At the sites where faith-based persons were well connected and closely involved with the schools, it was obvious from conversations that clergy played a significant role in the hours and days immediately following the crisis, and helped the community heal more quickly. As a result, the recommendation was made to initiate a school faith-based liaison to foster supportive relationships between clergy and area school officials. Clergy will be trained as part of the community crisis response team, and will participate in the Mitchell model of defusing and debriefing.[9] Police chaplains and hospital chaplains are to be included in this group.

Incident/Crisis
Trained clergy will be contacted to provide needed services.

Post-Incident Follow-Up
The police chaplain will plan a combined community-wide memorial service along with families of victims, other clergy affected by the crisis, school and law enforcement officials, media, and mental health representatives.

Implementation of the Phase One Recommendations

In summary, the recommendations were placed into three categories: the pre-plan, the incident or crisis, and the post-incident. It is obvious that clearly written plans utilizing the Incident Command System will provide operational procedures to deal with a crisis. Training is crucial. Prevention programs (from security to curricular programs) need to be established. During a crisis, communication among schools and agencies is critical. A media center concept is emphasized. The post-incident phase highlights a plan for debriefing and defusing students and other personnel involved in the crisis, and advocates for a community memorial service. In all of these phases, the task force insists that any plan be countywide, so that all parties involved will be operating uniformly. The plan will need to be systematically reviewed.

The task force designed a process whereby the recommendations would be brought to the township officials and tribal representatives, schools, law enforcement, fire and emergency response teams, clergy, mental health groups, media, the healthcare system, and community members. A sharing of information would allow for dialogue to take place, adjustments made to the plan if necessary, and the next step of implementation to begin. An assessment of training, materials, consultation, and workshops helped to develop a plan for the next step of implementation.

PHASE TWO OF THE PLAN

The need for further grant funding was identified as the plan was being implemented within the community. Over the next year, a variety of recommendations were carried out to the implementation phase, with adjustments to some. The need to continue this endeavor created the opportunity for a countywide intermediate school district to pick up the torch and move forward with phase three.

Members of the original task force offered time and expertise as they were called upon to share their findings with the community. Information from these groups provided data for suggestions to make the plan fit the community's desires better. At this point, the task force, in its eighteen-month journey, completed its original goals.

A decision was made to write another grant proposal for the continuation of the plan. The Saginaw Chippewa Indian Tribe awarded the grant, and a different group of key members was gathered to carry out the proposal. Public Safety Director Bill Yeagley approached the mayor of Mount Pleasant, Albert Kaufmann Jr., who was retiring soon from his position. Yeagley encouraged Kaufmann to continue with this project and see it through the second phase. Kaufmann agreed, and a consultant from Clear Direction Management Corporation, Deb Evans, was hired to facilitate this process, taking direction from Kaufmann.

Training became a major responsibility of this phase. Workshops trained school personnel in the BERT system; others attended media training. Along with this training, pieces of the plan were being implemented at the same time. Community members took the crisis response training, enabling them to be active members of a team to debrief anyone affected by an act of violence. Safety checks were established and security checks occurred in schools. Flip charts, tailor-made to each school setting and using a common design originally developed in Littleton, Colorado, were developed for schools.[10] Law enforcement underwent QUAD (quick action deployment) training. Schools implemented "go boxes," which carried numerous items listed earlier in this chapter. The red-green cards were adopted by school systems. The numbering system for schoolrooms and buildings began to be implemented.

The need to have school administrators and faculty understand the collaborative nature of the project and agree to the concept of the Incident Command System are not small undertakings. Systems thinking or systemic change is not understood by many school administrators, and few have had any training.[11] Systemic change tends to require more of a commitment than does compliance.[12] In order to be successful in their endeavors, their attitudes had to undergo a transformation, requiring continual effort and attention.[3] Creating BERTs and following the ICS are major changes in a school environment. Stakeholders had to

find new ways of learning from each other from within their organization and across organizational boundaries and beyond.[13] The ease with
which this part of the phase occurred leads directly to the collaborative
nature of Director Bill Yeagley, who sustained strong relationships with
school administrators throughout his career.

At the same time, the world changed for citizens of the United
States. The attack on the World Trade Center placed a different focus
on the plan for safer schools. Although a shift had already taken place
from 1999, from school violence to a more generic plan of school crisis,
this world event caused another shift. The threat of terrorism became
real. The overall plan needed to address terrorism as well.

As communication continued to increase across all disciplines with
the implementation of the plan, it was determined that the county
emergency services plan was an opportune tool with which to fold in
the plan for safer schools. The county emergency services coordinator
began to review the document and offer suggestions for a more seamless implementation.

Studies suggest that the challenge of leadership is about making connections—finding ways to connect stakeholders to each other in meaningful ways.[14] The structure, implementation, and overall project results
of the task force throughout phases one and two allowed for a collaborative style to be highly effective—not only with an effective plan that
showed strong promise for the community, but also with the possibility
that with choosing leaders who led collaboratively, the project would
continue to gain momentum.

As phase two wound down, the need for another group to carry on
the process surfaced. The phase one and phase two participants recommended passing on the commitment to a school-based group, which
resulted in offering this responsibility to a countywide intermediate
school district, which oversaw school-related services to area schools in
its jurisdiction. Director Bill Yeagley was instrumental in seeing to it
that this reliable organization, under the watchful eye of a responsible
and collaborative leader, would take over and continue the mission of
the project.

Phase three began with the creation of the School Safety Alliance
Committee.

PHASE THREE OF THE PLAN

The current phase three is directed by Byron Doty, school safety
consultant at the Gratiot Isabella Intermediate School District, who has

part-time responsibility for the budget and conducts monthly meetings of the committee. The new group is made of interested members from phases one and two, and some new members, including the county emergency services coordinator.

Since its inception, the group has accomplished significant tasks, including sections of school readiness plans, community readiness plans, and media plans, drawing from the recommendations. Workshops have been conducted, and school personnel have been trained. Flip charts were fine-tuned for school personnel. A close look at the county emergency services plan indicated overlap, which is being addressed to provide a more seamless plan.

One of the unique tasks of this group was to develop and implement a mock scenario of a terrorist attack on a local public elementary school. Three gunmen entered the school from a van loaded with a "bomb." The entire scenario took place on an early August morning in 2002, with more than 200 individuals and community groups who volunteered for half a day. School faculty, staff, administrators, university students, and others played the roles of victims and of children on the playground or in classrooms. Police, firefighters, mental health, clergy, and others were actively involved, and from this event they learned how to make the crisis plan better. The relationship-building style modeled by Yeagley, his public safety officers, and the wide-reaching network of task force members had a direct connection to the overwhelming positive response to the call for volunteers in the mock crisis.

At its most recent meeting in November 2003, an overall review of the mission of the group and a self study was conducted, to determine what pieces of the plan are close to being fully implemented and what still needs to be addressed. This will be the impetus for creating the next year's goals.

Through monthly meetings, this committee continues to encourage constant review, dialogue, and updating of the implementation of the plan. Its strengths include clear and open communication among committee members and the community at large, regular meetings, and a wide variety of roles represented by the committee members. The shift of the plan to incorporate terrorism has been a major focus of this group, and all aspects of the plan need to be reviewed to determine whether needed changes to reflect this shift are occurring.

The success of this endeavor from the idea stage to the present day relates directly to sustaining positive relationships developed and maintained over the years by Yeagley and the community at large. Research bears out the need for continual involvement of community members with any community-based project.[3] Yeagley's efforts to build collaborative relationships well beyond the scope of the law enforcement agencies obviously allowed this project its considerable success. Empowering the task force to have its voices heard and to develop a workable plan for this community further spread the power behind collaborative relationships in building a successful plan for school safety in the community. The task force truly became and still is a community of learners.

A strong sense of community and the ability to build and sustain relationships across disciplines are essential elements in the development of effective partnerships that utilize collaborative leadership.[15] Yeagley's overall plan to encourage commitment from the group and devote time to the task force to allow relationships to grow and meet the needs of all the members of the group are evidence that the Public Safety Director has a deep understanding of the elements research has shown to be successful in collaborative leadership.[16]

The continued success of the project from phase one through phase two and into phase three demonstrates the community's commitment to the leadership of many, guided by a few, in a nurturing culture of collaboration.

NOTES

1. Goals 2000: Educate America Act. 103rd Cong., H.R. 1804. Available from: www.ed.gov/legislation/GOALS2000/TheAct/index.html. Accessed November 25, 2003.

2. Stoto MA, Behrens R, Rosemont C, editors. Healthy people 2000: citizens chart the course. Washington, DC: National Academy Press, 1990. Available from: www.nap.edu/openbook/0309043409/html/. Accessed November 25, 2003.

3. Patterson J. Harsh realities about decentralized decision-making. School Administrator 1998;55(3):6–12.

4. Bass B, Stogdill R. The handbook of leadership: theory, research and managerial applications. 3rd ed. New York: Free Press; 1990; Bennis W. Managing people is like herding cats. Provo, UT: Executive Excellence Publishers; 1999.

5. Yeagley W, Lesiak WJ. Recommendations from the Isabella County community intervention task force on school violence. Mt. Pleasant, MI: Gratiot-Isabella RESD School Safety Alliances, 2001 Aug.

6. Wiseman R. The hidden world of bullying. Princ Leadership 2002 Dec:18–23.

7. Schneider T, Walker H, Sprague J. Safe school design: a handbook for educational leaders. Eugene, OR: ERIC Clearinghouse on Educational Management, College of Education, University of Oregon; 2000; Snoop R, Dunklee D.

Risk management. Princ Leadership 2002 Dec:28–32; Trump D, Lavarello C. No safe havens. Amer School Board J 2003 Mar:19–21.

8. Trump K. Classroom killers? Hallway hostages? How schools can prevent and manage school crises. Thousand Oaks, CA: Corwin Press Inc.; 2000.

9. Mitchell J, Everly G. Critical incident stress debriefing: an operations manual for CISD, defusing and other group crisis intervention services. Ellicott City, MD: Chevron Pub. Corp.; 2001.

10. Jefferson County Schools. Jefferson County School District quick reference chart emergency management plan. Littleton, CO: Jefferson County Schools; 2000.

11. Senge P. The fifth discipline: the art and discipline of the learning organization. New York: Doubleday; 1990.

12. Schlechty P. Shaking up the schoolhouse: how to support and sustain educational innovation. San Francisco: Jossey-Bass; 2001.

13. Fullan M. Leading in a culture of change. San Francisco: Jossey-Bass; 2001.

14. Sergiovanni T. Leadership: what's in it for schools? London: Routledge/Falmer; 2001.

15. Wagner T. Change as a collaborative initiative: a constructivist methodology for reinventing schools. Kappan 1998;79(6):512–7.

16. Rubin H. Collaborative leadership: developing effective partnerships in communities and schools. Thousand Oaks, CA: Corwin Press, Inc.; 2002.

14 Selecting an Effective Emergency Manager: A Key Player in the War on Terror

Kevin G. Love and
Svetlana V. Ivanitskaya

THE DAY BEGINS

Even though he is hard at work and his nose is buried in paper, the city's emergency manager keeps one eye on the clock. He has ninety minutes to handle a ton of paperwork before his first meeting of the day, one he is not excited about. It is a meeting with three county commissioners who want to discuss the job responsibilities of the emergency manager.

But he is busy right now reviewing the plans for a proposed shopping mall. It is easy to see why the developer wants to locate it as close as possible to the riverfront. Obviously the developer wants to take advantage of the beautiful riverfront vista. How else can they call it Riverview Mall? The developer's architectural plans look fine, but the emergency manager spots a problem with the site plan. The southern third of the mall parking area infringes into the flood plain of the Crystal River. The emergency manager knows that with a heavy rain, the rising water in the river coupled with the large runoff from the large asphalt parking lot may produce significant standing water. Water could back up into the storm sewers, overflow any holding ponds, and ultimately invade the mall itself. This is unacceptable.

Suddenly the administrative assistant bursts through the door. An explosion has ripped through the courthouse. No one is sure what caused it or how much damage occurred. The phone rings. Central Dispatch reports that a public works employee has reported a break-in at the water treatment plant. As he hangs up the phone, the administrative assistant returns with a damage report on the courthouse—five persons hurt and on their way to the hospital, smoke damage throughout the first floor, broken glass everywhere, and police officers on the scene and evacuating the building.

The paperwork will have to wait. It is time to mobilize the county emergency operations center and activate the disaster response protocol. The emergency manager shouts to the administrative assistant to get the city police chief, fire chief, and the county sheriff on the phone. "And get someone from the health department out to the water treatment plant on the double," he adds. "Call the director of public works and the water treatment plan supervisor. I need to know if anything has been stolen or destroyed at the plant. And call the state university. Find me someone who's an expert on waterborne biological contaminants."

One may wonder whether the above passage is an episode of a television series or a movie scene. What it actually represents is a realistic depiction of the job tasks performed by an emergency manager. The tasks, some of which may be associated with costly errors, demonstrate the complexity of this job—handling everyday routine responsibilities, responding to rare but important events, performing under time and physical pressure, coordinating efforts by multiple stakeholders, and other important tasks.

Individuals responsible for the selection, placement, and development of emergency managers must define the qualities that differentiate effective emergency managers from those who are not likely to meet the demands of the job. In this chapter, we provide research-based guidelines for analyzing the emergency manager position requirements and applying this knowledge to the design of state-of-the-art systems for selecting and training emergency managers. Industrial/organizational psychology is the discipline that contributes the most value to our discussion. For the last ninety years, industrial/organizational psychologists have engaged in applied research aimed at enhancing the job performance of employees in both public sector agencies and private for-profit organizations.

TODAY'S EMERGENCY MANAGER

With the advent of September 11, 2001, extreme scrutiny has been placed on the responsibilities and skills of individuals charged with safeguarding the public. For emergency management (EM) personnel, the pre-9/11 focus was on natural disasters and the commensurate mitigation or avoidance of dangerous conditions, planning for a quick response, and remediation and recovery in the aftermath. Today's perspective includes the strong possibility of organized attacks from a range of extremist organizations, both foreign and domestic. The public has become acutely aware of the important roles played by law enforcement, fire, and medical personnel in emergency preparedness and response. But most citizens have not been and currently are not aware of the critical role played by the EM, who must plan and coordinate emergency services before, during, and after a disaster. Once a position buried within the bureaucratic layers of a county sheriff's department or state emergency management division, today's EM is at the forefront of public security planning. But who are these EMs? What are the qualifications needed to perform this critical role? How should EMs be selected and trained?

METHODOLOGIES FOR DETERMINING THE COMPETENCIES REQUIRED FOR THE EMERGENCY MANAGER POSITION

The starting point for any analysis of position requirements is job analysis. An analysis of job requirements and accompanying competencies (knowledge, skills, abilities, and other personal characteristics [KSAOs]) must involve a systematic study of data on critical job duties, responsibilities, organizational roles, and training and education requirements. Job analysis can be defined as "the collection of data describing (a) observable (or otherwise verifiable) job behaviors performed by workers, including both *what is accomplished* as well as *what technologies* are employed to accomplish the end results, and (b) verifiable characteristics of the job environment with which workers interact, including physical, mechanical, social, and informational elements."[1] These data are gathered from authoritative sources such as subject matter experts, job incumbents, supervisors, certification standards, and others.

The data collected by job analysts are used to create a complete and legally defensible description of the essential job duties and, more important for hiring decisions, the KSAOs that underlie successful performance. According to Morgeson and Campion, a "job analysis forms the foundation upon which virtually every human resources system (such as selection systems, training programs, and performance management systems) is built." In addition to providing input into human resource activities and decisions, the use of job analysis helps defend these decisions from legal challenges.[2]

Tasks and duties performed on the job lead to job descriptions that specify *what* is done in the job, whereas a list of KSAOs is used to write job specifications that delineate *how* a job gets done.[2] A job description is created by developing a list of basic job units, which are called *task statements*. Subject matter experts are then asked to rate each task in terms of its importance, frequency of being performed, difficulty, and cost of errors. Most often, job analysts use job descriptions to identify relevant KSAOs, using a linkage analysis.[2] The linkage analysis is performed to determine which KSAOs are associated with important, frequently performed, difficult, and/or costly (in terms of potential errors) tasks. The outcome of this linkage analysis—a job specification—is used to design selection techniques, training programs, and compensation systems.

This commonly used approach, based on a combination of job-descriptive and job-specification inferences, has been called an *indirect* method for estimating job specifications. Many practitioners estimate job specifications *directly* by obtaining ratings of the level of importance of various KSAOs from subject matter experts; for instance, human resources staff or job incumbents.[3] However, this approach is based on the assumption that the identified KSAOs are strongly linked to actual on-the-job performance, which may or may not be true.[2]

Job information can be gathered using a variety of methods such as interviews, direct observations, and structured inventories.[1,4] A human resources staff member, manager, or outside consultant may interview a representative sample of job incumbents. They would ask the employees to describe a typical day from beginning to end. In addition, the interviewees would be asked to relate past situations in which other people in the same job (or themselves) performed extremely well and one in which performance was less than desirable. In some cases, the job analysts may capture actual on-the-job performance by recording observed behaviors. This is more than traditional "shadowing" of the employee. It involves developing a plan for systematic, timed periods of observation so that all aspects of the employee's job are documented. In some cases, the job analyst may even complete required job training or perform simplified tasks associated with the job under study. In-person interviewing and observation, however, can be costly and time-consuming. In many instances, a structured survey will be developed to provide the employee with an all-inclusive list of job duties. The employee rates each task on several scales (frequency of occurrence, importance, etc.). Using the survey method allows input from a wider range of employees and in some cases a more refined determination of the critical tasks of the job. Generally, it is recommended that several, if not all, of these data collection methods be used in developing job descriptions and subsequent job specifications.[5,6]

Several studies have compared the relative value and accuracy of different job analysis methods for a variety of jobs and cultures.[7-11] Collectively, these authors reached the conclusion that no one method of job analysis is superior to other methods in terms of accuracy of outcome data. Moreover, the researchers suggested that any method used by a well-trained job analyst involving motivated and highly knowledgeable subject matter experts and/or job incumbents would result in accurate job descriptions and job specifications. It is important to note that the opposite is also true. That is, an untrained job analyst, inexperienced subject matter experts, and/or unmotivated job incumbents are unlikely to provide accurate data, regardless of the job analysis method.

The importance of involving highly qualified job analysts and well-informed subject matter experts is further underscored by multiple factors that complicate the analysis of the EM position. These factors include:

1. *The lack of available EMs who are familiar with or who have had a chance to perform rare but critical tasks associated with extremely costly errors, such as those associated with potential loss of human life.* Examples of these tasks include the timely mobilization of an emergency operations center in response to a terrorism attack and consultation with regional or national experts for information to formulate an appropriate emergency response.

2. *The use of complex cognitive tasks as an integral part of the EM position.* These cognitively demanding tasks cannot be easily identified or studied via direct observation or interviewing, especially by untrained job analysts.

3. *The necessity for an effective EM to demonstrate a high level of interpersonal skill with a variety of persons, ranging from government officials to emotionally distraught citizens.* These social skills are difficult to describe and interpret through self-reports or even interview methods.

4. *The compressed time frame and accompanying pressure under which many rarely performed but critical tasks need to be executed by an EM that complicate the identification and accurate description of critical KSAOs.* In many instances, an individual capable of making accurate decisions under normal conditions may not be able to use the same good judgment under severe time pressures and when faced with many competing priorities and demands.

Compared to job analyses of more traditional manufacturing or clerical jobs where much of the work involves manual tasks, it is much more difficult to conduct an accurate job analysis for an EM position because of the greater inferential leap between their work output and the commensurate KSAOs. Therefore, it is critical that individuals well trained in job analysis techniques perform any job analysis of the EM position.

THE ROLE AND CRITICAL DUTIES OF THE EMERGENCY MANAGER

Generally, the EM position resides within a state or county public sector organization that provides protective services to the public. While some states mandate through law (state constitution, legislative public act, etc.) that an EM position be created at a specific government level (county, municipality, etc.), others may house an EM position within a state-level department so as to coordinate municipal, township, and/or county services. In any case, emergency services management as a position or a profession carries a mission "to foster, promote, and implement an emergency management system that protects communities and citizens from the effects of emergencies and disasters."[8]

This mission statement implies the following duties for an EM:

- Coordination of all necessary services at the federal, state, local, and private-sector levels.
- Dissemination of critical information regarding mitigation, preparedness, reaction, and remediation of emergency and disaster situations.
- Processing applications for aid at the state or federal level for planning and/or remediation of emergencies and disasters.
- Serving as a focal point for information regarding emergency preparedness and response capabilities.
- Applying the four phases of mitigation, preparedness, response, and recovery to natural, technical, and human-caused disasters and emergencies.

THE COMPETENT EMERGENCY MANAGER

Several comprehensive reviews of the EM position have been completed at the federal and state levels.[12-14] Subject matter experts at the National Coordinating Council of Emergency Management divided the tasks inherent in the EM position into two primary groups: tasks that are performed *before* an emergency and tasks that are performed *during* an emergency.[9] To ensure specificity, each primary task group was divided into related task categories, which were further subdivided into more specific units called task clusters. A detailed description of the two primary task groups follows.

Before an Emergency

Three task categories make up an EM's actions before a state of emergency is declared: (1) monitor and manage projects in-house, (2) conduct planning/mitigation exercises, and (3) maintain positive public relations. The first category includes the administrative tasks associated with managing current projects as well as developing new programs for emergency management. The second category involves assessing the potential for emergencies and planning for emergency situations. Finally, the last category involves establishing ties with the community to inform them of the emergency management program in their area and gaining their support and future cooperation.

During an Emergency

Three additional task categories represent an EM's actions, in chronological order, during an emergency: (1) preparation, (2) response, and (3) recovery. The first task category involves such actions as providing information to the public and other key players in the emergency management process and ensuring the availability of equipment and resources. The second category addresses the immediate response to the emergency—activation of an emergency operations center (EOC), declaration of a state of emergency, relocation of the populace, damage assessment, allocation of resources, coordination among government agencies, and preparation for recovery. This stage also involves information management processes such as addressing the public, keeping records, and controlling rumors. The last task category involves performing search and rescue, restoring vital facilities and services, coordinating a receiving center for relief supplies, and removing debris. The EM and/or an assigned staff member are responsible for gathering information about the nature of the emergency and the responses of the EM and other agencies. This responsibility is woven throughout all three task categories. At the conclusion of the emergency situation, the EM prepares a comprehensive report in which he or she evaluates how the situation was handled and provides recommendations for future improvements.

Task clusters or groupings and the corresponding KSAOs are shown in tables 14.1 and 14.2. A linkage analysis performed by the National Council on Emergency Management led to the identification of critical KSAOs that were associated with numerous task clusters.[13] Specifically, the Council determined that EMs must possess coordinating skills (linked to fourteen task clusters), writing skills (linked to eleven clusters), organizational skills

Table 14.1

**Primary Task Group "Before an Emergency": Task Categories,
Task Clusters, and Essential KSAOs**[13]

TASK CATEGORY: MONITOR AND MANAGE PROJECTS IN-HOUSE

Task Clusters	Knowledge	Skills
1. Conduct project briefings to external groups.	Group dynamics Instructional techniques	Research techniques Writing and public speaking skills
2. Communicate with staff and others.	Principles of effective meetings	Interpersonal skills Report writing
3. Develop a budget.	Organizational and power structure of jurisdiction Budgeting process Principles of fiscal management Grant management Creative methods Budget analysis	Research techniques Proposal writing Decision-making Leadership skills
4. Meet department goals.	Principles of management	Goal writing/setting Coordinating liaison skills
5. Complete projects on time.	Motivation methods Project management tools	Interpersonal skills
6. Develop new programs and/or enhance existing programs.	Computer systems Brainstorming and creative methods Emergency equipment and communication hardware	Facilitating problem-solving skills

TASK CATEGORY: CONDUCT PLANNING/MITIGATION ACTIVITIES

Task Clusters	Knowledge	Skills
1. Complete hazard vulnerability assessment.	Federal and state legislation Legislative process Principles of risk management Recordkeeping process of jurisdiction Generic hazards	Research skills Organizational skills Interviewing skills Analysis skills Writing skills
2. Develop local emergency operations plan.	Team-building methods Planning techniques Previous plan Group dynamics	Coordinating skills Liaison skills Motivational skills Leadership skills Writing skills Negotiation skills Diplomacy
3. Improve interagency cooperation.	Adult education principles and methods Exercise/simulation design Evaluation principles	Leadership skills
4. Test emergency equipment daily.	Emergency equipment	

Table 14.1

TASK CATEGORY: MAINTAIN POSITIVE PUBLIC RELATIONS		
Task Clusters	*Knowledge*	*Skills*
1. Develop community support for the emergency management program.	Media and media relations	Public speaking skills Marketing skills Dealing with the media Leadership skills Interpersonal skills
2. Disseminate info on what local emergency management is.	Adult education principles Principles of effective meetings Exercise/simulation design	Instructional skills
3. Help the public understand its responsibilities.	When to use prepared media information	Managing outside vendors/contractors Television/public speaking skills
4. Make the public aware of your capabilities.	Public protective actions	Writing skills Speaking skills Demonstration skills
5. Use volunteers.	Adult education principles Liability laws	Managing people Coordinating skills Interview skills Instructional skills Motivational skills Organizational skills

(linked to nine clusters), decision-making skills (linked to eight clusters), supervisory skills (linked to eight clusters), knowledge of specific plans and processes, such as damage assessment and emergency planning (linked to eight clusters), public speaking skills (linked to six clusters), research skills (linked to five clusters), and liaison skills (linked to five clusters).

In addition to the KSAOs shown in tables 14.1 and 14.2, the Council stated that the EM was either responsible for or managed others who were responsible for the areas of communication, radiological systems, hazardous materials, training, and logistics. Thus, EMs should also possess the requisite KSAOs to successfully perform tasks in these areas.

The Region V Advisory Committee for Training and Development, part of the Federal Emergency Management Administration,[10] surveyed a sample of EMs gathered for a professional training conference. Their survey identified the following core KSAOs for an EM: communication, coordination, leadership, planning, resource management, training, development, planning, implementation, business management, and evaluation. The Region V state emergency management training and exercise officers subsequently tied these KSAOs to FEMA training content domains for EMs. Table 14.3 shows these relationships. This

Table 14.2

Primary Task Group "During an Emergency": Task Categories, Task Clusters, and Essential KSAOs[13]

TASK CATEGORY: PREPARATION

Task Clusters	Knowledge	Skills
1. Prepare public information.	Joint and point information systems Emergency public relations plan Local media contacts	Data research and collection Writing skills
2. Disseminate public information.		Coordinating skills
3. Determine who is in charge and will speak for each agency.		Coordinating skills
4. Contact liaisons to be on standby.		
5. Prepare briefings for leaders.	Emergency plan	Public speaking skills
6. Assure proper recordkeeping.	Electronic data gathering system Public and private resources	Organizational skills Supervisory skills
7. Manage resources.	Contractual agreements	Judgment Decision-making skills Coordinating skills Liaison skills
8. Test emergency equipment.	Emergency equipment operation	
9. Checking availability of emergency supplies.		

TASK CATEGORY: RESPONSE

Task Clusters	Knowledge	Skills
1. Activate emergency operations center (EOC).	EOC SOP	Coordinating skills Supervisory skills Decision-making skills
2. Declare state of emergenecy.	Current state of emergency/disaster Media personnel hierarchy	Writing skills
3. Prepare additional public realtions releases as necessary.		Writing skills
4. Monitor field status.	Damage assessment process Incident Command System (ICS)	Map reading Decision-making Networking skills
5. Open shelters.	Shelter management	Coordinating skills Supervisory skills
6. Relocate the population.	Plan as related to annex groups such as Red Cross	Map reading Coordinating skills Negotiation skills

222

Table 14.2

TASK CATEGORY: RESPONSE		
Task Clusters	*Knowledge*	*Skills*
7. Assess damage and prepare for recovery considerations.	Forms	Supervisory skills Judgment Decision-making skills Supervisory skills
8. Assure proper recordkeeping.		Organizational skills
9. Conduct media briefings.		Public speaking skills
10. Allocate resources.		Decision-making skills Coordinating skills
11. Coordinate with various levels of government.		Coordinating skills Liaison skills
12. Establish rumor control.	Media channels and personnel	Supervisory skills Coordinating skills

TASK CATEGORY: RECOVERY		
Task Clusters	*Knowledge*	*Skills*
1. Maintian emergency information system.	Documentation requirements Local emergency plan Disaster Relief Act	Organizational skills Computer skills
2. Perform search and rescue.		Coordinating skills Organizational skills Map reading Counseling skills
3. Perform a preliminary windshield survey.	Damage assessment procedures	
4. Provide emergency access.	Two-way radio operation Perimeter control	Map reading
5. Begin restoration of vital facilities.	Resources available	Decision-making skills
6. Continue to gather information about the emergency/disaster.		Research skills Public speaking skills Leadership skills Coordinating skills Liaison skills
7. Implement site security and law and order provisions.	Disaster Assistance Act Disaster assistance process	Organizational skills Management skills Decision-making skills
8. Coordinate receiving centre for relief supplies.	Demographics of community	Organizational skills Supervisory skills
9. Begin debris removal.	Federal resources EPA source material and personnel	Negotiation skills Decision-making skills
10. Set up disaster application centre (DAC).	Disaster assistance process	Organizational skills Supervisory skills
11. Implement closing procedures for EOC.	Emergency operations management system	

(continued)

Table 14.2 (continued)

TASK CATEGORY: RECOVERY		
Task Clusters	*Knowledge*	*Skills*
12. Complete an "after action" report.		Writing skills
13. Critique the operation.		Writing skills

same group reviewed these KSAOs and indicated that communications, coordination, leadership, and planning were the most important ones for an effective EM.

In sum, the purpose of most attempts to identify EMs' competencies was personnel training and development. The KSAOs were defined in broad terms. However, the design of personnel selection, evaluation, and accreditation systems, as well as advanced training programs, should be based on much more detailed information regarding KSAOs. Unless KSAOs are stated in specific terms and measured precisely, it is hard to set objective cutoffs or passing scores that differentiate between successful and unsuccessful candidates.

The emergency management division of the Michigan Department of State Police conducted a comprehensive review of published works in order to identify specific task clusters, responsibilities, core competencies, and training content domains for EMs.[11] In addition, critical incident focus groups with over twenty EMs were conducted. Quite useful for the design of training and performance evaluation systems, the critical incident technique involves eliciting examples of particularly good and poor job performance.[12,13] Therefore, EMs provided actual scenarios in which they performed very effectively, as well as situations in which they performed ineffectively. A staff of four industrial/organizational psychologists with a background in the selection of police, fire, and public safety personnel content analyzed the scenarios to identify the critical behavioral dimensions that determined the EMs' on-the-job success versus failure. A written survey approach was used to refine their inferences. Specifically, thirty-five subject matter experts rated the importance of each behavior dimension as it related to success in the EM position. Combining the critical incident content analysis with EM performance requirements stated in prior published research led to the identification of ten core competencies (see table 14.4). The mean rating of importance, as provided by thirty-five subject matter experts, is also shown in table 14.4.

Table 14.3
KSAOs and Training Content Domains Matrix for the Emergency Manager Position[14]

Training Content Domains	Coordinating Skills	Writing Skills	Organization Skills	Decision-Making Skills	Leadership Skills	Job-Specific Knowledge	Public Speaking Skills	Research Skills	Liaison Skills	Communication Skills
Emergency management laws and authorities			X	X	X	X				
Hazard identification and risk assessment			X	X		X		X		
Capability assessment		X	X	X		X		X		
Hazard management	X	X	X	X	X	X		X	X	
Resource management	X	X	X	X	X	X		X	X	X
Planning	X	X	X	X		X	X	X	X	X
Direction, control, and coordination	X	X	X	X	X	X	X		X	X
Damage assessment	X	X	X	X		X		X	X	X
Communications and warning	X		X	X		X	X		X	X
Operations and procedures	X	X	X	X	X	X	X	X	X	X
Training	X	X	X	X	X	X	X	X	X	X
Exercises	X	X	X	X	X	X	X	X	X	X
Public education and information	X	X	X	X	X	X	X	X	X	X
Finance administration		X	X	X	X	X		X		

Table 14.4

Means and Standard Deviations of Importance Ratings Assigned by Subject Matter Experts to Emergency Manager's Competencies

Competency	Definition	Importance Ratings	
		M	*SD*
1. Coordination skills	The ability to effectively coordinate and manage available resources and the actions of a variety of a people, organizations, and local/state entities.	4.60	.60
2. Leadership skills	The ability to guide and manage people and organizations in order to achieve a common goal.	4.50	.71
3. Decision-making skills	The ability to analyze information in order to generate and support appropriate decisions.	4.46	.66
4. Oral communication skills	The ability to effectively and clearly convey (transmit and understand) information orally	4.34	.54
5. Liaison skills	The ability to foster positive relationships among diverse groups of individuals, providing appropriate and relevant information to all concerned stakeholders.	4.31	.76
6. Job-specific knowledge	Knowledge of specific and appropriate plans, procedures, and processes associated with effective emergency management practice (e.g., mitigation planning, damage assessment, and emergency preparedness planning).	4.29	.62
7. Organizational skills	The ability to systematically organize and structure information, finding ways to classify information in multiple ways in order to aid interpretation, analysis, and presentation.	4.26	.74
8. Writing skills	The ability to effectively and clearly convey (transmit and understand) information through writing.	3.89	.87
9. Public speaking skills	The ability to present ideas and information orally to groups of individuals in an interactive fashion, responding to their requests, comments, questions, etc.	3.83	.79
10. Research skills	The ability to locate, analyze, synthesize, and use information (e.g., data and research findings).	3.51	.78

USING THE ASSESSMENT CENTER METHOD TO SELECT AND DEVELOP COMPETENT EMERGENCY MANAGERS

An assessment center (AC) is a process in which individuals have an opportunity to participate in a series of situations (such as work sample exercises, job-related scenarios, and role plays) that resemble what EMs may be called upon to do as part of their job duties. AC participants may work alone in some situations or interact with role players in others. Several trained assessors observe the individual's performance in each situation. The assessors provide an evaluation of performance based solely on their observations of participants' actions within these situations. Generally, at the conclusion of the AC the assessors present evaluations of each participant they observed to the entire group of assessors. Each assessor gives a quantitative rating on each competency and, most importantly, provides a summary of behavioral observations that justify the rating. After an open discussion, the assessors reach a group consensus on the AC participant's performance within each competency. A final numerical rating is produced along with a summary of observed behaviors within each competency across the situations. The consensus decision process ensures a fair and impartial decision for each candidate. Any individual assessor's biases can be identified and dealt with by the group.

Originally developed by AT&T researchers in the 1960s to study the validity of predictors of management progress (promotion), over the years the AC method has gained support as one of the most accurate selection and promotion tools for a variety of professional positions.[14] The AC has demonstrated significant validity for a range of managerial and non-managerial positions within both the private and public sectors.[15] The original management/leadership dimensions assessed by AT&T were defined in broad and generic terms similar to today's competencies. Interestingly, many of these original dimensions and their operational definitions became part of the subsequent ACs that were created for a range of organizations and managerial jobs.[16] The similarities in important performance dimensions (competencies) among different managerial positions within a variety of corporate settings provided additional evidence that they were indeed *core* competencies.[17]

Two critical characteristics that determine the quality of ACs and other personnel assessment instruments are reliability and validity. Reliability, defined as measurement consistency or stability, is manifested when an AC exercise is used repeatedly and produces scores that are stable, both for a participant who repeats the AC and among a number of different participants. Validity indicates the extent to which an AC accurately predicts future on-the-job performance, and therefore is useful for drawing conclusions about an individual's level of KSAOs and commensurate job performance. Overall, ACs have shown exceptional reliability and validity in predicting the future success of management candidates. Moreover, ACs have withstood legal challenges to their fairness (such as lack of bias on the basis of race, gender, etc.), and have been limited in errors due to a candidate faking his or her abilities.[18] According to Caldwell and others, AC validity "is achieved because it combines the strengths of schema-driven observations, or frame of refer ence stimuli that evaluates knowledge globally, and behavior-driven observations that track specific details about events (p. 83)."[15] Research evidence suggests that AC scores are particularly good at predicting professional advancement, even over a long period of time.[17]

ACs, and the work sample exercises upon which they are based, are one of the only means of accurately assessing required *behavioral* competencies in organization selection and evaluation systems. Work samples, defined as measures that simulate important job-related tasks,[19] generally demonstrate high validity due to their lower susceptibility to rating errors as compared to more error-prone and subjective supervisor performance ratings.[20,21] Moreover, work samples have been shown to produce positive candidate reactions regarding the method itself and reduce adverse impact. That is a disproportionate rejection rate of one subgroup (race, ethnicity, gender, etc.) of candidates in comparison with other participants.[22]

Klimoski reported three recent trends related to the science and application of the AC methodology.[17] First, much attention has been recently devoted to the process that assessors use to make accurate judgments about an individual's performance. Second, an increasing number of ACs are used for personnel development (e.g., training and certification) rather than for administrative decision-making. Examples of administrative decisions made with the help of ACs are promotions, employee selection, and placement. Third, recent uses of ACs have involved large numbers of stakeholders—assessors, candidates, and other organizational members such as executives and board members. Consequently, human resource professionals must recognize that AC administrators have to be concerned with the interpretation of the AC method by all stakeholders and that perceptions of fair treatment are not limited to only those being assessed.[23] Concerns about equal treatment, perceptions of fairness, and proper development and use of ACs to maximize reliability and validity led to the creation and subsequent revisions of the article *Guidelines and Ethical Consideration for Assessment Center Operations.*[24]

Incorporating the AC Method into Personnel Decision-Making

Assessment centers provide an important complement to traditional written testing. If carefully constructed, written tests can be a valid, yet limited measure of certain facets of job knowledge. However, knowledge tests are poor indicators of how consistently and effectively an individual can apply relevant job knowledge. The measurement of knowledge application (which requires a basic ability or refined skill) involves eliciting relevant job behaviors of a candidate and having others observe and interpret that behavior, something that is impossible with a written test. A carefully crafted and administered AC can add valid measurement of requisite skills to the selection, evaluation, or certification process of EMs. When used in combination with a written examination, an oral board, or a one-on-one interview, the AC fills the behavior measurement gap caused by the indirect measurement of the underlying KSAOs. Therefore, AC measurement can provide added validity to any EM selection or certification process.

Participant Preparation for an Assessment Center

Preparation for an AC experience is a bit different from getting ready for a written test. The International Task Force on Assessment Center Guidelines[25] provides specific instructions as to what information should be shared with candidates. In particular, individuals should be informed about the purpose of the AC, how they were selected to participate in the AC, and choices regarding nonparticipation, staff qualifications, AC documentation, and use of results, performance feedback, and procedures for accessing the AC reports.

Because the AC measures skills that an EM candidate or job incumbent has developed through many years of experience and training, the best advice to a candidate is to rely upon his or her natural behavioral tendencies. In other words, if a candidate has handled these situations before, she or he can do it again. Common tips provided to AC participants about improving their performance include the following:

- *Read and utilize all background material provided within each exercise.* These documents and descriptions have been provided because they offer important pieces of information, which may be useful in solving the problems embedded in the exercise. Sufficient time is allocated for their review, and it should be used wisely.
- *Take on the role quickly.* While the role may describe a position within an agency or community that is not exactly similar to that of the EM candidate, it is in one's best interest to accept the parameters of the role and then behave as he or she would in an EM position.

- *Use every opportunity to show what can be done as an EM.* Assessment center exercises and the situations they describe are much like a soap opera episode on television. They are designed to elicit a range of behaviors that may occur over several events that in the real world may span months or even years on the job. These events are condensed into a single exercise and the series of exercises that are completed within a few hours. Therefore, the candidate is encouraged to handle all items in the time given within each situation. The candidate should not assume there are weeks or months to do things; he or she should do them within a short time frame.
- *Relate pieces of information together.* Sometimes several exercises are linked together, as they share background information and materials. The candidate should consider that the information given in one situation might help in another, just like in a real-life EM position.
- *Keep motivated!* Assessment centers are designed to measure job-related skills in a variety of situations. While a particular situation may not provide an opportunity to display all the relevant competencies of the EM candidate, there will be opportunities to demonstrate them in other exercises. The candidate should be encouraged to keep his or her level of motivation high and consistent throughout the assessment center. At the end of the AC, the candidate will be tired but satisfied that he or she had ample opportunity to demonstrate competence.

In their discussion of AC administration errors, Caldwell and others[20] emphasized the importance of good planning, adequate job analysis, well-defined and consistently observed behavioral performance dimensions, and carefully designed AC exercises that accurately measure these performance dimensions. The authors stressed the need to pre-test exercises, to use qualified and trained assessors who could make finely differentiated judgments, to prepare AC participants, and to appropriately use AC results. Finally, they highlighted the role of specific, objective scoring and documentation in maintaining an AC's validity, which tends to erode with time unless the administrators take steps to maintain assessor training, assessor motivation, and the AC's procedural integrity.

In an effort to further illustrate good practices of AC administration and its application to personnel development for EMs, the following section describes the Professional Emergency Manager Assessment Center (PEMAC) as developed for the emergency management division of the Michigan Department of State Police.[15] While the original impetus for the AC was professional certification, its use as a selection device by municipal and county administrators was seen as equally important.

THE MICHIGAN DEPARTMENT OF STATE POLICE PROFESSIONAL EMERGENCY MANAGER ASSESSMENT CENTER (PEMAC)

Overview of the Process

The PEMAC was designed as one component of the professional emergency manager (PEM) certification process for the state of Michigan (initial implementation of portions of the PEMAC began in 2002). The PEMAC was constructed to serve as a measurement tool that identified several job-related competencies for EMs. In so doing, it was important that the process provide detailed developmental feedback for each individual candidate.

After completion of required coursework and training in emergency management, a candidate for PEM certification completes a comprehensive written examination and the PEMAC. The PEMAC places a candidate in a series of job-related exercises in which he or she is asked to complete a variety of tasks (either alone or by interacting with other emergency management professionals and citizens) and review and absorb a significant amount of relevant data and background information.

Some exercises involve trained role players who interact with the candidates. For example, a role player may provide assistance to the candidate as an administrative aide or instruct the candidate about recent emergency-related information. As the candidate progresses through each exercise, trained assessors observe and record his or her behavior. Specifically, assessors interpret and categorize the candidate's behavior within each of ten core competencies that were identified through careful job analysis of the PEM position within the state of Michigan.

Upon completion of the PEMAC, assessors rate the candidate they observed on each of the ten performance dimensions. They use a five-point rating scale, where 1 indicates "improvement necessary" and 5 is "excellent." Researchers found that AC performance dimensions, represented by performance skills or interpersonal skills, should not be too numerous because of natural limitations in assessors' information-processing abilities.[25,26] Following the AC guidelines,[25] the number of dimensions in the PEMAC was limited to ten. Spychalski and others[27] reported that a large number of organizations measured more than ten dimensions. However, this practice minimizes the consistency and accuracy of ratings and encourages global evaluations of candidates in terms of their overall performance, not competency-specific behavior.[28]

Next, the assessors meet as a group and assign a final rating for each competency for the candidate, using a consensus decision-making process. The competency ratings are numerically weighted, based on the job analysis data collected from subject matter experts, in the form of ratings that show each competency's importance in relation to success as a PEM. A total score is computed by summing the weighted scores across competencies. Each candidate receives a numerical score and a short summary of his or her performance for each of the ten competencies. A brief developmental plan is provided to outline resources available to the candidate. Specifically, academic coursework, training sessions, experience, and other resources are suggested to candidates for increasing knowledge and/or skill within competencies rated as 2 ("fair") or 1 ("improvement necessary").

Qualification and Preparation for the PEMAC

In order to qualify for participation in the PEMAC, the candidates must complete all PEM coursework, training, and experience requirements. In advance of the PEMAC, the candidates are given a short written description of the process. In addition, they are provided a written guidebook that describes the assessment center method and gives several recommendations on maximizing one's performance. The candidates complete a written PEM certification examination the same day they participate in the PEMAC.

The PEMAC Experience

The PEMAC consists of approximately four hours of exercises scheduled in two blocks, either in the morning or in the afternoon (8 a.m.–12 noon or 1–5 p.m.). A summary of each AC work sample exercise can be found in appendix 14.A at the end of the chapter. Critical components of the PEMAC include the following:

- Four interrelated exercises, completed by each candidate
- Trained role player interaction, which is a part of each exercise
- Candidate observation and performance interpretation by trained assessors
- Ratings of exercise-specific performance dimensions
- Multiple measures of each performance dimension throughout the PEMAC
- Each assessor observing each candidate at least once during the PEMAC

- Final performance dimension ratings for each candidate, determined for ten performance areas using a consensus decision-making process

PEMAC Assessors and Assessor Training

Assessors are certified PEMs, that is, they are emergency management professionals who have completed the PEM certification process in the state of Michigan. In addition, having participated as candidates, all assessors have had direct experience with each exercise. Assessor training involves a classroom review of the development of the PEMAC, a description of the PEMAC process, an analysis of the behavioral definitions of each performance dimension through classroom discussions and reviews of videotaped candidate performance, hands-on practice assessing videotaped candidate performance, and calibration of assessor ratings aimed at enhancing measurement reliability. Appendix 14.B provides an example of an assessor-recording document, indicating observed behaviors associated with specific competencies.

PEMAC Role Players and Role Player Training

Role players are staff members of the emergency management division of the Michigan Department of State Police. As such, they are familiar with the PEMs' competencies. Role player training involves such activities as a classroom review of the development of the PEMAC, a description of the PEMAC process, an analysis of the behavioral definitions of each competency through classroom discussions, and reviews of videotaped candidate performance. In addition, role players are asked to review individual roles and associated role player scripts for each PEMAC exercise. A strong emphasis is placed upon the role player providing a consistent role performance with each candidate. Each role player then practices exercise-specific roles with other role players and critiques other role players' performance.

PEMAC Performance Dimensions, Rating Scales, and Competency Weighting

Ten competencies are measured within the PEMAC (see table 14.5). Using a thorough job analysis process, these competencies were identified as important for successful PEM performance.

Table 14.5
Competencies Measured within the Professional Emergency Manager Assessment Center (PEMAC) and Their Associated Weights

Competency	Weighting
1. Coordination skills	1.5
2. Leadership skills	1.5
3. Oral communication skills	1.5
4. Liaison skills	1.5
5. Job-specific knowledge	1.5
6. Organization skills	1.5
7. Writing skills	1.0
8. Decision-making skills	1.5
9. Public speaking skills	1.0
10. Research skills	1.0

Each competency is measured at least twice within the PEMAC. Specific exercises are designed to elicit behaviors categorized within particular performance dimensions. For a grid of PEMAC exercises and targeted competencies, see table 14.6. Exercise descriptions are included as appendix 14.A.

Each competency is rated on a five-point rating scale that ranges from 1 ("improvement necessary") to 5 ("excellent"). Table 14.7 illustrates behavioral anchors for one competency, *coordination skills*, defined as the ability to effectively coordinate and manage available resources and the actions of a variety of people, organizations, and local/state entities.

Table 14.6
A Grid of PEMAC Exercises and Corresponding Competencies

Competency	Exercise			
	Mitigation/ Planning	Emergency Response	Working with Key Players	Meeting with County Commissioners
1. Coordination skills	X	–	X	–
2. Leadership skills	–	–	X	X
3. Oral communication skills	X	–	X	X
4. Liaison skills	–	X	X	X
5. Job knowledge skills	X	X	X	X
6. Organization skills	X	–	X	–
7. Writing skills	X	–	X	–
8. Decision-making skills	X	X	X	X
9. Public speaking skills	–	–	X	X
10. Research skills	X	X	X	X

Table 14.7
A Sample Rating Scale for Coordination Skills

Rating	Definition	Behavioral Anchors
1.	Improvement necessary	Candidate failed to acknowledge information, which was provided as background material identifying resources available for his/her use. Therefore, the candidate did not incorporate or utilize these resources in the solution of problems, assignment of people, and so forth. This resulted in less-than-effective problem-solving, decision-making, etc.
2.	Fair	–
3.	Good	Actions taken or proposed by the candidate indicated that he/she had adequate knowledge of all available resources for problem solution and decision-making. Pieces of the background information were carefully incorporated into the ideas, actions, solutions, and so forth taken and/or proposed by the candidate.
4.	Very good	–
5.	Excellent	Almost every action or proposal was backed up by reference to available resources. The candidate utilized almost every available resource—people, organizations, etc.—in taking action, proposing solutions, directing others, and so forth. The candidate clearly absorbed all background material within the exercise.

Competency weighting is useful, as the PEMAC scoring may become part of a compensatory certification model. In contrast to a noncompensatory model that requires a candidate to reach a minimally acceptable level on *each* competency in order to be certified (referred to as multiple cutoffs or hurdles), a compensatory model is one in which a low score on one competency can be compensated for by a high score in another.[29] In PEMAC's compensatory model, ratings are summed or averaged across the ten competencies, and a candidate is required to achieve a specific total score for the PEMAC as a whole. According to *Principles for the Validation and Use of Personnel Selection Procedures*, whereas both compensatory and noncompensatory models may be used for personnel decision-making, they may have unequal reliability and lead to different decisions regarding candidate selection and/or certification.[30] Because PEM certification is a voluntary process, a compensatory model was chosen initially for the PEMAC. That is, it is not required for an EM in the state of Michigan to complete the PEMAC to enter or retain his/her position. The compensatory model creates a developmental atmosphere in which candidate improvement is emphasized. The PEM board of the state of Michigan has decided that after several years of PEMAC data collection, it may be possible to move toward a noncompensatory, multiple cutoff competency mode.

The weight assigned for each competency is shown in table 14.5. The dimension weights are based on subject matter expert ratings ($n = 35$) of the perceived importance of the competency in predicting success as a PEM. The range of possible weighted total scores, summed across the ten performance dimensions, is 13.5 (low) to 67.5 (high). The passing score for certification as a PEM is 40.5, which corresponds to a weighted average of 3 in each performance dimension. If a candidate scores below this level, he or she can repeat the PEMAC until a passing grade is attained. The passing grade is used for developmental purposes (accreditation); however, it can be equally useful for making personnel selection decisions and conducting performance evaluations.

REPORTING OF CANDIDATE SCORES AND FEEDBACK IN THE PROFESSIONAL EMERGENCY MANAGER ASSESSMENT CENTER

Each candidate receives a report, which provides a numerical rating in each of the ten competencies. A short summary describes the candidate's performance within each competency across exercises. A listing of development activities (e.g., coursework, experiences, and seminars) is provided for those performance areas rated as "improvement necessary." Appendix 14.C presents a sample candidate report.

SUMMARY AND RECOMMENDATIONS

This chapter highlighted the critical competencies for effective performance as an emergency manager (EM). In our review of these competencies, we emphasize the important role the EM plays in preparing for and responding to potential terrorist attacks and civic emergencies of all kinds. Many behaviors critical to EM success are hard to observe and measure. Therefore, a carefully crafted and systematically executed study of the EM's position is needed in order to accurately identify and measure the EM's core competencies. Job analysis is the key to the design of effective and legally defensible systems for selecting and developing EMs. Typically, a proper job analysis will involve data collection and analysis from a variety of individuals, ranging from job incumbents to subject matter experts to industrial/organizational psychologists.

A review of several competency models for EMs concludes that the majority of these models are too broad and vague to be useful to the design of human resource management systems such as selection, accreditation, and performance evaluation. To overcome this problem, we provide a framework of ten behaviorally defined core competencies for the EM position. Identified through a comprehensive review of published studies and an analysis of critical incidents, the core competencies incorporate observable (and therefore measurable) aspects of the EM position and reflect actual job tasks described by subject matter experts. The assessment center method can be used as an accurate means of selecting, developing, and evaluating EMs' performance. The Professional Emergency Manager Assessment Center (PEMAC), as designed by the emergency management division of the Michigan Department of State Police,[15] provides a concrete example of an appropriate application of the assessment center (AC) method to the evaluation of EMs' competencies.

The AC's predictive value will be compromised if it is not properly designed and administered. Of particular concern is the accuracy of observation and measurement of EMs' critical competencies. Therefore, it is important that those charged with the selection, training, development, and evaluation of EMs follow these recommendations:

1. Competencies should be identified through the use of systematic job analysis techniques. Whenever possible, job incumbents (practicing EMs) should be involved in providing job analysis data. Appropriate measures, such as work sample exercises, organized within a comprehensive assessment center should be used to generate accurate behavioral descriptions of EMs' performance within each competency. More traditional measures such as written tests and interviews should be used as only one component in the EM selection or evaluation process. Written tests and interviews are very limited in their measurement of behavioral competencies.
2. High reliability and validity of AC measurement of EM competencies is only possible if trained assessors are used in the process. Experienced EMs should be included in the assessor pool. All assessors must complete training that addresses techniques of systematically observing and recording relevant candidate behaviors, the potential bias of common rating errors, how the work sample exercises and assessment center were developed (e.g., the job analysis methodology and resulting KSAOs identified for the position), behavioral definitions of the competencies to be assessed, and how to prepare candidate reports.
3. ACs should measure each competency in at least two ways—using at least two different work sample exercises.

4. Exercises should provide job-related scenarios that incorporate typical emergency management tasks, as opposed to generic management situations. This strategy is likely to increase candidates' motivation to perform and to enhance job relatedness of the AC exercises.

5. Each candidate should be aware of the purpose and nature of the AC. If possible, candidates should be informed as to what to expect from the work sample exercises, how the AC results will be used, and whether they are able to repeat the AC if their performance is below standard. Candidates can be referred to background literature and books to provide assistance in their preparation for the AC.

APPENDIX 14.A: PEMAC EXERCISE DESCRIPTIONS

1. Mitigation/Planning exercise

This exercise presents the candidate with a variety of written documents, memos, reports, and forms. The candidate must read and organize significant amounts of background material to identify the important elements of the relationship among emergency response units in the county, available resources, potential for future growth, and past successes and failures in emergency management. The candidate is required to develop a county plan for the mitigation and planning activities so as to ensure readiness for possible emergency situations.

2. Emergency response exercise

The purpose of this exercise is to present the candidate with a real-time emergency situation. The candidate is provided pieces of information orally and in written form through an administrative assistant as an emergency situation unfolds. The candidate is expected to formulate quick decisions as to actions and react appropriately to each piece of new information. Along with responsiveness, the candidate must provide ongoing debriefings with the media, who may challenge his decisions and remind the candidate of past successes and failures in the county.

3. Working with key players

The candidate must meet with fire, law enforcement, and public works officials and handle an ensuing group interaction that becomes fairly heated. The candidate is instructed to implement a plan for coordinating these critical elements should an emergency situation arise. Key players bring with them a unique perspective as to their roles in an emergency response and demonstrate a strong desire to maintain control over their resources.

4. **Meeting with county commissioners**

The candidate must explain the role of a professional emergency manager to elected county officials who, through their positions, control important resources of emergency management (budget, staffing, etc.). Therefore, the candidate must inform and persuade, at the same time working toward a goal of building support from these commissioners (for example, a local business leader and human services provider). Each commissioner has a specific platform upon which his or her constituency is based and uses that to provide a narrow perspective about emergency management responsiveness.

APPENDIX 14.B: SAMPLE ASSESSOR RATING DOCUMENT FOR THE "WORKING WITH KEY PLAYERS" EXERCISE

Candidate: [Candidate's name]
Assessor: [Assessor's name]   Date:

Rating scale for a "working with key players" exercise:

1	2	3	4	5
Needs improvement	Fair	Good	Very Good	Excellent

I. Coordination skills: The ability to effectively coordinate and manage available resources and the actions of a variety of people, organizations, and local/state entities.
Rating: 4
Comments:

* Candidate stressed working together.
* Candidate made reference to incident command structure as a model for coordination.
* Candidate knew his role as an emergency manager.

II. Leadership skills: The ability to guide and manage people and organizations in order to achieve a common goal.
Rating: 4
Comments:

* Candidate interjected between role players, kept control of the meeting.

- Used "team emphasis" to assert control.
- Candidate clearly expressed a goal for the meeting and continued until goal (that is, stated agreement to cooperate from key players) was met.

III. Oral communication skills: The ability to effectively and clearly convey (transmit and understand) information orally.

Rating: 4

Comments:

- Candidate provided a cordial greeting of others and stated the purpose of the meeting.
- Oral presentation was smooth.
- Clear, concise commentary, with a direct style of delivery.
- Eye contact and body posture were positive and effective.

IV. Liaison skills: The ability to foster positive relationships among diverse groups of individuals, providing appropriate and relevant information to all concerned stakeholders.

Rating: 4

Comments:

- Candidate acknowledged the expertise of others (role players): "might be the same plan you had."
- Highlighted the necessity of good communication among departments.
- Offered his services, such as a detailed call list.

V. Job-specific knowledge: Knowledge of specific and appropriate plans, procedures, and processes associated with effective emergency management practice (mitigation planning, damage assessment, emergency preparedness planning, etc.).

Rating: 5

Comments:

- Reacted to all pieces of information contained in the exercise:
- Outlined areas of interest on the maps.
- Provided appropriate points to raise during the meeting, based on the exercise needs.

VI. Organization skills: The ability to systematically organize and structure information, and finding ways to classify information in multiple ways in order to aid interpretation, analysis, and presentation.

Rating: 5
Comments:

- Used written outline to organize materials and presentation to key players.
- Followed written outline during presentation to key players to make sure he covered all the important areas.
- Referred to outline to guide discussion.
- Candidate frequently pointed to areas highlighted on overheads to emphasize main points of his discussion and for impact.

VII. Writing skills: The ability to effectively and clearly convey (transmit and understand) information through writing.
Rating: 4
Comments:

- Written outlines used for presentation purposes were clear and detailed.
- Candidate recorded notes regarding background information, which were used in meetings with subordinates and others.
- When reaching decisions, the candidate clearly demonstrated an understanding of the written background material by citing specific facts and figures, referring to particular geographic locations on maps, and so forth.
- Written plans for mitigation and preparatory exercises were clearly written at a level commensurate with staff understanding.

VIII. Decision-making skills: The ability to analyze information in order to generate and support appropriate decisions.
Rating: 4
Comments:

- Written materials created by the candidate indicated coverage of all background material.
- The candidate turned the action plan development back to the fire department when challenged.

IX. Public speaking skills: The ability to present ideas and information orally to groups of individuals in an interactive fashion, responding to their requests, comments, questions, and so forth.

Rating: 4
Comments:

- Candidate provided structure to the presentation.
- Control of the presentation was maintained in spite of role player arguments.
- Candidate style was direct and controlling, yet open to the input of others.

X. Research skills: The ability to locate, analyze, synthesize, and use information (data, research findings, etc.).
Rating: 4
Comments:

- Decisions in exercises indicated that the candidate understood the background materials as they were based on the facts presented.
- The candidate cited specific background data in oral presentations and written work.
- When questioned by others, the candidate was able to quickly reference the relevant background material and use it to further explain his decision.
- In each exercise, relevant background information was physically grouped together and summarized as the basis for the decision at hand.

APPENDIX 14.C: A SAMPLE PEMAC CANDIDATE REPORT

Candidate report for: [Candidate's name]
This report contains brief, yet detailed information on the candidate's performance as seen by assessors across all PEMAC exercises.

For the PEMAC evaluations, the candidate has been given a final rating for each performance area based on a consensus judgment among all assessors who evaluated that candidate. This final rating is based on the sum of relevant behaviors exhibited by the candidate through performance in all PEMAC exercises.

In providing the ratings, the following scale is used:

5 – Excellent
4 – Very good
3 – Good
2 – Fair
1 – Improvement necessary

For each performance area, a quantitative rating using this scale is shown accompanied by a description of candidate behaviors that supports and documents the consensus rating. These descriptions are based on the recorded observations of the assessors across PEMAC exercises.

The information contained in this report should be considered CONFIDENTIAL and treated in a manner consistent with personnel information-reporting guidelines and standard operating procedures.

This information has been designed for use in emergency manager certification decisions. The sponsoring agency (county, township, municipality, etc.) bears the responsibility of using the candidate information contained within this report in a nondiscriminatory, job-related, ethical manner. To maximize the utility of the PEMAC information, it is highly recommended that candidates receive detailed feedback from the agency regarding their performance in the PEMAC. The agency is further encouraged to provide appropriate training or development opportunities for candidate improvement in performance areas designated as "improvement necessary."

I. Coordination skills: The ability to effectively coordinate and manage available resources and the actions of a variety of people, organizations, and local/state entities.

Rating: 4

Observations:

Whenever needed, the candidate identified a variety of other agencies, key players, and contact options so that coordination of services could occur. The information to be collected from each agency was clearly identified and used effectively when available. In developing plans and solutions to problems, it was clear that the candidate understood the necessity of having agencies prepared in advance to interact with one another effectively under emergency conditions.

II. Leadership skills: The ability to guide and manage people and organizations in order to achieve a common goal.

Rating: 4

Observations:

When working with others, the candidate was quick to take charge of the situation by outlining his plan of action and then explaining important background facts, the situation at hand, etc. While he was fairly directive in his approach to guiding others, his guidance was based on information he possessed through research and planning using the background materials. When needed, the candidate used interpersonal persuasive techniques, such as acknowledging the power of various local government officials, in an attempt to build a positive working relationship.

III. Oral communication skills: The ability to effectively and clearly convey (transmit and understand) information orally.
Rating: 3
Observations:
The candidate was very clear when speaking with others, and the information he wished to emphasize was easily identified. Eye contact, voice inflection, and body posture added to the impact of his oral presentations. While the candidate listened to others, at times he was not able to incorporate their comments into his own statements or reflect back that they were heard and understood.

IV. Liaison skills: The ability to foster positive relationships among diverse groups of individuals, providing appropriate and relevant information to all concerned stakeholders.
Rating: 4
Observations:
The candidate was quick to identify and reflect the understanding of the importance of building positive relationships with other agencies, key players, and so forth. He often stated the political necessity of building strong relationships with local officials and others who were integral parts of any effective emergency management system. The candidate knew the various important stakeholder groups for an emergency manager and knew how to keep them informed so that they would work together in a cooperative fashion.

V. Job-specific knowledge: Knowledge of specific and appropriate plans, procedures, and processes associated with effective emergency management practice (mitigation planning, damage assessment, emergency preparedness planning, etc.).
Rating: 5
Observations:
The candidate impressed role players with his comprehensive understanding of the background material and the decisions he made. In each scenario the candidate identified the important pieces of information, and every agency and affiliated action that he could take was stated either orally or in writing. Each scenario was handled by applying appropriate emergency management procedures.

VI. Organization skills: The ability to systematically organize and structure information, and finding ways to classify information in multiple ways in order to aid interpretation, analysis, and presentation.

Rating: 4

Observations:

When faced with a large amount of written background information, the candidate was able to organize the information in a manner that facilitated his and others' understanding. The organization of materials assisted in the candidate's ability to convey important pieces of information to others. Whenever needed, actual and potential problems were identified and appropriate action plans were constructed. The candidate easily prioritized the important pieces of information and handled each in turn.

VII. Writing skills: The ability to effectively and clearly convey (transmit and understand) information through writing.

Rating: 3

Observations:

The candidate provided brief yet clear written commentary, directions, and so forth when required to do so. At times, however, the candidate's written directions were somewhat lacking in detail. This lack of detail may lead to confusion or questioning down the road. All required information was provided in writing for each scenario, especially in mitigation/planning. He clearly identified important features and areas on maps, tables, figures, and so forth to increase the clarity of his presentations and thereby make them easier to understand. When needed, the candidate used written outlines to summarize and assist in presenting data and his ideas (plans, actions, etc.) to others.

VIII. Decision-making skills: The ability to analyze information in order to generate and support appropriate decisions.

Rating: 4

Observations:

When faced with a problem situation, the candidate always provided an appropriate decision. The candidate was forceful and direct in communicating decisions to others. At times, however, it seemed as though he could have given more detail in providing background or a rationale for his decisions. Nevertheless, the candidate's decisions were well accepted by others.

IX. Public speaking skills: The ability to present ideas and information orally to groups of individuals in an interactive fashion, responding to their requests, comments, questions, and so forth.

Rating: 3

Observations:

At times the candidate was fairly abrupt and overly direct in his demeanor when working with role players. While there was no doubt that he was going to control the situation, the abruptness could be interpreted as the candidate attempting to be overbearing. In most exercises, the candidate presented a clear outline of his intentions as a means of starting the interaction. He generally provided only basic information to others and was somewhat hesitant to field questions or add clarification.

X. Research skills: The ability to locate, analyze, synthesize, and use information (data, research, findings, etc.).

Rating: 4

Observations:

The candidate knew which pieces of background information were most appropriate to formulating a plan of action and/or response within each scenario. He was able to identify where to gather needed information from the background materials, as well as data and other facts that he would have liked to have, but were not part of the exercise. The candidate used significant detail within each exercise so that his responses were well supported by available facts, findings, and so forth.

NOTES

1. Harvey RJ. Job analysis. In: Dunnette MD, Hough LM, editors. Handbook of industrial and organizational psychology. 2nd ed. vol. 2. Palo Alto, CA: Consulting Psychologists Press; 1991. p. 71–163.

2. Muchinsky PM. Psychology applied to work. 7th ed. Belmont, CA: Wadsworth/Thomson Learning; 2003.

3. Robertson IT, Smith M. Personnel selection. J Occ and Org Psych 2001;74:441–72.

4. Gatewood RD, Field HS. Human resource selection. Mason, OH: South-Western; 2001.

5. Ash RA. Job elements for task clusters: arguments for using multi-methodological approaches to job analysis and a demonstration of their utility. Pub Personnel Manag 1982;11:80–90.

6. Levine EL, Ash RA, Hall H, Sistrunk F. Evaluation of job analysis methods by experienced job analysts. Acad Manag J 1983;26:339–47.

7. Morgeson FP, Campion MA. Social and cognitive sources of potential inaccuracy in job analysis. J Appl Psych 1997;82:819–27.

8. Emergency Management Division, Michigan Department of State Police. Emergency services management. Lansing, MI: Author; 2000.

9. National Coordinating Council on Emergency Management. Emergency program manager: knowledges, skills, and abilities. Falls Church, VA: Author; 1999. Information in tables is adapted from the National Coordinating Council on Emergency Management.

10. Region V Advisory Committee for Training and Development, Federal Emergency Management Administration. Emergency Management Training and Development Survey Summary Report. Washington, DC: Author; 2000. Information in table is adapted from the FEMA Region V Advisory Committee for Training and Development Survey Summary Report.

11. Love KG, Holland S, Linton L, Wolcott-Burnam S. An assessment center for the evaluation of emergency program managers: development, pilot testing, and assessor training/calibration. Lansing, MI: Michigan Department of State Police, Emergency Management Division; 2001.

12. Bownas DA, Bernardin HJ. Critical incident technique. In: Gael S, editor. The job analysis handbook for business, industry, and government. New York: Wiley; 1988.

13. Flanagan JC. The critical incident technique. Psych Bul 1954;51:327–58.

14. Jaffee CL, Sefcik JT. What is an assessment center? Personnel Administrator 1980 Feb;25:40–3.

15. Caldwell C, Thornton GC III, Gruys ML. Ten classic assessment center errors: challenges to selection validity. Pub Personnel Manag 2003;32:73–88.

16. Shippmann JS, Hughes GL, Prien EP. The use of structured multidomain job analysis for the construction of assessment center methods and procedures. J Bus and Psych 1987;1:353–66.

17. Jansen PG, Stoop BA. The dynamics of assessment center validity: results of a 7-year study. J Appl Psych 2001;86:741–53.

18. Klimoski RJ, Brickner M. Why do assessment centers work? The puzzle of assessment center validity. Personnel Psych 1987;40:243–60.

19. Schmidt FL, Hunter JE, Outerbridge AN. Impact of job experience and ability on job knowledge, work sample performance, and supervisory ratings of job performance. J Appl Psych 1986;71:432–40.

20. Hunter JE, Hunter RF. Validity and utility of alternative predictors of job performance. Psych Bull 1984;96:72–98.

21. Reilly RR, Israelski EW. Development and validation of minicourses in the telecommunication industry. J Appl Psych 1988;73:721–7.

22. Robertson IT, Kandola RS. Work sample tests: validity, adverse impact and applicant reaction. J Occup Psych 1982;55:171–84.

23. Caldwell C, Gruys ML, Thornton GC III. Public safety assessment centers: a steward's perspective. Pub Personnel Manag 2003;32:229–49.

24. International Task Force on Assessment Center Guidelines. Guidelines and ethical considerations for assessment center operations: international task force on assessment center guidelines. Pub Personnel Manag 2000;29(3): 315–31.

25. Gaugler BB, Thornton GC III. Number of assessment center dimensions as a determinant of assessor accuracy. J Appl Psych 1989;74:611–8.

26. Sagie A, Magnezie R. Assessor type, number of distinguishable dimension categories, and assessment center construct validity. J Occup and Org Psych 1997;70:103–8.

27. Spychalski AC, Quinones MA, Gaugler BB, Pohley K. A survey of assessment center practices in the United States. Personnel Psych 1997;50: 71–90.

28. Sackett PR, Tuzinski KA. The role of dimensions and exercises in assessment center judgments. In: London M, editor. How people evaluate others in organizations. Mahwah, NJ: Erlbaum; 2001 p. 111–34.

29. Society for Industrial and Organizational Psychology, Inc. Principles for the validation and use of personnel selection procedures. 4th ed. Bowling Green, OH: Author; 2003.

30. Sackett PR, Roth L. Multi-stage selection strategies: a Monte Carlo investigation of effects on performance and minority hiring. Personnel Psych 1996;49:549–72.

15 Public Health Ethics, Business, and Terrorism

Irene O'Boyle and Michele Simms

With the events of September 11, 2001, a dramatic and immediate shift in focus on terrorism forced the role of public health into the spotlight. Although terrorism is an international and globalization concern, and it portends broad environmental consequences, medical emergencies will fall "first and hardest" on local communities.[1] For the local healthcare systems, clinical ethical dilemmas have already and are increasingly shifting to the institutional/systemic level. The additional response to terrorism now required by these systems raises issues of how public health will define their role and function to "conduct themselves in an ethical manner that emphasizes a basic community service orientation and justifies the public's trust."[2] How do we view health in the context of terrorism and biotechnology? Are there assumptions that we have a strong public health infrastructure? Can we redefine business in this role? What is the ethical relevance of emergent new epidemics and ecological threats worldwide?[3]

This chapter examines the role of public health in understanding the threat of terrorism and warfare in the context of international and global concerns while also requiring an ethical response locally and from the community, of which the business enterprise is a part. The chapter posits that a continued focus on the basics of the public health infrastructure—community assessment, policy development, and assurance—will form and inform the "new" ethics of sustainability, human rights, and community health and practice. The chapter concludes with implications and suggested roles for public health institutions.

BACKGROUND

The events of the recent past influence and guide public health decision-making. The relationships among medicine, public health, ethics, and human rights are evolving in response to a series of events, including political, economic, and social experiences. Human rights thinking and actions, closely aligned to public health and human rights-related roles and responsibilities for healthcare professionals, are receiving increased attention.

Recent public health trends include substantial growth in organized healthcare delivery systems, including managed care organizations, increasingly "purchaser driven" healthcare services, an aging population, rapid changes in technology, emerging new infectious diseases and re-emerging old ones, a shift from infectious/communicable diseases to chronic disease, increased importance of behavioral risk factors and impact on community health, a decline in the percentage of healthcare expenditures dedicated to public health core services, low levels of trust in public institutions, and the growing importance of community involvement and collaboration activities.

Public health ethics maintains a population-based perspective whose function is to understand disease from a group or community perspective. The goal then becomes to measure and improve the health status of these populations. This perspective views the "patient" as the whole community or population, in contrast to the medical model, which views and treats a "patient" as an individual. The public health methodological approach results from this perspective, with focus on the epidemiology and etiology of health and disease in communities.[3]

The population-based focus leads some to assert that public health is paternalistic (that is, it relies on state and government involvement to promote community health and safety). "Yet the ethical disputes in public health are far more extensive than the debates over paternalism would suggest. What is the nature of the population? Of the community? Does the community share a common good? Who bears the burdens of prevention?" (p. 23).[3] Raising such questions is at the core of how public health continues to assess and gain role clarity and illuminates the future in medical ethics, of which the public's health is a part.

ROLE CLARITY: HOW DO WE VIEW HEALTH IN THE CONTEXT OF BIOTECHNOLOGY AND TERRORISM?

As an integrative and interdisciplinary field, public health is based on principles of social justice. It encompasses biology, environment, lifestyle, and health service organization. Justice is a dynamic concept that relates the allocation of one's fair share of collective burdens and benefits. Social justice maintains that social class distinctions, heredity, racism, and ethnicity often preclude fair distribution of these benefits in society.[4] It is the philosophy of social justice that provides a firm foundation to public health and attracts practitioners who believe they can "make a difference" by contributing to the health and welfare of communities.

"Health" is tied to population-based prevention and the three core functions of assessment, policy development, and assurance.[5] Assessment aims at detecting and analyzing emerging trends in infectious and noninfectious disease and environmental hazards. Policy development focuses on primary prevention for target populations. Assurance focuses on community capacity to prevent disease and injury, with much of the public health funding for these services as categorical and linked to clinical services.[6] Within these core functions, the Centers for Disease Control and Prevention (CDC) has identified basic public health practices integral to the operation of state and local health agencies, with the core functions as the foundation for prevention, surveillance, and intervention.[7]

The biggest advances in public health in the last century were interventions primarily focused on sanitation and hygiene: clean food, clean water, and immunizations, which are concerns at the forefront of sustainability. Public health efforts also helped expand health and life expectancy in the United States from forty-seven years in 1900 to seventy-eight years in 1995.[7] The field has contributed to the quality of life within a managed care system, yet less than 1 percent of the prevention money is used for programs that impact public health. Therefore, one of today's major challenges for health leaders is to bring together the perspectives and resources of the medical care industry, the population-based public health sector, and the community to develop community-based health systems that work.[8]

This challenge is compounded when considering the overwhelming advances in biomedicine, with the 1990s introducing 148,000 patents as part of the mapping and sequencing of the human genome. Advances in biotechnology, such as prenatal genetic testing, new reproductive technologies, and DNA data banks, displace the less-provocative public and social issues of gun control, immunization, employee leave programs to assist care for dying relatives, emergency room use as primary care sites by the uninsured, and medical care for the homeless.[9] Further, the very advances in biotechnology make possible the reality of terrorism.[10] Due to the urgency that terrorism poses, preventive medicine, social medicine, and the core competencies of public health concerns receive less, if any, attention.

What if public health were to go beyond these core functions, mobilize communities, and act as a "catalyst" or community facilitator/architect for healthier communities—an effort that would truly impact the overall health of communities? An assessment by the Institute of Medicine in 1988 highlights the need to improve essential public health functions. The IOM proposal includes monitoring efforts to achieve the national health objective to "increase to at least 90 percent the proportion of people who are served by a local health department that is effectively carrying out the core functions of public health."[11] This would include some technological linkages to state and local health departments, ongoing workforce training, and an integrated reporting surveillance system that included environmental indicators. Key to this three-pronged approach is that it ensures commitment to core competencies while providing a mechanism for public health response to advances in biotechnology and the shifting focus the geopolitical realities of terrorism bring.

PUBLIC HEALTH AND 9/11

The public health focus shifted with the events of September 11.[12] One result is greater communication and new partnerships between public health personnel and emergency responders. While the nation's public health system is better prepared to respond to a terrorist attack than it was a year ago, the system is still behind in areas such as training, coordination, and education, according to a report card released in September 2002 by the American Public Health Association (APHA). The year's successes included a reinforced public health infrastructure, expanded public health laboratories, improved surveillance, and strengthened communication.[13] The report highlights strides made in increased funding for readiness and programs aimed at responding to emergencies. Yet, the report also states that public health is behind in a number of areas such as regional coordination of response activities, education and training for public health professionals, protection of food and water supplies, and ensuring the safety of chemical plants.

Many advocates, however, are concerned that terrorism may overshadow and siphon funding from the broader mission of protecting and improving the public's health. This shift in priorities has been especially apparent at the CDC, with preparedness funding shifting to the states.

Because of these efforts, state agencies have increased laboratory capacity, instituted new training and procedures, recruited new personnel, and strengthened surveillance. CDC Director Julie Gerberding states, "We are building terrorism capacity on the foundation of public health, but we are also using new investments in terrorism to strengthen the public health foundation—and these two programs are inextricably linked, and I think both will benefit from the efforts and the investments we intend to make on an ongoing basis."[14]

Despite the potential conflict between building terrorism capacity and strengthening public health foundations, the question remains: who should shoulder the burden of caring for the sick and dying following a major terrorist attack, when the public health infrastructure is already suffering from personnel shortages and financial woes? Knowing that successful prevention efforts have an effect on lower utilization of healthcare services, there is a way to conceptualize and present prevention services and their outcomes that reinforces their value in a managed care environment. This moves from a "needs assessment" mentality to an outcomes mentality. This transition takes time as organizations learn from each other. Knowing that successful community prevention efforts have an effect on lower utilization of healthcare services, it is possible that community prevention efforts and their outcomes are presented in a way that reinforces their value in a managed care environment. This is seen as blending a "needs assessment" mentality with a mentality that addresses the management of access, utilization, cost, and quality.[13]

Developing a model for reinforcing prevention and health promotion in a managed care environment can be a vision. This vision includes high-quality, cost-effective healthcare that focuses on prevention and wellness and results in the highest level of health possible for all residents. The mission includes development and implementation strategies through a community-based process to prevent physical and mental health problems and promote the optimum physical and mental health for each person in our community. The goal of this model would be to develop and present a view of community prevention services (as distinct from clinical prevention services) and their outcomes in a way that underscores their value in a managed care environment. Below are some key tenets of this model:

- *Beyond traditional customer definition*: Traditionally managed care organizations have focused their attention on the enrolled membership of their plans, while healthcare providers have focused on their patients

when defining the constituency or customer group. This model broad-
ens the customer or member base to include the community at large.
• *Beyond traditional clinical prevention services*: This model further expands
  the range of activities to be addressed through prevention efforts to
  include primary and secondary prevention efforts, community prevention efforts targeted at substance abuse, teen pregnancy, community
  and domestic violence, tobacco use, family dysfunction, and environmental health.

These efforts go beyond the clinical prevention efforts outlined
in HEDIS[15] and those traditionally pursued by managed care organizations and public health departments, including reduction in
incidence of low-birth-weight infants, vaccinations, mammography,
screenings for cervical cancer and cholesterol, prenatal care, and
retina examinations for persons with diabetes. This model calls for
collaboration of public and private (for-profit and nonprofit) sectors
in integrating these community prevention efforts into managed
care plans operating within communities. The public partners would
be local health departments and community mental health boards.
The private partners would include managed care organizations/
health maintenance organizations, traditional indemnity insurers,
and employers.[16]

This model is based on seven assumptions. First, as society reduces
public funding for community prevention, the health-related needs
that initiated those efforts still remain. Second, community prevention
efforts have not been an integral part of managed care plans, given the
view that they do not "pay off" for managed care organization (MCO)
in the immediate reduction in the expenditure of acute care dollars,
given that membership has churned through the MCO fairly rapidly.
Third, a maturing managed care environment (both physical and
behavioral health), will result in care management plans that cover
stable and large populations of enrolled members (with less churning
of membership). A fourth assumption examines a stable and broad
enrolled membership base. The healthcare costs borne by payers
(managed care organizations and employers) will be impacted by a
wide range of factors traditionally not addressed by private and public
payers, factors that are community-wide in scope. Fifth, to control
costs associated with these factors in the moderate and long term,
healthcare plans will need to incorporate community prevention efforts
into a comprehensive managed care approach. The sixth assumption
is that those parties with significant and long-standing expertise in

addressing these issues are the local public health and community health boards. Finally, bringing players into the healthcare community to understand the need for community prevention efforts and the value of its integration into a managed care system is as important to health promotion as are both traditional clinical prevention efforts and acute care.[17]

This view of leadership understands that "community" is a powerful force. Healthy communities can be created. The most important factor in building and strengthening healthy communities is "community visioning": the process of effectively stating what we, as a community, really want to be. The sign of strengthened community is that its citizens have made choices as to what they realistically want to be.[18] Leadership that incorporates community includes working within the organizational or system boundaries and distinctly contrasts traditional, romantic views of leaders as isolated, often enigmatic, idiosyncratic heroes. Leadership will result in revising the meanings given to preventive health, comprehensive managed care plans, and the work of local public and mental health departments.

Understanding policy in the context of managed care illuminates how public health/mental health systems must evolve from an integration of the dynamics of government, community, provider, and consumer and agency relationships while keeping core values.[16] Defining what those core values are is the task of those in public health today. The field is served well to consider these cross-sector relationships as part of a public health response to terrorism that is built upon the foundation of core competencies. Further challenges for public health officials include balancing the goals of promoting and protecting public health while protecting against human rights violations.[3] The ethical dimensions of public health practice become of great significance as public health seeks to "ensure the conditions in which people can be healthy," and "as those conditions are societal, to be engaged in public health necessarily involves a commitment to societal transformation."[19]

When assessing human rights and dignity, the questions of ethics naturally ensue. For example, public health is expected to respond to difficult issues, like HIV/AIDS, even when no cure is yet available, while also being expected to respond to its call to not abandon vulnerable populations. Beauchamp and Steinbock[3] note that the current approach of public health will require major changes in public health reflection, analysis, action, and education in order to engage the major health challenges of today's globalized world.

PUBLIC HEALTH AND WORKFORCE CHALLENGES

Historically, public health focused on containing communicable diseases (plague, smallpox, etc.). Today, public health concentrates on chronic disease, yet has limited training and skills to prepare the public health workforce to concentrate on biological agents and toxins that terrorize populations. Some of these health threats have been recognized for years as potential threats yet not addressed due to the strain on the public health system.[20]

The Institute of Medicine and Centers for Disease Control and Prevention detail new challenges for the next decade. These include moving back to science as the basis of public health policy. The goal is to stimulate state and local governments to review the organization, delivery, payments, and evaluation of health services in order to create a healthier population. Current public health efforts identify priorities of acquiring funds for health promotion and health education, negotiating state and federal cuts in health promotion and health education other than those earmarked for terrorism, developing partnerships in today's dynamic healthcare environment, and addressing mandates for future health initiatives, which range from immunizations to terrorism.

In the assessment role, public health concentrates on monitoring trends, economics, and demography. Recently, public health has initiated practice scenarios for various conditions (such as terrorism), producing community "report cards," and acting as a clearinghouse for health information (informatics). The advocacy role is accomplished by working with diverse populations to assess present challenges in preventive healthcare services through social marketing and acting as experts by policy makers in interpreting policies. In this role, public health continues to be sensitive to social, cultural, economic, and political influences. The assurance role is aimed at developing, initiating, and implementing programs and services through collaborative efforts with business, church, and the community in which it serves. "To effectively create the future, mastering the process of anticipatory thinking is vital. Anticipatory thinking is the process of using scanning and what-if scenarios to anticipate the future conditions that may exist. But the anticipatory thinking process must also be inclusive and involve a significant amount of grassroots input" (p. 20).[21]

Recent insight into what is called "the tipping point" offers an additional way to monitor the environment. The Tipping Point is that magic moment when an idea, trend or social behavior crosses a threshold, tips and spreads like wildfire. Just as a single sick person can start an epidemic of the flu, so, too, can a small but precisely targeted push cause a fashion trend, the popularity of a new product, or a drop in the crime rate. This is changing the way people throughout the world think about selling products and disseminating ideas.[22] A tipping point framework provides a way to understand phenomena ranging from the emergence of fashion trends to the rise of teenage smoking and suicides. This phenomenon is based on epidemiology principles that ideas and behaviors spread just like viruses do.[23] This is relevant to the practice of public health as an idea and a product, and also public understanding of its role.

A survey conducted by Kathleen Phalen[23] called "Public Health: A Victim of Its Own Success?" found that 57 percent of respondents could not define public health. A study by the Harvard School of Public Health called "Survey Shows Americans Not Panicking over Anthrax"[24] indicated that local community sources considered reliable in disseminating information in the event of a health and/or terrorist outbreak were fire departments (61 percent), police departments (53 percent), health departments (52 percent), and one's own physician (77 percent).

Accordingly, "the public health workforce lacks adequate training to ensure the protection of the public's health."[25] This may be attributed to the changing workforce:[26]

1. The existing workforce is aging.
2. Fewer people are joining the public health professions.
3. The role of the public health workforce is changing.
4. More work than staff means that some employees are not getting paid for all their work.
5. There are large turnovers due to nurse shortages.
6. Significant amounts of time and money are spent on training staff.
7. Hiring nurses without experience or bachelors' degrees increases training costs.

According to CDC and Health Resources and Services Administration (HRSA) data, as much as 80 percent of the public health workforce is without formal, academic training in public health, although this may not reflect practice expertise. This does suggest, however, a clear need to maintain a consistent level of performance among all public health workers nationwide.

One way this need is being met is through funding from the Health Alert Network as part of terrorism emergency funding from Congress.

Initial start-up monies are expected to serve all states on a continuing basis. Four areas of support include:

- Replacing of outdated IT equipment in local health departments.
- Linking local and state public health jurisdictions, community partners, and federal health organizations via the Internet, resulting in high-speed, full-time connections.
- Providing ongoing workforce training in information management and technology.
- Integrating reporting and electronic surveillance systems that include environmental health surveillance.[25]

This effort strengthens the public health infrastructure by incorporating the three areas of organizational capacity, workforce development, and information technology, each area being addressed in the Healthy People 2010 Objectives for Improving Health. "In fact, Healthy People 2010 for the first time includes an entire chapter on 'Public Health Infrastructure' (Chapter 23) that should be given consideration."[25]

This challenging public health workforce parallels and signals formidable public health challenges. "Whether preparing for terrorism or preparing for emerging and resurging infectious diseases, it is not always possible to know when and where an event may occur. The challenge is to be adequately prepared for the unimaginable at all times, in all places."[27] Infectious disease has no boundary of race, ethnicity, or socioeconomic status and continues as a common cause of death and suffering with great burden on society.

Despite advances in the control of some diseases with the advent of antibiotics and vaccines, new diseases—such as SARS—are constantly appearing. At the same time, infections like tuberculosis and bacterial pneumonias are now resistant to drug treatments. "As our world grows ever more connected, public health must change and adapt to meet our new challenges. [The] CDC's systems to detect and diminish harm are our nation's safety net. By preparing for the worst, we make America's response to ongoing health threats, infectious and chronic diseases, injuries, environmental exposure to toxins and others more comprehensive and effective."[27] It is the interconnected world that expands public health into areas of national safety and security as part of its public health agenda.

PUBLIC HEALTH AND NATIONAL INTERESTS

National questions of safety, security, health, and human rights propelled President Bush's initiative to shift some of the nation's public health responsibilities to the Department of Homeland Security (DHS). This has met with concern from some public health experts, who worry that the plan will compromise the nation's overall public health system.[28] Under the Bush plan, the security, protection, and emergency response activities of the Centers for Disease Control and Prevention, The Department of Health and Human Services, and the Health Resources and Services Administration are one department. Many public health experts express concern that this will hinder overall effectiveness of a broad-based public health system. This is especially true given that the DHS was created to respond directly to terrorist activity and threatens to take resources from other public health activities/threats.

Senator Henry Waxman (D-California) testified at a hearing of the House Energy and Commerce Committee's Oversight and Investigations Subcommittee on June 25, 2002, stating, "If we attempt to protect ourselves at the expense of our nation's public health system, we may find that we have undermined, rather than enhanced, our nation's true security."[29] Under this proposal, the function is moved out of the Department of Health and Human Services into a new department in the Bush cabinet that includes oversight of pharmaceutical stockpiles, medical supplies, transfer of dangerous pathogens and toxins, and the Office of Public Health Emergency Preparedness, created in 2001. The concern is that removing certain public health activities from the Department of Health and Human Services could disrupt public health activities and investigations, which depend on the same communications structure, resources, and infrastructure. Accordingly, the American Public Health Association opposes transfer of public health program management, research, and funding to the new department.[28] Despite the creation of the DHS, many public health departments, organizations, and universities across the country continue to use public health competencies to help strengthen their workforce and programs. The core competencies for public health professionals, developed by the Council on Linkages between Academia and Public Health Practice,[30] outline the skills, knowledge, and attitudes required to carry out and improve the practice of public health. These competencies are built around ten essential public health services, which include monitoring health status, investigating health problems, and enforcing regulations and laws. They blend theory and practice and create a consistent protocol by clearly identifying what skills and abilities professionals need, a practice that itself supports sustainable development. There is wide buy-in that focus on core competencies is necessary for workforce development and is being used at the local levels as a standard that health department staffs must meet in leadership and cultural awareness.[31]

Focus is also placed on the three factors of agent, host, and environment, which directly affect the public's health. Public health officials need to ask: how does this complex system interact with health promotion/ prevention activities to protect the ability to react to disease, the environment, and the community? Successful protection of the public's health includes efforts at interrupting this agent, host, and environment cycle— the fundamentals of public health—while protecting the quality of life.

The deliberate attention to the agent-host-environment cycle best serves the public health role in addressing terrorism, as well. Secretary of Health and Human Services Tommy Thompson sent letters to governors in all states,[32] detailing how much each state would receive of the $1.1 billion in appropriated acts intended to develop comprehensive terrorism preparedness plans, upgrade infectious disease surveillance and investigation, enhance the readiness of hospital systems to deal with large numbers of casualties, expand public laboratory and communication capacities, and improve the connectivity between hospitals and local and state health departments to enhance disease reporting. The secretary reported that the money was sent to states and local communities to build strong public health systems for responding to terrorism attacks. "These funds are just the start of our efforts to help states and communities build up their core public health capabilities. We must do everything we can to ensure that America's ability to deal with terrorism is as strong as possible."[32] The expected outcomes include improved preparedness to respond to public health emergencies, including those resulting from terrorist actions by hospitals and emergency medical service (EMS) systems; assessment and capacity upgrades for hospitals and medical control authorities that involve training, equipment, surveillance, medical supply, or communications upgrades; and multitiered systems to triage, isolate, treat, stabilize, and refer multiple casualties of a terrorist incident. These outcomes will coordinate and communicate responses from public health, law enforcement, and emergency management resources in the event of a terrorist attack.

This shifting burden on public health comes at a time of a declining health status within a fragile public health system. The Future of Public Health Committee,[20] a bipartisan multi-issue coalition in Michigan, recommends in part:

- Rebuilding public health capacity for surveillance, assessment, investigation, and policymaking at the state and local levels.

- Applying public health science in selecting, designing, and implementing public health policies and programs.
- Building partnerships that mobilize talents of community-based organizations, business, academia, managed care, healthcare providers, and other stakeholders into powerful coalitions that can approach our complex health issues from every angle.
- Initiating science-based, multi-sectored efforts to close the gap between the healthiest and least-healthy population groups.
- Integrating public health and managed care to maximize synergies in addressing disease prevention and health promotion.
- Aligning the public health functions within state government under a structure for accountable performance.

The Committee further states that strengthening Michigan's public health system requires a three-pronged approach to planning that actively involves (1) local communities, (2) emphasis on prevention of illness and accidents, and (3) a statewide infrastructure able to track and monitor progress at every level. This approach may well serve as a national model as well.

Implications: Public Health, Sustainability, and the Role of Partnering

Responding to the myriad of challenges in the age of terrorism requires developing innovative partnerships among business, international and local human rights groups, labor unions, religious institutions, and charitable foundations. This trend of cross-sector partnering recognizes community health in its broadest dimension: creating webs of relationships among individuals, communities, and the environment that are tied to sustainable development practices.[33] Business involvement is vital to the success and impact of many community health initiatives. Engaging business in such activities is challenging, and most community health development efforts lack effective partnerships with local businesses. A recent survey by Project Access, a national initiative to assist local communities in developing and sustaining efforts that promote universal healthcare access, reported that only 25 percent of community coalitions had businesses involved in their community efforts. The Institute of Medicine's recent study of improving community health through performance monitoring[5] finds that most communities have limited experience with collaborative efforts among the diverse mix of stakeholders that make up community health.[34]

Engaging business in community health efforts requires a rethinking of the role that market forces have traditionally played in determining what constitutes healthy communities in the first place. What is the proper balance between the cultural or moral spheres and the public's health, knowing that how we answer that question shapes any future response?[33] Beauchamp and Steinbock[3] continue to raise relevant questions that drive a new ethic:

> What are the boundaries and limits for free discussion and speech, and for the public's health? These topics require consideration of not just what each individual deserves and needs but of what will help whole communities hold together and what will encourage people to consider themselves a community given to powerful forces on health policy from abortion to national health reform that tend to pull a community apart. (p. ix)

At a time of emerging new epidemics and international ecological threats, the focus shifts not only to who is responsible for prevention but to whether healthcare becomes a common good tied to community efforts.

As public health strives to promote those conditions that keep communities healthy, and as those conditions are societal, the work of public health quite naturally involves a commitment to societal transformation.[19] Business faces an equal charge of creating sustainable environments linked to social transformation that ensures quality of life now and for future generations. The triple bottom line, broadening accountability to include economic, environmental, and social impacts,[35] is the cornerstone of a sustainable future.

This focus on sustainability manifests trends in business toward human rights practices and healthy society perspectives that create long-term benefits.[33] Just as public health is moving away from the biomedical language of death, disease, and disability to one of well-being and health related to underlying societal conditions, so, too, is business acknowledging its relationship and responsibility to society. With the interdependencies and ramifications of environmentalism and globalization tied to sustainable development and clearly related to public health practice as well, new business models are emerging. Examples include how disease and the environment affect economies, biocentric and eco-model approaches, nongovernmental organizations (NGOs), and corporate humanism.[36-41] There is an "inextricable link with promoting and protecting health" (p. 89),[19] and business has a role to play.

What emerges across the disciplines of public health and business are universal themes of sustainability and sustainable development, the common good, community health and healthy societies, the ensuing progression to human rights practices, and personal responsibility. The business community can partner with public health and thus shape the cross-industry/cross-discipline dialogue on terrorism and health, strengthen the roles of public health and business in society, educate biotechnology industry leaders on the range of values questions generated by the times, and ensure public health and business ethics as core practices.[33]

CONCLUSION

What does this mean for institutions in the business of health? Eight areas are provided as ways to reinforce public health's role as a leader in "communities of concern."[42] Health institutions, both public and private, must

1. Commit to a more holistic view of the inter-rational impact of factors that influence health outcomes at both individual and community levels.
2. Work to establish genuine relationships with communities built on mutual respect and an appreciation for community strengths and needs.
3. Learn how to be involved in community activities that may not appear to have a direct impact on their point of interest, but are identified as community priorities (issues of safety, housing, crime, etc.).
4. Engage in empowerment and capacity-building of communities as an integral part of any community planning health education and health research.
5. Allocate resources directly to communities to address health issues. Herein lies a role for business in resource procurement.
6. Learn how to serve as technical advisors and provide leadership when requested by the community.
7. Establish trusted relationships and mechanisms for decision-making with the community long before the grant application process and/or implementing actions that create unnecessary conflict.
8. Provide education and training to BOTH health providers and communities on topics of empowerment, conflict resolution, negotiation, and consensus-building.

What does this require of public health leadership? In order to develop new solutions to both population-based and community health problems, with terrorism and national security as part of their agenda, the public health leaders of tomorrow will be required to unite and work with multicultural groups. These leaders need to embody a visionary leadership style that inspires and motivates others and, in the process, seeks new solutions, culminating in a sense of shared ownership. Public health is a complex field requiring organizations, especially public health departments, to create partnerships and collaborations that maximize capacities and resources of all stakeholders, of which the business enterprise is a part, to improve community health.[9]

NOTES

1. U.S. Department of Health and Human Services Factsheet. 2001 Aug 16. Available from: www.hhs.gov. Accessed August 10, 2003.

2. American Hospital Association. Management advisory ethical conduct for healthcare institutions. 2001. Available from: www.aha.org. Accessed August 10, 2002.

3. Beauchamp DE, Steinbock B. New ethics in public's health. Oxford, UK: Oxford University Press; 1999.

4. Turncock BJ. Public health: what it is and how it works. Frederick, MD: Aspen Publishers; 1997.

5. Institute of Medicine. The future of public health. Washington, DC: National Academy Press; 1988.

6. Berkowitz B. Health system reform: a blueprint for the future of public health in Washington state. Lead in Pub Health 1994 Fall;3:11–5.

7. CDC forecasts top ten challenges of 21st century. Medical letter on the CDC and FDA. 2000 Oct 22.

8. Bloom B. The future of public health. Harv Pub Health Rev. 2000 Fall. Available from: www.hsph.harvard.edu/review/review_2000/specialfoph.html. Accessed February 4, 2004.

9. Woltring CS, Barlas C. Journey to leadership: profiles of women leaders in public health. Seattle, WA: Artists-Writers Publishing; 2001.

10. Turner L. Bioethics, public health, and firearm-related violence: missing links between bioethics and public health. J Law, Med and Eth 1997;25(1):42–8.

11. Simms M. On linking bioethics, bioterrorism and business ethics. J Bus Eth [special edition]. 2003 (in press).

12. Public Health Service. Healthy people 2000: National health promotion and disease prevention objectives—full report, with commentary. DHHS publication no. (PHS) 91-50212. Washington, DC: U.S. Department of Health and Human Services, Public Health Service; 1991.

13. American Public Health Association. One year later: public health system improved overall. Nation's Health Series 2002 Oct.

14. American Public Health Association. Principles for a public health response to terrorism. Presented at the 129th Annual Conference; 2001 Nov; Atlanta, GA.

15. Mientka M. West Nile a gauge for CDC's bioterrorism response. U.S. Medicine. 2002 Oct. Available from: www.usmedicine.com/article.cfm?article ID=514&issueID=43. Accessed February 3, 2004.

16. O'Boyle I, Glandon R, Sheehan R, St. Germain J. Providing prevention through a public-private partnership. Document prepared for Michigan Community Health Leadership Institute. 1997 Aug 12.

17. Three frameworks that provide more systematic accounts of community benefits that managed care might produce include the following: community health emphasizes roles/responsibilities that inform practice and performances; a healthy community paradigm emphasizes sociology and epidemiology factors that affect populations; and market failures based on economic model emphasize harm and benefit for communities not enrolled in managed care. Tasks needed to increase community benefits include establishing more accountability by measuring HMOs' activities, the need of state and federal agencies to develop criteria similar to HEDIS for health promotion, and incorporating concerns into public health policies. See Schlesinger M. Trends in public health and inconsistencies. 1998.

18. Bargen D. Community visioning and leadership. J Leadership Stud 1996;3(3)135–62.

19. Mann J. Medicine and public health, ethics and human rights. Hastings Center Rep 1997 May/June:6–13.

20. Future of Public Health Committee. The health of the public in Michigan: a vision for the twenty-first century. 2002 Sep. Available from: www.mipha.org/futurepubhlth.pdf. Accessed February 3, 2004.

21. Barlow ED. Preparing for the future through anticipatory thinking. Forum 2001 Jan/Feb;85(1):20.

22. Gladwell M. The tipping point: how little things can make a big difference. Boston: Back Bay Books. Little, Brown and Company; 2000.

23. Phalen K. Public health: a victim of its own success? Amednews 2002 Dec 31. Available from: www.ama-assn.org. Accessed February 3, 2004.

24. Blendon RJ, Benson JM, DesRoches CM, Herrmann MJ. Survey shows Americans not panicking over anthrax: but starting to take steps to protect themselves against possible bioterrorist attacks [press release]. Harv Sch Pub Health 2001 Nov 8.

25. Milne T. Institute of Medicine testimony to the Health Committee on Assuring the Health of the Public in the 21st Century. Washington, DC; 2001 Feb 8. Available from: www.naccho.org. Accessed February 4, 2004.

26. Minnesota Department of Health, State CHS Advisory Committee, Healthcare Workers. A shortage revisited: employment outlook for the future of the healthcare industry. Minn Ec Trends 2003 Apr. Available from: www.mnworkforcecenter.org/lmi/pdfs/healthapril2003.pdf. Accessed February 3, 2004.

27. Centers for Disease Control and Prevention. The state of the CDC, fiscal year 2003: challenges in preventing new and old threats. Available from: www.cdc.gov/od/oc/media/. Accessed February 4, 2004.

28. American Public Health Association. Homeland department plan may undermine public health. Nation's Health Series 2002 Aug.

29. Waxman H. Subcommittee on Oversight and Investigations of Committee on Energy and Commerce, U.S. House of Representatives. Creating the Department of Homeland Security: consideration of the administration's proposal. 107th Congressional House hearings from the U.S. Government Printing Office. DOC ID: f:80680.wais. 2002 June 25.

30. Public Health Foundation. Council on linkages between academia and public health practices. Available from: www.phf.org/Link.htm. Accessed February 4, 2004.

31. American Public Health Association. Nation's Health Series 2002 Sep.

32. Thompson T. Secretary Thompson to release $100 million to assist states with smallpox vaccination programs [press release]. U.S. Department of Health and Human Services. 2003 May 5. Available from: www.hhs.gov/news/press/2003pres/20030505a.html. Accessed on February 3, 2004.

33. Simms M. Trends in corporate social responsibility. A broader vision for managed care, Part 1: measuring the benefit to communities. 2003 May/June;17(3).

34. Britt M, Sharda C. The business interest in a community's health. 2000.

35. Whiting M, Bennett C. The road to sustainability: business' first steps. New York: The Conference Board; 2001.

36. Mele D. A humanistic framework of the corporation of the 21st century. Paper presented at the Center for Business Ethics, University of St. Thomas; 2002; Houston, TX.

37. Simms M. Catholic insight on workplace human rights and corporate humanism. In: Miller PJ, Fossey R, editors. Mapping the Catholic cultural landscape. Lanham, MD: Sheed & Ward; 2004. p. 217–29.

38. Mele D, Sison A. Corporations and the social contract: a reply to Professor Thomas Donaldson. Barcelona, Spain: IESE Publishing, University of Navarra; 1993.

39. Hoffman M. Business and environmental ethics. In: Heath E, editor. Morality and the markets: ethics and virtue in the conduct of business. New York: McGraw-Hill; 2002. p. 667–73.

40. Panayoutou T. Globalization and environment. CID working paper no. 53. 2000 July. Available from: www.cid.harvard.edu. Accessed July 10, 2001.

41. Elkington J. The chrysalis economy: how citizen CEOs and corporations can fuse values and value creation. Oxford, UK: Capstone; 2001.

42. McManus P. Incorporating other voices: facilitating the dialectic between traditional epidemiologic measures of health and the contextual concerns of the community. In: A dialogue between private and community partners. Presentation at Community Health 2000; 1998 Oct 9; Wayne State University, Detroit, MI.

16 Bioterrorism, Medical Readiness, and Distributed Simulation Training of First Responders

Dag K. J. E. von Lubitz and Marvis J. Lary

BIOTERRORISM AND MEDICAL READINESS

The alleged threat represented by the Iraqi weapons of mass destruction (WMD) was the principal cause of the "Third Gulf War" (Operation Iraqi Freedom). While the actual presence of WMD in Iraq is now the subject of intense debate, and the veracity of the original intelligence data and their interpretation increasingly doubtful, the threat posed by WMD in the hands of terrorist organizations remains as real as ever.[1] Worldwide destabilization caused by regional conflicts is, unquestionably, the most significant factor that amplifies the plausibility of employing WMD in acts of national and international terror.[2,3] Among the considerable range of "tools" available on the legal and illegal international markets, the biological agents are the most readily accessible and, at the same time, potentially most devastating form of weaponry suitable for terrorist action. Easily manufactured, concealed, and transported across borders, biological agents can be disseminated among the unsuspecting target population with minimal difficulties. Incubation periods of days to weeks allow the perpetrators sufficient time to escape immediate capture, and the virulence of many of the pathogens suitable for bioterrorist use may lead to massive casualties.[4,5] Importantly, in addition to the immediate consequences of the bioterrorist acts, their long-term and indirect health and economic effects present a continuously unexplored challenge.[6]

Despite the events of September 11, 2001, U.S. plans of defense against biological and other forms of terrorism remain in disarray,[7-9] even if billions of dollars continue to be spent on the improvement of readiness against a likely attack.[10-12] With singular exceptions (such as Israel),[13,14] similar lack of coordination of effort can be found among other nations that may be potential targets.[15-17] Not surprisingly, efforts at national and international levels are made to address these deficiencies.[18-28] The results of studies performed as part of these efforts show persistent concern in the areas affected by the anthrax outbreak in 2001, and indicate substantial fear and confusion (particularly among media personnel)[29] indicating, at the same time, reliance on the advice from family physicians if another outbreak of an infectious disease occurred.[30] Other studies show substantial deficiencies in national and international triage systems that would be used following mass-casualty events.[31-36] All reports consistently stress two essential elements among the measures proposed as responses to the ever-growing threat of bioterrorism—the needs for education and continuous training.[37-52]

Unquestionably, the strongest rationale for establishing training to address preparedness against bioterrorist assault rests on the fact that, despite unceasing efforts to change the current status quo, America is essentially still unprepared either for bioterrorism or any other large-scale public health emergency.[53-59] A study conducted in 2002 showed that in the United States alone, the number of civilian public health professionals (physicians, nurses, physician assistants), who constitute the first line of defense against bioterrorism, reached 448,254.[58] An additional 3 million personnel provide relevant medical support (emergency medical technicians, police, firefighters, etc.). Hence, it is an alarming fact that 70 percent of responders to a recent survey[60] indicated they would be unable to help victims of chemical or biological terrorism. Clearly, a bioterrorist attack against the United States may have devastating consequences.[61]

INCREASING DEMAND FOR MEDICAL TRAINING

The past fifty years have witnessed the most explosive growth of medical knowledge in the history of medicine. This growth has imposed dramatic changes on the practice of healthcare.[62,63] Unsurprisingly, the issue of lifelong medical learning rose to unprecedented prominence. It also intensified exploration of the means to improve efficiency of medical education and postgraduate training that often involve very sophisticated technologies.[64-66] Yet, while most advanced training is routinely practiced at the major medical training centers,[67-69] the access to even relatively simple continuous medical education (CME) is often difficult in rural and remote regions of the globe.[70-73] Isolation, inadequate funds, inconsistent quality of training programs, and variation in the allocation of training resources have been often described as the principal issues that need to be addressed to produce measurable changes.[74]

The emergence of new medical threats such as bioterrorism introduced a new challenge to educate the large numbers of pre-hospital and emergency room personnel needed to ensure a maximum level of readiness.[75-78] Medical professionals who typically do not participate in EMS operations may have an active role in interventions following an act of bioterrorism.[78] This clearly indicates that the required training must account for the existing differences in the baseline knowledge. Moreover, the required training programs must be highly standardized and conducted at a consistently high-quality level if they are to develop and sustain adequate preparedness against emerging threats of bioterrorism or mass casualty events.[79-84] In summary, even a perfunctory review of the existing literature clearly indicates the persistent and rapidly growing need for continuous education and training of both pre- and in-hospital personnel,[85-87] and also the significant role of federal, state, local, and non-governmental agencies in developing robust tools and systems that will be sufficient to provide both continuous and "just in time" medical training.[88-90]

FIRST RESPONDERS AND CURRENT TRAINING DEFICIENCIES

Changes in medical practice, increasing specialization, and multi- or cross-disciplinary approaches to the treatment of disease[91-98] require a very wide range of sophisticated postgraduate education programs at both pre- and in-hospital levels of medical operations. Problems ranging from communication and definition of professional identities and roles within the medical management team,[99-102] through procedure difficulties,[102-104] missed or wrong diagnoses,[105-108] to errors in medical command of EMS operations or even fundamental inadequacies in training of pre-hospital and in-hospital healthcare providers have been described in a large number of publications.[106,109-114] One unifying trend that emerges from those studies is inadequate training of non-specialist healthcare workers in adult and pediatric emergency and trauma medicine[113-123] and also in surgery.[124-128] This is particularly pronounced in rural and remote regions worldwide.

Clinical and procedural errors resulting from training deficiencies at the first responder/paramedic level[129,130] are as common as those at the higher echelons of care providers, and pose similar major concerns. The adverse effects of less-than-optimal teamwork that is caused by poor team training,[131] substandard mastery of essential (even basic) diagnostic skills and resuscitation procedures,[132-136] and unreliability in the delivery of commonly encountered services such as advanced cardiac life support[137] have been well documented. Even more problematic are the substantial inadequacies in pediatric resuscitation skills resulting from both inadequate initial training and infrequent refresher education that combine with a relatively rare exposure to pediatric emergencies.[138-141] The intense need for continuous education and training is emphasized even more strongly by the recently reported lack of reliability in performance rating during EMT licensing examinations[142]—a failure that allows operational entry of personnel with less-than-optimal knowledge and skills. Cumulatively, the inadequate entry-level preparation combined with the demonstrated skills decay[140,141,143] are not only the sources of major concerns, but argue further for vigorously maintaining clinical competence through life-long learning by all healthcare professionals.[144-153]

Trivial in comparison to the often life-and-death repercussions of medical errors, the expenditure that accompanies each incident of faulty patient management constitutes another significant motive for sustained training of medical personnel. It is estimated that the average cost of a resuscitation attempt varies between $3,000 and $10,000, depending on whether it started as an in-hospital or pre-hospital event.[154-156] Clearly, any error resulting in a serious aggravation of the presenting complaint will automatically increase the final cost of care by making it more complex and more resource demanding.[157] Thus, while the argument "I am certified" may still be heard, the wealth of existing data on errors indicates that the presence of certification alone may offer very false security in one's own medical prowess. The real cost of such (possibly unwarranted) certitude may indeed be quite extreme both in the medical outcomes and in the expenditure.

TRADITIONAL TRAINING PATTERNS

Presently, medical education at all levels of expertise is conducted in a manner that, despite a host of advances in technology, has not changed significantly during the recorded history of medicine. Training of healthcare professionals is conducted either as a totally passive assimilation of the existing body of knowledge, such as through books[158,159] or lectures,[160-162] or through an active, bedside-based approach. The latter may involve either the combination of passive and active methods or the hands-on methods alone.[162-164] Significantly, while it is often claimed that electronic dissemination of medical knowledge provides "interactivity," many existing platforms represent nothing but technologically advanced forms of traditional (essentially passive) training based on traditional didactic principles.[165-167] The primary advantage of information technology in the didactic e-training packages rests with the ease of access to the appropriate sources of latest information, rapid cross-referencing of information and the supporting data, and the ability to organize information derived from various resources into easily catalogued logical units that assist in assimilation and solidification/retention of the acquired knowledge.

Rapid growth of Internet connectivity in the technologically advanced countries is associated with the most important attribute of electronic healthcare knowledge dissemination: erosion of distance as the main obstacle in accessing postgraduate professional education among healthcare personnel in rural and remote regions of the world. The existing Internet/web-based medical training and/or consultation programs cover a wide range of topics, satisfy almost every need for specialized knowledge, and, with the increasing sophistication of the existing protocols, may involve a large variety of approaches spanning from e-mail exchange to videoconferencing and multimedia offerings.[168-180] The main disadvantage of didactic distance learning is its essentially static nature, which fails to reflect the dynamism of medical specialties such as emergency/trauma medicine, military medicine, and surgery.[181] The existence of inaccurate, obsolete, or incomplete content of many medical information sites provides another major problem that affects the overall quality of many Internet-based learning resources.[182,183]

Hands-on training based on the trainee-patient contact, while highly effective in developing the necessary clinical skills,[184,185] is associated with a number of challenges[186-190] and risks.[191] Facing equally daunting issues of hands-on training, the aviation community (where both training and operations are associated with many characteristics similar to the high-paced tempo of medical specialties such as emergency medicine, trauma medicine, and perioperative care) in the past eighty years used simulation devices both to increase the efficiency of training and to minimize associated dangers.[192-195] Although the history of simulation in medicine is significantly shorter, both its role in education and training and its level of sophistication increase very rapidly.[196-200] Presently, high fidelity patient simulators (or HFPS, previously known as human patient simulators) serve as highly complex "medical flight simulators" in a wide variety of training tasks. The use of HFPS units in hands-on training eliminates all risk factors of similar training on living patients, permits improvement of diagnostic skills by allowing practical understanding of the involved steps, hones interactions of medical teams, and promotes punishment-free learning based on one's own errors.[201-207] Training based on or in virtual reality environments[181,207-210] is technologically the most sophisticated level of medical simulation and has proven to be particularly suitable in surgery and emergency medicine.[182,211]

SIMULATION TRAINING—GOOD BUT INACCESSIBLE

A rapidly increasing number of publications describe preeminent applicability of medical simulation in training of healthcare personnel in a variety of medical specialties.[212-223] However, in the majority of cases, studies of simulation efficacy were performed in large training institutions that could easily supply the required significant fiscal resources for acquiring the simulation equipment, and these institutions could provide both the space and personnel necessary for successfully operating a simulation center.[224,225] Not surprisingly, then, the target audience of simulation-based training consists typically of students and residents associated with the institution that already has its own simulation center, that is, the trainees who are also exposed to the essentially maximal concentration of the traditional educational resources. In contrast, both pre- and in-hospital healthcare professionals, particularly in rural and remote regions, are largely excluded from the benefits of simulation-based training predominantly conducted at the large academic medical education centers. The cost of attending and of the training itself, the ease of accessing the training site, and the difficulty in fitting training into professional schedules appear to be the predominant obstacles.[181] Thus, it is paradoxical that the economical and logistics issues may prevent simulation technology from reaching the audiences where it may have a far greater impact than at the established centers of medical learning.

Simulation-Based Distributed Medical Training

In our previous publications,[226-230] we extensively discussed the need for simulation-based training of medical personnel and the problems associated with such training. Despite its obvious advantages in simultaneous and uniform training of large numbers of students, the combination of advanced distributed learning and simulation imposes challenges. In order to circumvent these obstacles, we developed and operationally tested a series of models for distributed simulation-based training targeted at widely dispersed, large numbers of medical personnel. The models are based on the concept of Med-ASP[231] combining the principles of distributed interactive simulation[232] and the application service provider (ASP). Practical implementation of the Med-ASP concept permits effective access to and utilization of a sophisticated, central simulation facility by remote learners, who may be separated from the facility by several thousand miles.[227-229] The Med-ASP concept is associated with several other attributes: (1) dissemination of highly realistic, interactive training aimed at a large number of learners performed in the complex and stress-filled environment that effectively prepares for the challenges of field emergency and trauma medicine; (2) independence from the geographical distribution of multiple learner groups;[230,233] and (3) suitability for real-time, wide-area dissemination of world-class medical training expertise in the form of practical "patient demonstrations" rather than the commonly encountered didactic format of a theoretical lecture.[231,232] As a result, pre-hospital and in-hospital personnel in rural and remote regions with demonstrated difficulties in accessing arguably the most sophisticated form of medical learning can now derive measurable training benefits based on an easy access to advanced training technology and expertise, and on the customized teaching/training services that may be provided whenever these are required. Significantly, the demonstrated value of simulation-based distance training[226,228,229] is also of a special importance for EMS and military healthcare providers, particularly in situations of increased need for "just in time" training of a large number of personnel deployed to several geographically dispersed sites[226,227,233] seen during chemical/biological terrorism or warfare threats, military conflicts, or large-scale rescue operations (figure 16.1).[234-237]

Simulation Platforms

Medical accuracy based on physiological versatility, relatively accurate modeling of the relevant aspects of human anatomy, sophistication of a broad range of the incorporated pharmacological responses, and the relative programming ease make high-fidelity patient simulators (HFPS) excellent for education and training.[215-217] Advanced HFPS units faithfully reproduce the majority of sounds and signs relevant to field and emergency

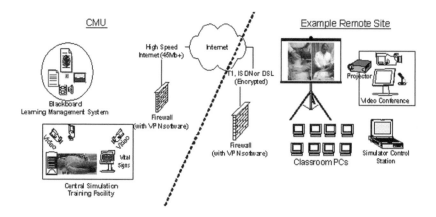

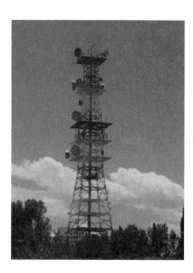
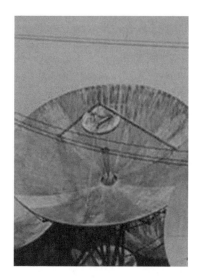

Figure 16.1

A diagram of the principles involved in distance-based simulation training
(upper photograph). Simulators, together with the expert trainer, are located
at the central simulation facility. Their view, simulator-generated vital signs,
diagnostic data, and all other pertinent information are transmitted to the
trainees at the remote site. The imagery and all data are transmitted using
any available telecommunication platforms (wireless, ISDN lines, or, on a
few occasions, POTS). The trainees have full control of the simulators from
their site, a facility that allows them remote execution of several procedures
(establishment of airway, placement of IV lines, administration of drugs,
defibrillation, etc.). During each training session, the trainees are presented
with a completely unknown case. Their task is to stabilize the patient,
perform initial diagnosis, initiate treatment, and make decisions on the

room diagnosis, stabilization, and initial treatment.[238] Moreover, all vital signs can be monitored either on the screen of a monitor (either brand-name or an emulated version) or assessed directly through the physical interaction with the simulator. Finally, the most sophisticated HFPS units permit execution of several often-complex resuscitation and field stabilization procedures, such as noninvasive or surgical insertion of a wide range of airway maintenance devices, establishment of intravenous (IV) access and infusion of IV fluids, placement of catheters, placement of chest tubes, pericardiocenthesis, and so forth. Also, the machines can be defibrillated using standard defibrillating devices (including AEDs) and defibrillation procedures and cardiac pacing. Both manual procedures and drug treatment are accompanied by appropriate physiological responses. Hence, incorrect or delayed intervention may result in complications or a fatal outcome. The medical veracity of HFPS exposes the student to all aspects of a clinical encounter with a severely ill patient who demands immediate response based on intellectual and technical resources available to the trainee.

Multi-Platform Environments

When several dispersed HFPS units are controlled from a central training facility or accessed by the remote learners, the only means to ensure uniformity of training is to make it independent of both physical and operational characteristics of the simulation devices. This is particularly important when the training center has the overriding remote control of all distributed HPFS units, or when it serves as the "expertise center"[228,239] during simultaneous training of large numbers of learners isolated by geographical distances, for example, in multi-simulator training of dispersed medical intervention teams (just-in-time preparation for mass casualties caused by the acts of terrorism, natural disasters, etc.).[230,233,235]

Figure 16.1 (continued)

subsequent management (e.g., discharge, transfer to ICU, surgery). Errors in management may result in a fatal outcome (and often do)—a valid and sobering training element. At the end of the exercise, the scenario is debriefed by the expert instructor, mistakes are discussed, and the scenario is then repeated with the trainees following a clinically correct approach. During each training period, cosmetically disguised scenarios (changed circumstances, modified age or sex of the victim, etc.) are rerun in order to consolidate the retention of the knowledge acquired by the trainees.

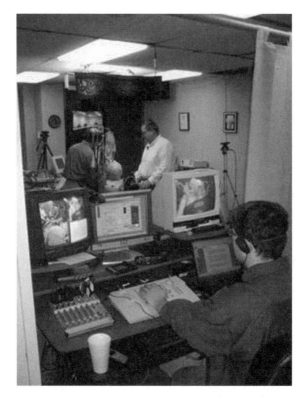

Figure 16.2
The central simulation facility in Ann Arbor, Michigan (MedSMART).
Two expert instructors (an emergency medicine physician and a paramedic)
provide training in trauma management to the Italian group of family
practitioners and medical students (photograph above). The engineer in the
foreground has full control of the simulators, visualization, and data transmission at both sites. The photograph on the opposite page shows one of
the world's most advanced control rooms at the Herbert H. and Grace A.
Dow College of Health Professions at Central Michigan University (CMU).
The engineers at CMU can provide real-time dissemination of the training
session in progress to any location in the United States or overseas. The
CMU facility is also capable of video recording and converting the training
sessions into widely accessible Web-based, on-demand training resources.

While the two principal HFPS systems in existence (Laerdal and
METI) have practically identical anatomical features and generate very
similar profiles of training-relevant output, the conceptual basis of
their software/hardware interaction differs significantly. As a result of
these differences, combining both systems into a unified, remotely

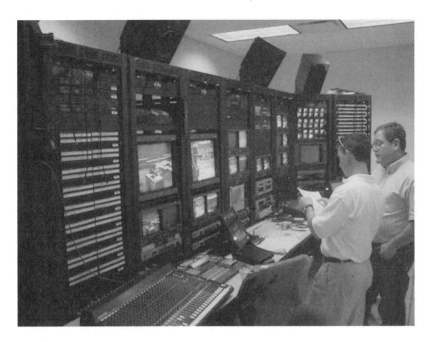

accessible training environment poses practical difficulties. In the simplest setting of multiple simulators produced by the same manufacturer, all devices can be easily slaved to the same high-speed CPU/high-RAM control computer located at the central training facility, allowing simultaneous or individual remote operation of the federated HFPS units (figure 16.2). However, simultaneous remote control of dispersed, collaborating simulators built by different manufacturers is severely impeded due to software incompatibility of the machines. From the medical point of view, voice commands given by the remote trainee to the personnel at the simulator host site (e.g., the central training facility) are the most realistic solution to this problem: the procedure approximates the routine approach of medical team personnel during real-life activities. The use of separate computers dedicated solely to the control of the identical brand federation of HFPS units provides another simple solution. Yet, it must be also remembered that in a fast-paced environment of a multi-patient scenario, such control, particularly if remotely executed by the trainees with little or no background in computer operations, may become very cumbersome. Consequently, trainees' attention may rapidly shift from the main subject (medical training) to the frantic attempts at mastering unfamiliar technology that will, in turn, significantly erode the realism of and deteriorate the effectiveness of training. Simulator-bridging software that automatically translates commands given from the control interface of one system into the commands that are understood by the simulator of a different and otherwise incompatible brand is the most effective solution. It is also technically the most complex since, in the absence of commercially available products; the software bridge must be developed as a private venture of the competent staff at the user's facility. It becomes readily apparent that, from the technical and fiscal points of view, the most suitable placement of the software bridge is at the central (hub) control facility at which all signal processing takes place. In summary, implementation of the ASP concept simplifies signal traffic and, by providing its more effective processing, results in the elimination of the annoying time lags that may render distance-based simulation training exceedingly unrealistic. The Med-ASP concept assures that only the meaningful commands are passed within the simulator federation and also that exchange occurs at the maximum speed allowed by the available bandwidth. The concept has been implemented and validated during pilot multi-simulator training conducted at one of the U.S. military facilities during which both Laerdal and METI units were used.[230,233]

Visualization

The most essential aspect of simulation-based distance training is visualization (figure 16.3). Both the quality of the image and the field of vision at the remote site must be identical to the direct view at the simulator site. Even if endowed with pan/tilt/zoom capacity, single-view cameras do not offer such capability. Hence, multiple camera systems under remote control from the central operating station must be used. Moreover, the controlling system must be capable of both independent and simultaneous operation of any and all onsite and remote cameras, a highly complex operation that can be facilitated by the use of the commercially available multi-camera control systems. Albeit the use of such systems is unquestionably the most practical solution, it is also the most expensive, technologically demanding, and requires expert staff for operation and maintenance. Bandwidth erosion allows only a specific number of the remote sites to be served by a single set (assembly) of cameras. When limited image transmission resources such as typical videoconferencing systems are available, a single camera set (typically consisting of three units giving lateral and overhead views) can provide optimum service to a maximum of three or four sites. Addition of further remote sites fragments the available bandwidth and results in substantial deterioration of the remote image quality.

Another critical aspect of camera operation is calibration of the field of view provided by individual assemblies of cameras during multisite activities in which a centrally located simulator is both operated and viewed by a large number of remote sites (figure 16.4). During such activities, each remote site must have an identical field of view, which is difficult to obtain when a large number of camera assemblies is involved. Mounting camera sets in the angle of view-corrected racks provides a simple but rather cumbersome solution. The solution to all these problems is provided either by the use of wavelet compression software such as WINVICOS[231] or integration with comprehensive medical communication systems.[232] While such approach is both an optimal and operationally robust approach, it must be remembered that the compression takes place at the transmission site—a problem that limits its use to the more technologically advanced remote sites. Furthermore, integration of compression software with the preexisting transmission systems at the remote site will require ready access to the telecommunications experts and frequent expert monitoring of the remote platform performance within the context of the entire training network. Naturally, in the environments (rare at present) where the available bandwidth is of limited or no concern, substandard bandwidth allocation to each camera set ceases to be an overriding issue.

Access and Remote Simulator Control

Access from the periphery to the central facility and vice versa can be obtained either by using point-to-point connectivity, with each remote site having its own IP address and an allocated fast Internet connection, dedicated ISDN lines, or through a web-based portal hosted at the central training facility. The Internet-based access without quality of service, although the simplest one, may become unreliable during extended (more than one hour) continuous transmission due to frequent connection interruptions and slowdowns, or upload and download loss of transmission speed. These problems are particularly annoying during long- or very-long-distance operations (e.g., transcontinental or global). Work in which ISDN lines are routinely used is also the most expensive. Access through a Web portal necessitates its creation—a matter of technical complexity that is best accomplished by the technical personnel at the central simulation facility serving as a Med-ASP organization. However, with the portal located at the servers of the training facility,

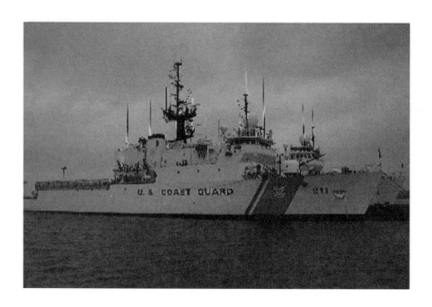

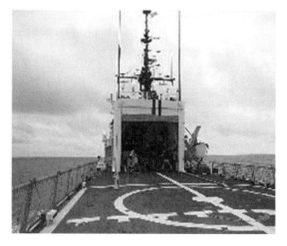

Figure 16.3

The first example of distance-based simulation training at sea conducted during Operation Unitas in the summer of 2001 aboard USCGC *Forward* (top photograph). The simulator was placed in the empty hangar of the ship adjacent to the flight deck (bottom photograph)—the area where casualties would be landed and triaged (photograph on opposite page). During this pioneering exercise, the shipboard system and a portable satellite e-mail system were used to program the simulator to present signs of exposure to the nerve agent (VX). Crew training was conducted in the Atlantic, approximately 1,500 miles off shore, under the direction of two emergency medicine physicians (one stationed in Ann Arbor, MI; the other embarked as the member of the training team).

and with the significant part of the operational software necessary for the efficient training (HFPS control/translation software, remote camera control software, training scenario programs, etc.) accessible through such a portal, multi site activities become greatly facilitated. The peripheral sites are provided with a simple, intuitively understood simulator control interface displayed at the remote computer monitor, and the operation of the simulator is performed either via point-and-click mouse interaction or, at a more sophisticated level, by touching appropriate controls on the touch-sensitive screen.

In summary, one of the principal roles of the central training facility is that of a broad-concept ASP that, in addition to standard training activities aimed at a large number of distributed learners, provides simulation-centered software and supplies supporting electronic training elements, such as access to more traditional didactic tools, archives of previous simulation-based courses, testing materials, and so forth. In such a configuration, prior experience indicates that transmission speeds of 128 kilobytes per second are adequate to fulfill all the required tasks without any deterioration in the quality of image/voice/data elements.

THE TRAINING CONCEPT: OODA

In 1965 four F-105 Thunderchief fighters of the U.S. Air Force were attacked by technologically vastly inferior North Vietnamese MIG 17 aircraft. Two U.S. airplanes were immediately shot down. Two others, badly damaged, got away. The encounter was the beginning of the

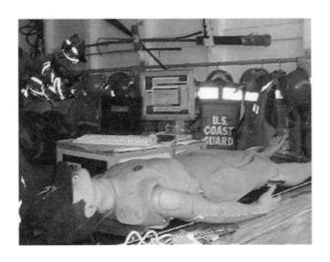

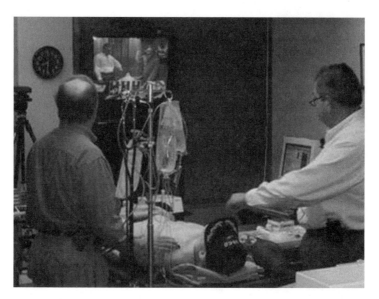

Figure 16.4
Multipoint training using several simulators (Laerdal and METI) located at
two separate sites (MedSMART, Ann Arbor, MI, and Air National Guard
Station, Alpena, MI). The experts in Ann Arbor (photograph above) train
military and civilian personnel in L'Aquila in Italy and in Alpena and Ann
Arbor in Michigan (upper photograph, opposite page) in management
of terrorism-related blast injuries and in recognition and management
of a bioweapons victims. The simulators are centrally controlled by the
engineer at the Ann Arbor site. The imagery, voice, and data are recorded
at the control room at CMU in Mt. Pleasant, Michigan, and relayed from
there to Italy and Alpena. The entire event is conducted in real time,
and all participants in the exercise (altogether nearly 100 lay and medical
participants at all involved sites) are in contact with each other, and may,
if needed, interact with the simulators. The technological requirements
for the satisfactory conduct of complex, multipoint training operations
are very substantial as indicated by the photograph on the opposite page
showing the switches and routers at the Italian site (at the training facility of
Telecom Italia in L'Aquila). Large-scale operations as the one depicted here
require significant resources and the participation of telecommunications and
IT experts. Yet, they also allow highly effective training of large numbers of
geographically dispersed participants.

"OODA" concept created by the notoriously abrasive but brilliant U.S.
Air Force pilot John Boyd.[239] Boyd's philosophy of aerial combat was
based on four words: observe, orient, determine, act. Within a brief
period, Boyd's approach became the mantra of fighter pilots all over the

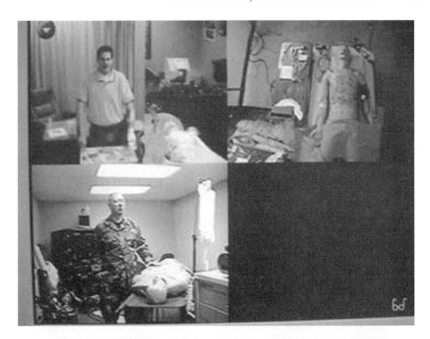

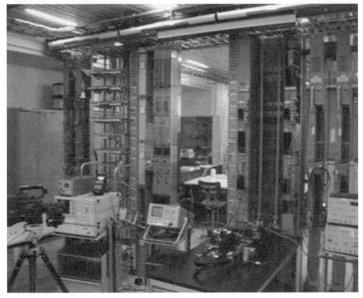

world. Boyd recognized that neither size nor speed mattered in aerial warfighting. It was the pilot's ability to change the state of the aircraft from one to another—transient—that was the key to victory. Furthermore, Boyd advocated removal of all cumbersome, heavy, and (under the majority of circumstances) unnecessary equipment to allow maximum transient exploitation within the entire flying envelope of the aircraft. Finally, Boyd advocated intensive training of fighter pilots in the exploitation of transients—that is, immediate response to the threatening situation based on the combined ability of the pilot to think, fly the aircraft, use its characteristics to his advantage, and combine all these independent attributes into a coherent plan of action that would ultimately lead to placing the aircraft behind the tail of the enemy—the ultimate "kill position."[240]

The concept of OODA applies, in similarity to many other notions recognized by aviation as critical for flying or its safety, to medicine.[241] In medicine, as much as in fighter combat, the dictum "Observe, orient, determine, act" has a cardinal importance to the outcome—particularly in those specialties where operational patient "transients" are frequent: emergency and trauma medicine, and surgery. From the first moment of contact with the patient, the healthcare practitioner must observe in order to assess the immediate condition of the patient. *Observation* must be continuous—a transient may occur at any time, and often entirely unpredictably. *Orientation* means that the preliminary diagnosis and stabilization are equally essential. *Determination* is the act of refining diagnosis through the process of differential approach, that is, elimination of probable other causes of the present disease. *Action* is the time when definitive treatment begins. At all stages, the physician, nurse, or paramedic must combine a vast range of theoretical and practical knowledge, much of the latter based on experience, and manual skills needed at any particular stage of the process. The task may be daunting, particularly for those who do not specialize in the branches of medicine that at times require almost instantaneous "brain-eye-hand" coordination. The difficulties compound when a series of logically consecutive decisions must be made and appropriate actions taken under stress amplified by the ever-present probability of "transients" that present the greatest subconscious challenge to one's confidence and preparedness.

Incorporation of OODA as the fundamental principle of distance-based simulation training exposes trainees to a multitasking, unpredictable, and stressful environment[241] and permits rapid development of critical cognitive and leadership skills under eminently realistic conditions. The approach developed by us is based on frequent training sessions—at least once a month. The remote trainees are never aware of the subject, and simulated patients always present as they would in real life—suddenly, with a variety of signs and symptoms that need to be analyzed using the rules of differential diagnosis before the concept of the definitive pathology can be developed (figure 16.5). Action in the simulated environment is never interrupted by the instructor, whose role is that of a critical observer only, and the instructor-directed debriefing sessions are performed *after* the trainees declare the definitive transfer of the "patient" to another unit (e.g., ICU, surgery, discharge home) or the patient dies. Unpredictable events are always possible during each session but not always present. Essentially, training based on the mixture of OODA and distance-based simulation is "lean" and concentrates on two critical aspects of medicine—rapid, critical thinking followed by rapid, well-conceived, and directed action.[229-233,235] Its primary goal is to free the "fighter" from cumbersome pondering on countless possibilities and their repercussions, assisting instead with narrowing the focus of treatment, based on the continuous information input and on rapid disease identification.

CURRICULUM

Development of a suitable training curriculum is among the most essential elements contributing to the success of distributed simulation-based training. Although the approach combines the most effective elements of purely didactic and hands-on training methods, it does not allow the practice of relevant procedures, which can be trained only in a direct, physical contact with the simulator. Nonetheless, although provisions for such exposure must be made as a part of the course, distributed training provides solid grounding in the practical principles of overall management of a seriously ill patient. It also hones diagnostic skills and prepares for the appropriate procedure selection. It teaches the true relevance of the selected procedures to the particular medical condition. Finally, simulation-based distance training permits viewing of complex procedures as performed by an expert.[229,235,237] In the latter context, stepwise explanation of the correct approach, analysis of pitfalls in the context of a highly realistic behavior of the "simulated" patient in response to inappropriately performed procedure, and the ongoing commentary on the actions that must be taken to ensure its success are among the important elements facilitating subsequent learning of the relevant motor skills.[228]

The principal goal of the distributed simulation-based training is the maintenance of maximum medical realism and a rapid practical preparation of the trainees for the challenges of real-life operations. Hence, the curriculum must incorporate a significantly higher pace and impose significantly higher demands on the active participation of

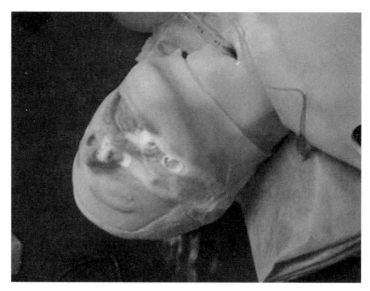

Figure 16.5
Simulation of the acute exposure to the chemical warfare agent sarin
(photograph above). Despite obvious and clearly visible signs of poisoning
(excessive, frothy salivation and eye irritation, swollen tongue, seizures), only
very few civilian participants in the exercise recognized the symptomatology or
knew how to initiate treatment. Most diagnosed the patient in the photograph
on the opposite page as suffering of smallpox despite clearly non-smallpox
distribution of skin eruptions (pustules). The simulator has been moulaged
to show the characteristic distribution of skin lesions that accompany
chicken pox (concentrating on the area of the chest rather than arms, face,
and soles of the feet as would be the case in smallpox). The failure to provide
proper diagnosis is disturbing in view of the considerable attention paid to sarin
and smallpox as bioterrorism agents by both lay and professional medical media.

individual trainees than in the didactic or the nonsimulated hands-on
environments. In the didactic setting, the principal burden of action is
placed on the teacher, while the possibility of harm to the patient that
may occur in the nonsimulated hands-on training demands frequent
interventions and guidance by the training expert. In simulated encounters, the burden of action is placed directly on the trainee and allows
errors of omission and commission to take place without the risk of
adverse consequences or punitive instructor response. The expert's role
is not to interrupt and explain while mistakes take place but, once the
scenario runs to its end, to repeat it while providing a thorough
debriefing and instruction on correct approaches. Hence, the curriculum

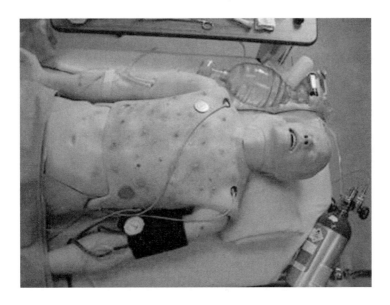

must not shy from incorporating the common patient management errors or the role of human factors and their relation to adverse outcomes. Contrary to real life, the death of a "patient" is not a traumatic but potentially very intense learning experience that needs not be avoided. The curriculum must also allow for both individual and team training—an essential aspect of modern medical operations. Finally, the need for a focused curriculum cannot be overemphasized. Because each of the potentially involved disciplines has its own training needs, the curriculum must be very specific in its objectives: field management of trauma must concentrate on that topic rather than elements of perisurgical crises that may affect the survival of a traumatized patient. Unless specific goals of simulation-based training are strictly pursued, the training can easily degrade into a highly theatrical demonstration of medical emergencies similar to the numerous television shows that vividly depict the bloody nature of field and emergency medicine but are completely useless as training tools.

INTERDISCIPLINARY EDUCATION MODEL

Emergency medical education would be a valuable core component for all students in health professions, including physicians, nurses, physician assistants, physical therapists, and others who work with patients and high-risk populations. Distributed simulation-based training is an ideal method of facilitating team learning across health professions education. It can be delivered to remote clinical training sites or can be provided onsite with collaboration between schools/colleges of health professions (HP). While various HP disciplines have individualized education requirements, a standardized curriculum for simulation-based emergency medical education could be incorporated across professional curricula. Competencies to be mastered are the same for all trainees; therefore, curricular aspects remain the same regardless of previous education/training or experience of the students.

A strong attribute of the simulation-based training is the learner-centered design of the curriculum and the delivery method. Outcomes can be quickly assessed to allow trainees to have individualized attention and ample opportunity to master competencies. To ensure that trainees in larger classes are uniformly engaged, participatory exercises, such as question/discussion instruments, can be completed by students during the training session for use in later interdisciplinary discussions. This type of exercise lends itself to a variety of educational models such as case-based training, problem-based learning, and traditional interdisciplinary discussion models.

In times of local or national disaster, those in health professions are the first to be sought out for assistance. This makes a strong case for including simulation-based emergency training as a core component in the educational process for all students in health professions. The numbers of health care personnel who are competent in pre-hospital emergency care could be dramatically increased without significant cost added to health professions education.

OPERATIONAL USES OF SIMULATION-BASED DISTRIBUTED MEDICAL TRAINING

Practical implementation of the concept of simulation-based distributed learning allows execution of highly realistic training in the often complex and stress-filled environment of field operations that obviates the need for the physical presence of the trainees at the simulation facility (figure 16.6).[226,233] Another major advantage of this form of training is its preeminent suitability for real-time dissemination of world-class medical training expertise[229] in the form of practical "patient demonstrations" rather than the commonly encountered didactic format of a theoretical lecture.[237] Consequently, pre-hospital learner audiences in rural and remote regions benefit from both advanced training technology and expertise and from the customized training services that may be provided whenever needed.

We have performed numerous operations that utilized and validated the concept of distance-based simulation training at all levels of medical expertise. Courses in ACLS, ATLS, and CTLS were given to U.S. and NATO military personnel,[236] medical students, and physicians[230,233] and first responders, with the distance between the simulation facility in Ann Arbor and the trainees from 140 to nearly 8,000 miles (transatlantic training in France and Italy).[242] In two instances of transatlantic training, highly innovative peri- and intraoperative decision-making and team training were the main subjects of the courses.[229] Finally, crew responses to a chemical warfare threat were practiced aboard a U.S. Coast Guard vessel (USCGC *Forward*) during its operational deployment in the south Atlantic.[228] The demonstrated efficacy and ease of such training combined with the high level of interactivity and readily

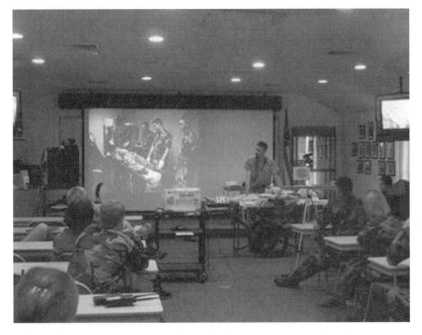

Figure 16.6
Multipoint training of military (Air National Guard and Air Force) personnel. The participants in the audience and at the remote site must deal with two seriously wounded victims, one of whom (the simulator in the foreground) may be also affected by an unknown chemical agent. The trainees practice medical leadership skills without which both victims would rapidly die. Such skills can be trained only by means of simulation.

available remote access to the advanced simulation facility and world-class training expertise are of special significance for EMS and military healthcare providers. In situations of increased tension, when the need for "just in time" training of a large number of personnel deployed to several geographically dispersed sites[226,228] as seen during bioterrorist threats, military conflicts, or large-scale rescue operations[236,237] is pre-eminent, distance-based simulation training may provide one of the most effective and realistic methods available.

QUO VADIS?

The recently concluded international exercise Global Mercury[243] demonstrated once again what has been already known from the very large number of studies that emerged since "the anthrax assault" of 2001: we are still largely unprepared to deal with the consequences of bioterrorism. Complacency, political wrangling, lack of imaginative uses of the existing technologies, dogmatism, and interagency fighting combine to produce this startling failure. Billions of dollars have been spent, yet the report published by the Trust for America's Health[244] in November 2003 shows that only four states rate as well-prepared, scoring seven points on the ten-point evaluation. The vast majority of the United States continues to hover in the atmosphere of "it cannot happen to us" pre-9/11 bliss.

The inability to address the issues of bioterrorism in a less-than-obvious manner (such as vaccine stockpiling) is surprising in view of a very gloomy CIA report that clearly indicates a "bright future" for bio-terrorism. Advances in microbiology and genetic engineering exploded upon the world and made bioweapons a cheap and effective means of exercising pressure on the world community.[245] Today, high school students perform experiments that ten years ago would be considered the cutting edge of biomedical sciences. The same can be done by the forces intent not on curing but on making infectious diseases more vicious. Genetic modification of the existing biopathogens can be done with minimum funding, using fairly unsophisticated facilities, and with the knowledge derived from the detailed scientific reports openly available in journals and on the Internet. Yet, rather than being one step ahead in the war against bioterrorism, we continue to be several steps behind, mired in the traditional "fighting the last war" mentality. We faithfully repeat conceptual mistakes of the past when, despite clear advance warnings, the meaningful response to the assault arrives only after it has taken place.

Presently, bioterrorism is even viewed by some as the means of unleashing another Armageddon. Many of the currently contemplated scenarios envisage thousands of casualties, the public health system completely overwhelmed, and chaos spreading first throughout the nation, then the world. A catastrophe of such magnitude is possible. Realistically, though, it belongs to the Hollywood sphere of cliffhanger thrillers. As pointed out in a recent book,[4] terrorism is not about inflicting the maximum number of casualties but about destabilizing the adversary. It is about forcing the society to legitimize the terrorist's demands and then convert it into a bona fide political agenda where terror will become a seemingly benign effort to redress grievances. Seventy years ago, Germany legitimized Adolf Hitler. Forty years later, Saddam Hussein was accepted as president of Iraq. Even today, attempts are made to portray the actions of Osama Bin Laden as an attempt to liberate the Islamic world from decades of oppression.

Almost all people will have difficulties accepting terrorism associated with a very large number of casualties as the "struggle for freedom" or an effort to gain national or ethnic identity. Since such a form of terrorism will never reach the level of Western sympathy necessary for recognition and legitimization of terrorist demands, from the guerrilla's point of view anything involving true mass casualties is counterproductive as the means of "converting" the Western society. On the other hand, a series of minor, nonlethal, but visible events perpetrated across the country in several places at the same time will cause the required disruption and panic as effectively as the employment of a lethal, mass casualty-inducing agent in a single event. The same significant economic consequences will ensue, as will the same polarization of the society, and the same mistrust of the government and its way of handling the problem. Ultimately, and after a few repetitions of synchronized but dispersed attacks, the society's will to fight back will start to erode. The very moment a public voice will declare "there might be something to their demands, after all," a new Munich crisis will be on our hands. Like then, "peace in our time" will be long in coming. Rapid dissolution of unity within the seemingly monolithic block of NATO, based on the divergence of national economic interests, immediately prior to Operation Iraqi Freedom may serve as a serious warning of such likelihood. As frightening as the concept may be, at the time of bioterrorism-induced, large-scale crisis, the "jointness of purpose" may rapidly convert into "everyone for himself." At that time, the degree of national preparedness will be the determinant between survival and demise.

Synchronicity, geographic dispersal of the assault sites, and the essential crudeness of the employed technology are the hallmarks of al Qaeda "conventional" operations. The same philosophy can be readily applied to actions involving bioweapons. Any assault using such means, even if involving exposure to relatively benign agents, would be extremely costly, particularly if the terrorist group made a clear announcement of the "ownership" to dispel any notions about the possibility of a coincidental nature of contamination/disease outbreaks. The unpredictability of time and place of the attacks would rapidly induce and sustain the Pimpernel Effect ("He is here, he is there, he is everywhere"), imposing upon the authorities the demand for continuous maintenance of maximum vigilance everywhere. Realistic simulations of bioterrorism uniformly indicate the logistic, fiscal, and political nightmare of the need to simultaneously address allocation of suddenly inadequate healthcare and disease-containment resources, introduction and maintenance of strict quarantine rules, and the concomitant control of panic that complicates disease containment even further. The very likely closure of state and national borders will lead to the rapid decline of the local and national economy, inducing long-lasting hardships among the affected population. Significant political instability will be the ultimate consequence. As outlandish as such visions may seem, the national and international consequences of the outbreak of SARS or the stress imposed upon the U.S. public health system during the influenza pandemic in 2003 indicated how catastrophic the consequences of a coordinated but *essentially nonlethal* multipoint bioterrorist attack may be.

Prevention of such events is the principal task of the national and international intelligence, law enforcement agencies, and, whenever needed, armed forces—particularly their special operations units. However, once the assault has taken place, healthcare authorities assume the dominant role in management of its consequences. From the onset, first responders and emergency medicine services constitute the mainstay of the defense, which, in order to be effective, must be based on a very close cooperation of public health officials, medical personnel, healthcare administrators, law enforcement, and public information media. The issues that need to be confronted in the event of a major bioterrorism event are highly complex and may be contradictory. While the efficiency of outbreak containment and elimination will depend on real-time solutions to the stream of rapidly presenting and frequently unforeseen dilemmas, attempts to find such solutions *during* the outbreak are doomed to failure. Trivial as it may sound, only very careful operational preparation will guarantee success, and the level of such preparation can be attained only through a very rigorously implemented and sustained training at all levels, culminating in regularly scheduled "combined operations" exercises.

As indicated in the introduction, with a few striking exceptions (chiefly at the federal or Department of Defense level), the counter-bioterrorism training of medical personnel is largely inadequate.[60] Much of the problem rests with the fact that routine exposure to the infectious diseases and their recognition and treatment is provided only at the large medical centers. The exposure of the physically remote medical communities remains theoretical and is based primarily on the data and fact sheets published on the Internet, in medical papers, in information pamphlets, or through onsite or webcast lectures. All of these methods are passive, and none assures the ability to implement the acquired knowledge in practice and on demand. Moreover, the reliance on web-based information may have its own dangers, as pointed out by the East Coast blackout in 2003, when much of e-based communication systems were either fully or partially disabled. The disruption accompanying a purposeful downing of a few strategically placed high-voltage masts will result in medical information chaos—despite the millions spent on infrastructure, it is unlikely that the generators will be available at all EMS centers, rural hospitals, community clinics, and so forth in the nation. Hence, all training must concentrate on the development of diagnostic and patient management skills combined with the ability to implement such preexisting knowledge and skills instantaneously, under most likely very austere circumstances, in the atmosphere of unpredictability and essential randomness, and with limited or nonexistent sources of outside help. Training must test the ability to act in a stressful, constantly changing, adversarial environment. It also must clearly indicate the state of current readiness, mercilessly point out its deficiencies, and indicate what needs to be done to improve it. Such training is costly, imposes rigorous demands upon the participants, and disrupts routine activities. However, the only benefits of preparing for the obvious, where training is based on the execution of well-scripted events predetermined long before the exercise start, where everyone knows everything and every action is defined *a priori* to assure success, and the outcome is always laudatory, are political accolades and positive press comments. Operationally, it is the surest way to disaster.

Military history is replete with incidents where orthodoxy of preparation or anticipation led to major defeats. German offensives in Ardennes in 1940 and then in 1944, Pearl Harbor, and the Japanese campaign in Malaya in 1941 serve as some of the most glaring recent examples of catastrophes caused by anticipating the obvious and by the failure to prepare for the unexpected. Yet, the basic operational philosophy of terrorism is that of the unexpected strike. Hence, all preparatory measures—and that includes training of medical personnel, their interaction with personnel from other agencies, communications, logistics, and so forth—must contain a large dose of spontaneous chaos, unpredictability, and must be based on a high-operation tempo. The ability to deal with the "fog of war"[235,246] is one of the critical aspects of managing a bioterrorism-related disease outbreak, and would be critical in situations where a number of incidents occurred synchronically at several dispersed sites.

Too often, training exercises are executed poorly: the participants know exactly what to expect, the personnel from all relevant agencies are not involved, and the script is based on a highly unimaginative action that would never be contemplated for real-life implementation by any terrorist group worth its name. Even in the exercise as serious as the Global Mercury, the infected attacker conveniently developed suspicious symptoms in front of the quarantine officer. In real life, the perpetrators would assure that the disease carrier entered the country undetected, managed to infect a number of others, and collapsed in the manner precluding recognition either as a terrorist or the source of the outbreak. The "ownership" would be announced through anonymous contacts in much the same way the "Osama tapes" are forwarded to the Western media, reinforcing the Pimpernel Effect and the associated uncertainty of all countermeasure-involved agencies. Large-scale multinational exercises (such as Global Mercury) demand a very sophisticated level of coordination and logistics that limits (but not excludes) spontaneity and true unpredictability. On the other hand, exercises at the community level will hardly disclose any of the existing deficiencies if the principal goal is either to go through the motions or merely prove the high readiness level of all involved. Among the most likely best examples of how an unannounced and unpredictable test can discover major problems in operational readiness are the exploits of CDR Richard Marcinko and the Red Cell team under his command, whose unorthodox stealth tactics revealed striking lapses in the security procedures of the U.S. Navy.[247] The same approach, based on suddenness and lack of prior preparation of the participants, has been used in a series of international training events that demonstrated the essential lack of readiness to cope with the victims of bio- and chemical terrorism (smallpox and sarin) among medical (civilian and military) and lay participants.[229-233] The observed deficiencies were even more striking when viewed in the context of almost incessant exposure of both professionals and the general public to the issues of detecting and dealing with smallpox and nerve gas contamination.

There is no question that the issue of training is of paramount importance if bioterrorism is to be efficiently countered. However, training must be realistic and based on plausible, but unorthodox, real-life scenarios. It must anticipate the terrorist mindset rather than the mindset of a CDC or state public health bureaucrat. As already pointed out, even at the theoretical level the current extent of preparation to cope with victims of bioterrorism may be inadequate. The only way to investigate whether or not the practical approaches fall into the same category is not through placid questionnaires and web-based multiple choice tests but through the rigorous conduct of unannounced exercises whose scripts are not revealed to the participants, that involve interdisciplinary/interagency effort and participation, and that test several aspects of performance instead of merely one (medical knowledge, communications, materiel readiness, etc.) Finally, since skill deterioration over time is a well-known phenomenon,[248-251] major practical drills need to be performed at least twice a year while procedure drills (such as diagnostic training and disease management) must be performed at two- to three-month intervals.

There is absolutely no doubt that exercises such as those outlined in the preceding paragraphs are costly and highly disruptive to the routine functions of all participants, and that they demand time at their preparatory stages and even more time for analysis and implementation of the required changes and improvements. Practical requirements (travel, expenses, time) make frequent training in physical reality impractical even at the level of a relatively small county. The combination of virtual reality, rapidly spreading broadband Internet access, availability of Internet 2, and the decreasing cost of distributed interactive simulation offer the ideal substitute for the traditional forms of field training. Many academic institutions of the country have or are developing superb e-education facilities that are frequently either underutilized or applied solely in intramural education. Yet, it is these types of facilities that can serve as the nodal points in a counterterrorism training network. Hence, they ought to be made available to the local communities in a community-academia partnership arrangement sponsored by state/federal authorities. The authors of a seminal yet largely ignored paper published one year prior to the events of September 11, 2001, proposed a national network of such training centers that would allow the use of advanced information technology as the essential foundation for distributed training leading to improved medical readiness.[235] Implementation of the concept would allow simultaneous training of large numbers of multispecialty personnel in dealing with a wide variety of problems associated with a suddenly occurring large-scale medical crisis. The network would permit easy incorporation of a broad range of issues starting from crisis management at the national level, through the complexities of logistics and local management, to the problems associated with medical staff exhaustion at the level of a rural ER, or their ability to manage individual patients. The fusion of distributed interactive simulation and Med-ASP concepts obviates many of the difficulties, while introducing, at the same time, a robust platform for the development and testing of many solutions to the hitherto unsolvable dilemmas.

CONCLUSION

The threat of bioterrorism increases rather than diminishes, requiring dramatic change in the current attitudes at all levels of politics, administration, health care, and law and its enforcement. Among the principal aspects of such change is the need for a dramatic change in training, particularly of the first responders—starting from individuals, through counties, states, the nation, and ultimately ending at the international health authorities and law enforcement community. It is imperative that advanced information and simulation technologies be utilized to the full extent of their capabilities rather than continue to be used in a parochial manner, as is often practiced today. Multidisciplinary/multi-agency approaches need to be developed and practiced with the goal of fighting bioterrorism rather than individual turf, and funds must be used on the initiatives that have potential for providing effective solutions to the currently burning issue of training very large numbers of frontline personnel—the first responders. Vegetius was as correct in the fourth century as he is today: *si vis pacem, para bellum*—if you want peace, prepare for war.

ACKNOWLEDGMENTS

To CDR Richard Marcinko, U.S. Navy (ret.) and the Red Cell Team for pointing out that preparing for the unexpected is the only way to train for winning the war.

This chapter presents our vision of how simulation can be employed as a highly effective training modality in the setting of advanced distributed learning. Much of the work quoted has already been done, and the vision would not be possible without our colleagues, whose effort was instrumental in making the present analysis. Hence, the authors wish to express their gratitude for the superb contribution of all their colleagues and collaborators who, even if not named as the authors, were directly involved in providing background to the present paper: Ms. Y. Acosta-Arbona, Mr. B. Carrasco, F. Gabrielli, J. Hawayek, Ms. M. Leigh, H. Levine, T. Ludwig, T. Pletcher, C. Poirier, F. Patricelli, S. Richir, and G. Wroblewski. Tim Pletcher also drew the diagram used in figure 16.1. Several institutions were also extremely generous in their support. The faith of Laerdal USA and MPL, Inc., particularly of Mr. David Johnson and Mr. Rick Ritt, was unprecedented. Citrix Systems, Inc. provided the initial financial support, whose acquisition was greatly facilitated by Ms. J. Moskowitz and T. Gruen-Kennedy. Digital Realm, Inc. unfailingly provided the most generous technical and materiel assistance, while Mr. G. Scigliano of Pentax USA allowed us to use their sophisticated fiber optic equipment. Telecom Italia offered their facilities in Italy together with connectivity for the transatlantic operations, while ISTIA at the University of Angers did the same in France. Medical School of L'Aquila, particularly its department of surgery, did not hesitate to allow us to use their senior students and staff as our experimental subjects, while CPT A. French, USCG, facilitated our shipboard activities and at the Innovation Exhibition organized by USCG in Baltimore in 2002. Last, but by no means least, BG C. A. Fausone, NG, and MAJ J. Kirk, USAF, and his staff at Alpena ANG Station were instrumental in allowing us to conduct the "impossible" at their training facilities. Participation of Central Michigan University in some of the experiments that provided the basis for the present paper was made possible by a grant from the HHS Office for the Advancement of the Telehealth. To all of them, our gratitude.

NOTES

1. Hutchinson R. Weapons of mass destruction. London, UK: Weidenfeld & Nicholson; 2003. p. 1–283.

2. Yaukey J. Gannett News Service. 2003. Available from: theolympian. gannettonline.com/gns/wmd/index.html.

3. Croddy E. Chemical and biological warfare: a comprehensive study for the concerned citizen. New York: Springer Verlag; 2002. p. 1–306.

4. von Lubitz DKJE. Bioterrorism: field guide to disease identification and initial patient management. Boca Raton, FL: CRC Press; 2003. p. 1–188.

5. Noah DL, Huebener KD, Darling RG, Waeckerle JF. The history and threat of biological warfare and terrorism. Emerg Med Clin North Am 2002;20:255–71.

6. Hyams KC, Murphy FM, Wessley S. Responding to chemical, biological, or nuclear terrorism: the indirect and long-term effects may present the greatest challenge. J Health Polit Policy Law 2002;27:273–91.

7. Kates B. U.S. bioterror defense plans need coordinated effort, critics say. CentreDaily.com. 2003 Oct 14. Available from: www.centredaily.com/mld/centredaily/news/7010075.htm.

8. Clark R. State emergency plans don't allow for terrorist threat. The Clarion Ledger. 2003 Sep 10. Available from: www.clarionledger.com/news/o309/10/m03.html.

9. GAO-03-1155T. Washington, DC: 2003.

10. Department of Health and Human Services. 2003. Available from: www.hhsgov/new/press/20030912d.html.

11. Centers for Disease Control and Prevention. 2003 July 6. Available from: www.cdc.gov/od/oc/media/pressrel/r031003a.htm

12. U.S. House of Representatives. 1st session. 2003 September. Available from: thomas.loc.gov/cgi-bin/cpqueryT?&report+hr280&dbname+cp108&. Accessed October 10, 2003.

13. Oren M. Bioterrorism. Harefuah 2002;141(Spec. no. 13-5):124.

14. Robenshtok SR, Katz LH, Reznikovich S, Hendler I, Poles L, Hourvitz A, et al. Preparedness of the Israeli health system for a biologic warfare event. Isr Med Assoc J 2003;4:495–7.

15. Ansley G. U.S. alliance drawing Canberra into the mire. NZ Herald 2003 Oct 21.

16. Reuters News Service. NAFTA partners fear new U.S. rules on bioterrorism. 2003 Oct. 11.

17. Wilson N, Lush D. Bioterrorism in the Northern Hemisphere and potential impact on New Zealand. NZ Med J 2002;115:247–51.

18. Jortani SA, Snyder JW, Valdes R Jr. The role of the clinical laboratory in managing chemical or biological terrorism. Clin Chem 2000;46:1881–93.

19. Krenzlok EP. The critical role of the poison center in the recognition, mitigation and management of biological and chemical terrorism. Przegl Lek 2001;58:177–81.

20. Burkle FM Jr. Mass casualty management of a large-scale bioterrorist event: an epidemiological approach that shapes triage decisions. Emerg Med Clin North Am 2002;20:409–36.

21. Scharoun K, van Caulil K, Liberman A. Bioterrorism vs. health security—crafting a plan of preparedness. Health Care Manag (Frederick) 2002;21:74–92.

22. Sacra JC, Murphy M. Oklahoma City and Tulsa Metropolitan Medical Response System. J Okla State Med Assoc 2002;95:281–5.

23. Kaplan J. CDC strategic plan for bioterrorism preparedness and response. Pub Health Rep 2001;116(suppl. 2):9–16.

24. Salinsky E. Will the nation be ready for the next bioterrorism attack? Mending gaps in the public health infrastructure. NHPF issue brief 2002 Jun 12;(776):1–19.

25. Ponco de Leon-Rosales S, Lazcano-Ponce E, Rangel-Frasto MS, Sosa-Lozano LA, Huerta-Jimenez MA. Bioterrorism: notes for an agenda in case of the unexpected. Salud Publica Mex 2001;43:589–603.

26. Kuhr S, Hauer JM. Intergovernmental preparedness and response to potential catastrophic biological terrorism. J Public Health Manag Pract 2000;6:50–6.

27. Poles I. The Israeli medical response plan for an unusual biological event. Harefuah 2002;141(spec. no. 22-8):122–3.

28. Arnold JL. Disaster medicine in the 21st century: future hazards, vulnerabilities, and risk. Prehosp Disaster Med 2002;17(1):3–11.

29. DiGiovanni C Jr, Reynolds B, Harwell R. Community reaction to bioterrorism: prospective study of simulated outbreak. Emerg Infect Dis 2003;9:708–12.

30. Blendon RJ, Benson JM, DesRoches CM, Pollard WE, Parvanta CM, Herrmann MJ. The impact of anthrax attacks on the American public. Med Gen Med 2002;17:1.

31. Kilner T. Triage decisions of prehospital emergency care providers, using a multiple casualty scenario paper exercise. Emerg Med J 2002;19:348–53.

32. Belman S, Murphy J, Steiner JF, Kempe A. Consistency of triage decisions by call center nurses. Ambul Pediatr 2002;2:396–400.

33. Ihlenfeld JT. A primer on triage and mass casualty. Dimens Crit Care Nurs 2003;22:204–7.

34. Nocera A, Garner A. Australian disaster triage: a colour maze in the Tower of Babel. Aust NZ J Surg 1999;69:508–602.

35. Schuftan C. Triage management in the Third World health ministries. Trop Doct 1996;26:90–1.

36. Wildner J. Emergency assessment—the Italian experience: color codes determine priorities. Pflege Z 2001;54:427–32.

37. Salzar MK, Kelman B. Planning for biological disasters. Occupational health nurses as "first responders." AAOHN J 2002;50:174–81.

38. Eitzen EM Jr. Education is the key to defense against bioterrorism. Ann Emerg Med 1999;14:221–3.

39. Mothershead JL, Tonat K, Koenig KL. Bioterrorism preparedness III: state and federal programs and response. Emerg Med Clin North Am 2002;20:477–500.

40. Flowers LK, Motherhead JL, Blackwell TH. Bioterrorism preparedness II: the community and emergency medical services systems. Emerg Med Clin North Am 2002;20:457–76.

41. Schultz CH, Motherhead JL, Field M. Bioterrorism preparedness I: the emergency department and hospital. Emerg Med Clin North Am 2002;20: 437–55.

42. Keim M, Kaufmann AF. Principles for emergency response to bioterrorism. Ann Emerg Med 1999;34:177–82.

43. Karva M, Bronzert P, Kretan V. Bioterrorism and critical care. Crit Care Clin 2003;19:279–313.

44. Blazes DL, Lawler JV, Lazarus AA. When biotoxins are tools of terror. Early recognition of international poisoning can attenuate effects. Postgrad Med 2002;112:89–92, 95–6, 98.

45. Becker SM. Meeting the threat of weapons of mass destruction terrorism: toward a broader conception of consequence management. Mil Med 2001; 166(suppl. 12):13–6.

46. Morse A. Bioterrorism preparedness for local health departments. Comm Health Nurs 2002;19:203–11.

47. Silvagni AJ, Levy LA, McFee RB. NOVA Southeastern University— College of Osteopathic Medicine Task Force on Bioterrorism and Weapons of Mass Destruction. J Am Osteopath Assoc 2002;102:491–9.

48. Franz DR, Zajtchuk R. Biological terrorism. Dis Mon 2003;48:493–564.

49. Dudley JP. New challenges for public health care: biological and chemical weapons awareness, surveillance and response. Biol Res Nurs 2003;4:244–50.

50. Crichton M, Flinn R. Training for emergency management: tactical decision games. J Hazard Mater 2001;88:255–66.

51. Jones J, Terndrup TE, Franz DR, Eitzen EM Jr. Future challenges in preparing for and responding to bioterrorism events. Emerg Med Clin North Am 2002;20:501–24.

52. Tyre TE. Wake-up call: a bioterrorism exercise. Mil Med 2001;166(suppl. 12):90–1.

53. Lorenti A, Leus X, Van Holsteijn B. Relevant in times of turmoil: WHO and public health in unstable situations. Prehosp Disast Med 2001;16: 184–91.

54. GAO-02-6211. Washington, DC; 2002.

55. GAO-02-5481. Washington, DC; 2002.

56. GAO-02-1601. Washington, DC; 2001.

57. GAO-01-1621. Washington, DC; 2001.

58. GAO-01-909. Washington, DC; 2001.

59. Lichtveld M, Hodge JG, Gebbie K, Thompson FE, et al. J Law Med Ethics 2002;30(suppl. 3):184–8.

60. Chen FM, Hickner J, Fink KS, Galliher JM, Burstin H. On the frontlines: family physicians' preparedness for bioterrorism. J Fam Pract 2002;51: 745–50.

61. Rose MA, Larrimore KL. Knowledge and awareness concerning chemical and biological terrorism: continuing education implications. J Contin Educ Nurs 2002;33:253–8.

62. Ingleby TV, O'Toole T, Henderson DA. Preventing the use of biological weapons: improving response should prevention fail. Clin Infect Diseases 2000;30:926–9.

63. Porter R. The greatest benefit to mankind: a medical history of humanity. New York: W. W. Norton & Co.;1997. p. 3–831.

64. Colliver JA. Educational theory and medical education practice: a cautionary note for medical school faculty. Acad Med 2002;77:1217–20.

65. Hans K. Global standards in medical education for better health care. Med Educ 2002;36:1116.

66. Billingham K, Howe A, Walters C. In our own image—a multidisciplinary qualitative analysis of medical education. J Interprof Care 2002; 16:379–89.

67. Leitch RA, Magee H, Moses GR. Simulation and the future of military medicine. Mil Med 2002;167:350–4.

68. Harter P, Krummel T, Reznek M. Virtual reality and simulation: training the future emergency physician. Acad Emerg Med 2002;9:78–87.

69. Letterie GS. How virtual reality may enhance training in obstetrics and gynecology. Am J Obstet Gynecol 2002;187:S37–40.

70. Hoyal FM. "Swallowing the medicine": determining the present and desired modes for delivery of continuing medical education to rural doctors. Aust J Rural Health 1999;7:212–5.

71. Davis P, McCraken P. Restructuring rural continuing medical education through videoconferencing. J Telemed Telecare 2002;8:108–9.

72. Delaney G, Khadra MH, Lim SE, Sar L, Sturmberg JP, Yang SC. Challenges to rural medical education: a student perspective. Aust J Rural Health 2002;10:168–72.

73. Booth B, Lawrance R. Quality assurance and continuing education needs of rural and remote general practitioners: how are they changing? Aust J Rural Health 2001;9:256–7.

74. Rourke JT, Rourke LL. Rural family medicine training in Canada. Can Fam Physician 1995;41:993–1000.

75. Darling RG, Huebner KD, Noah DL, Waeckerle JF. The history and threat of biological warfare and terrorism. Emerg Med Clin North Am 2002;20:255–71.

76. Brocato CE, Miller GT. The next agent of terror? Understanding smallpox & its implications for prehospital crews. J Emerg Med Serv 2002;27:52–5.

77. Williams B. Bioterrorism: are we prepared? Tenn Med 2001;94:413–7.

78. Cunha BA. Anthrax, tularemia, plague, Ebola or smallpox as agents of bioterrorism: recognition in the emergency room. Clin Microbiol Infect 2002;8:489–503.

79. Fahlgren TL, Drenkard KN. Healthcare system disaster preparedness, part 2: nursing executive role in leadership. J Nurs Adm 2002;32:531–7.

80. Guay AH. Dentistry's response to bioterrorism: a report of consensus workshop. J Am Dent Assoc 2002;133:1181–7.

81. Rubinshtein R, Robenshtok E, Eisenkraft A, Vidan A, Hourvitz A. Training Israeli medical personnel to treat casualties of nuclear, biologic, and chemical warfare. Isr Med Assoc 2002;4:545–8.

82. George G, Ramsay K, Rochester M, Seah R, Spencer H, Vijayasankar D, et al. Facilities for chemical decontamination in accident and emergency departments in the United Kingdom. Emerg Med J 2002;19:453–7.

83. Baker DJ. Management of respiratory failure in toxic disasters. Resusc 1999;42:125–31.

84. Peleg K, Reuveni H, Stein M. Earthquake disasters—lessons to be learned. Isr Med Assoc J 2002;4:361–5.

85. Cowley RA, Myers RA, Gretes AJ. EMS response to mass casualties. Emerg Med Clin North Am 1984;2:687–92.

86. Doyle CJ. Mass casualty incident. Integration with prehospital care. Emerg Med Clin North Am 1990;8:163–75.

87. Watterson AE, Thomas HF. Acute pesticide poisoning in the UK and information and training needs of general practitioners recording a conundrum. Pub Health 1992;106:473–80.

88. Lalich RA. The role of state government, local government, and non-governmental organizations in medical innovative readiness training. Mil Med 2002;167:367–9.

89. Koplan J. CDC's strategic plan for bioterrorism preparedness and response. Pub Health Rep 2001;116(2):9–16.

90. Levi L, Michaelson M, Admi H, Bregman D, Bar-Nahor R. National strategy for mass casualty situations and its effects on the hospital. Prehosp Disast Med 2002 Jan–Mar;17(1):12–6.

91. Donini-Lenhoff FG, Hedrick HL. Growth of specialization in graduate medical education. JAMA 2000;284:1284–9.

92. Schroeder SA. Primary care at a crossroads. Acad Med 2002;77:767–73.

93. Gulesen O. Specialization of doctors, general practice and the training system. Cah Sociol Demogr Med 2001;41:386–96.

94. Buckingham CD, Adams A. Classifying clinical decision making: a unifying approach. J Adv Nurs 2000;32:981–9.

95. Connor M, Ponte PR, Conway J. Multidisciplinary approaches to reducing error and risk in a patient care setting. Crit Care Nurs Clin North Am 2002;14:359–67.

96. Scheen AJ, Rorive M, Letiexhe M, Devoitille L, Jandrain B. Multidisciplinary management of the obese patient: example from the Obesity Center at the University of Liege. Rev Med Liege 2001;56:474–9.

97. Hazard RG. The multidisciplinary approach to occupational low back pain and disability. J Am Acad Orthop Surg 1994;2:157–63.

98. Schriefer J, Engelhard J, DiCesare L, Miller M, Schriefer J. Merging clinical pathway programs as part of overall health systems mergers: a ten-step guide. Spectrum Health. Jt Comm J Qual Improv 2000;26:29–38.

99. Burd A, Cheung KW, Ho WS, Wong TW, Ying SY, Cheng PH. Before the paradigm shift: concepts and communication between doctors and nurses in a burns team. Burns 2002;28:691–5.

100. Sherwood G, Thomas E, Bennett DS, Lewis P. A teamwork model to promote patient safety in critical care. Crit Care Nurs Clin North Am 2002;14:333–40.

101. Lingard L, Reznick R, DeVito I, Espin S. Forming professional identities on the health care team: discursive constructions of the "other" in the operating room. Med Educ 2002;36:728–34.

102. Cooper JB, Newbower RS, Long CD, McPeek B. Preventable anesthesia mishaps: a study of human factors. Qual Saf Health Care 2002;11: 277–82.

103. Ruppert M, Reith MW, Widmann JH, Lackner CK, Kerkmann R, Schweiberer L, et al. Checking for breathing: evaluation of the diagnostic capability of emergency medical services personnel, physicians, medical students, and medical laypersons. Ann Emerg Med 1999;34:720–9.

104. Lefrancois DP, Dufour DG. Use of the esophageal tracheal combitube by basic emergency medical technicians. Resusc 2002;52:77–83.

105. De Lorenzo RA. Prehospital misidentification of tachydysrhythmias: a report of five cases. J Emerg Med 1993;11:431–6.

106. Trzeciak S, Erickson T, Bunney EB, Sloan EP. Variation in patient management based on ECG interpretation by emergency medicine and internal medicine residents. Am J Emerg Med 2002;20:188–95.

107. Herlitz J, Hansson E, Ringvall E, Starke M, Karlson BW, Waagstein L. Predicting a life-threatening disease and death among ambulance-transported patients with chest pain or other symptoms raising suspicion of an acute coronary syndrome. Am J Emerg Med 2002;20:588–94.

108. Linn S, Knoller N, Giligan CG, Dreifus U. The sky is a limit: errors in prehospital diagnosis by flight physicians. Am J Emerg Med 1997;15: 316–20.

109. Bair AE, Filbin MR, Kulkarni RG, Walls RM. The failed intubation attempt in the emergency department: analysis of prevalence, rescue techniques, and personnel. J Emerg Med 2002;23:131–40.

110. Holliman CJ, Wuerz RC, Meador SA. Medical command errors in an urban advanced life support system. Ann Emerg Med 1992;21:347–50.

111. Chiara O, Scott JD, Cimbanassi S, Marini A, Zoia R, Rodriguez A, et al. Trauma deaths in an Italian urban area: an audit of pre-hospital and in-hospital trauma care. Injury 2002;33:553–62.

112. Cupera J, Mannova J, Rihova H, Brychta P, Cundrle I. Quality of prehospital management of patients with burn injuries—a retrospective study. Acta Chir Plast 2002;44:59–62.

113. Cone KJ, Murray R. Characteristics, insights, decision making, and preparation of ED triage nurses. J Emerg Nurs 2002;28:401–6.

114. Hodgetts TJ, Kenward G, Vlackonikolis I, Payne S, Castle N, Crouch R, et al. Incidence, location and reasons for avoidable in-hospital cardiac arrest in a district general hospital. Resusc 2002;54:115–23.

115. Tye JB, Hartford CE, Wallace RB. Survey of continuing needs for nonemergency physicians in emergency medicine. JACEP 1978;7:16–9.

116. Luiz T, Hees K, Ellinger K. Prehospital management of emergency patients after previous treatment by general practitioners—a prospective study. Anasthesiol Intensivmed Notfallmed Schmerzther 1997;32:726–33.

117. Tollhurst H, McMillan J, McInerney P, Bernasconi J. The emergency medicine training needs of rural general practitioners. Aust J Rural Health 1999;7:90–6.

118. Somers GT, Maxfield N, Drinkwater EJ. General practitioner preparedness to respond to a medical disaster. Part I: skills and equipment. Aust Fam Phys 1999;28:S3–9.

119. Johnston, CL, Coulthard MG, Schluter PJ, Dick ML. Medical emergencies in general practice in south-east Queensland: prevalence and practice preparedness. Med J Aust 2001;175:99–103.

120. Dick ML, Schluter P, Johnston C, Coulthard M. GP's perceived competence and comfort in managing medical emergencies in southeast Queensland. Aust Fam Phys 2002;31:870–5.

121. Dick ML, Johnston C, Schluter P. Managing emergencies in general practice. How can we do even better? Aust Fam Phys 2002;31:789–90.

122. Simon HK, Steele DW, Lewander WJ, Linakis JG. Are pediatric emergency medicine training programs meeting their goals and objectives? A self-assessment of individuals completing fellowship training in 1993. Pediatr Emerg Care 1994;10:208–12.

123. Simon HK, Sullivan F. Confidence in performance of pediatric emergency procedures by community emergency practitioners. Pediatr Emerg Care 1996;12:336–9.

124. Mil'kov BO, Shamrei GP, Stashchuk VF, Deibuk GD, Kulachek FG. Training of the general physician in the problems of emergency surgical care. Sov Zdravookhr 1988;7:46–8.

125. Kelly L. Surgical skills for family physicians. Do family physicians make the cut? Can Fam Physician 1998;44:476–7.

126. Reid SJ, Chabikuli N, Jaques PH, Fehrsen GS. The procedural skills of rural hospital doctors. S Afr Med J 1999;89:769–74.

127. Sohier N, Frejacques L, Gagnayre R. Design and implementation of a training programme for general practitioners in emergency surgery and obstetrics in precarious situations in Ethiopia. Ann R Coll Surg Engl 1999;81:367–75.

128. Girgis A, Sanson-Fisher RW, Walsh RA. Preventive and other interactional skills of general practitioners, surgeons, and physicians: perceived competence and endorsement of postgraduate training. Prev Med 2001; 32:73–81.

129. Linder G, Murphy P, Streger MR. You did what? Clinical errors in EMS. Emerg Med Serv 2001;30:69–71.

130. Cayten CG, Herrmann N, Cole LW, Walsh S. Assessing the validity of EMS data. JACEP 1978;7:390–6.

131. Williams KA, Rose WD, Simon R. Teamwork in emergency medical services. Air Med J 1999;18:149–53.

132. Eberle B, Dick WF, Schneider T, Wisser G, Doetsch S, Tzanova I. Checking the carotid pulse check: diagnostic accuracy of first responders in patients with and without a pulse. Resusc 1996;33:107–16.

133. Coontz DA, Gratton M. Endotracheal rules of engagement. How to reduce the incidence of unrecognized esophageal intubations. J Emerg Med Serv 2002;27:44–50, 52–4, 56–9.

134. Bradley JS, Billows GL, Olinger ML, Boha SP, Cordell WH, Nelson DR. Prehospital oral endotracheal intubation by rural basic emergency medical technicians. Ann Emerg Med 1998;32:26–32.

135. Hubble MW, Paschal KR, Sanders TA. Medication calculation skills of practicing paramedics. Prehosp Emerg Care 2000;4:253–60.

136. Liberman M, Lavoie A, Mulder D, Sampalis J. Cardiopulmonary resuscitation: errors made by pre-hospital emergency medical personnel. Resusc 1999;42:47–55.

137. Peacock JB, Blackwell VH, Wainscott M. Medical reliability of advanced prehospital cardiac life support. Ann Emerg Med 1985;14:407–9.

138. Seidel JS, Henderson DP, Ward P, Wayland BW, Ness B. Pediatric prehospital care in urban and rural areas. Pediatrics 1991;88:681–90.

139. Seidel, JS. Emergency medical services and the pediatric patient: are the needs being met? II. Training and equipping emergency medical services providers for pediatric emergencies. Pediatrics 1986;78:808–12.

140. Su E, Schmidt TA, Mann NC, Zechnich AD. A randomized controlled trial to assess decay ion acquired knowledge among paramedics completing a pediatric resuscitation course. Acad Emerg Med 2000;7:779–86.

141. West H. Basic infant life support: retention of knowledge and skill. Paediatr Nurs 2000;12:34–7.

142. Snyder W, Smit S. Evaluating the evaluators: interrater reliability on EMT licensing examination. Prehosp Emerg Care 1998;2:37–46.

143. Zautcke JL, Lee RW, Ethington NA. Paramedic skill decay. J Emerg Med 1987;5:505–12.

144. Graber M, Gordon R, Franklin N. Reducing diagnostic errors in medicine: what's the goal? Acad Med 2002;77:981–92.

145. Elkin PL, Gorman PN. Continuing medical education and patient safety: an agenda for lifelong learning. J Am Med Inform Assoc 2002;9: S128–32.

146. Sultz HA, Sawner KA, Sherwin FS. Determining and maintaining competence: an obligation of allied health education. J Allied Health 1984;13:272–9.

147. Taylor HA, Kiser WR. Reported comfort with obstetrical emergencies before and after participation in the advanced life support in obstetrics course. Fam Med 1998;30:103–7.

148. Hall WL, Nowels D. Colorado family practice graduates' preparation for and practice of emergency medicine. J Am Board Fam Pract 2000;13: 246–50.

149. Wise AL, Hays RB, Adkins PB, Craig ML, Mahoney MD, Sheehan M, et al. Training for rural general practice. Med J Aust 1994;161:314–8.

150. Forti EM, Martin KE, Jones RL, Herman JM. An assessment of practice support and continuing medical education needs of rural Pennsylvania family physicians. J Rural Health 1996;12:432–7.

151. Orient JM, Lindsay D, Whitney PJ. Educating primary physicians in emergency surgical procedures. South Med J 1982;75:852–4.

152. Kanz KG, Sturm JA, Mutschler W. Algorithm for prehospital blunt trauma management. Unfallchirurg 2002;105:1007–14.

153. el-Tobgy E, Rupp T. Anaphylaxis. Vicious chain reaction. J Emerg Med Serv 2002;27:84–8, 90–3.

154. Gage H, Kenward G, Hodgetts TJ, Castle N, Ineson N, Shaikh L. Health system costs of in-hospital cardiac arrest. Resusc 2002;54:139–46.

155. Ronco R, King W, Donley DK, Tilden SJ. Outcome and cost at a children's hospital following resuscitation for out-of-hospital cardiopulmonary arrest. Arch Pediatr Adolesc Med 1995;149:210–4.

156. Rosemurgy AS, Norris PA, Olson SM, Hurst JM, Albrink MH. Prehospital traumatic cardiac arrest: the cost of futility. J Trauma 1993;35:473–4.

157. Zack JE, Garrison T, Trovillion E, Clinkscale D, Coopersmith CM, Fraser VJ, et al. Effect of an education aimed at reducing the occurrence of ventilator-associated pneumonia. Crit Care Med 2002;30:2407–12.

158. Lancaster T, Hart R, Gardner S. Literature and medicine: evaluating a special study module using the nominal group technique. Med Educ 2002;36:1071–6.

159. Fritsche L, Greenhalgh T, Falck-Ytter Y, Neumayer HH, Kunz R. Do short courses in evidence based medicine improve knowledge and skills? Validation of Berlin questionnaire and before and after study of courses in evidence based medicine. BMJ 2002;325:1338–41.

160. Murphy AW, Bury G, Dowling EJ. Teaching immediate cardiac care to general practitioners: a faculty-based approach. Med Educ 1995;29:154–8.

161. Rourke JT. Rural advanced life support update course. J Emerg Med 1994;12:107–11.

162. Loutfi A, McLean AP, Pickering J. Training general practitioners in surgical and obstetrical emergencies in Ethiopia. Trop Doct 1995;25(1):22–6.

163. Sanson-Fisher RW, Rolfe IE, Jones P, Ringland C, Agrez M. Trialing a new way to learn clinical skills: systematic clinical appraisal and learning. Med Educ 2002;36:1028–34.

164. Moseley TH, Cantrell MJ, Deloney LA. Clinical skills center attending: an innovative senior medical school elective. Acad Med 2002;77:1176.

165. Gold JP, Verrier EA, Olinger GN, Orringer MB. Development of a CD-ROM Internet hybrid: a new thoracic surgery curriculum. Ann Thorac Surg 2002;74:1741–6.

166. De Leo G, Krishna S, Balas EA, Maglaveras N, Boren SA, Beltrame F, et al. WEB-WAP Based Telecare Proc AMIA Symp; 2002. p. 202–4.

167. Dornan T, Carroll C, Parboosingh J. An electronic learning portfolio for reflective continuing professional development. Med Educ 2002;36:767–9.

168. Greengold NL. A web-based program for implementing evidence-based patient safety recommendations. Jt Comm Qual Improv 2002;28:340–8.

169. Tichon JG. Problem-based learning: a case study in providing e-health education using the Internet. J Telemed Telecare 2002;8:66–8.

170. Mann T, Colven R. A picture is worth more than a thousand words: enhancement of a pre-exam telephone consultation in dermatology with digital images. Acad Med 2002;77:742–3.

171. Casebeer L, Allison J, Spettell CM. Designing tailored web-based instruction to improve practicing physicians' chlamydial screening rates. Acad Med 2002;77:929.

172. Poyner A, Wood A, Herzberg J. Distance learning project-information skills training: supporting flexible trainees in psychiatry. Health Info Libr J 2002;19:84–9.

173. Fieschi M, Soula G, Giorgi R, Gouvernet J, Fieschi D, Botti G, et al. Experimenting with new paradigms for medical education and the emergence of a distance learning degree using the Internet: teaching evidence-based medicine. Med Inform Internet Med 2002;27:1–11.

174. Deodhar J. Telemedicine by email—experience in neonatal care at a primary care facility in rural India. J Telemed Telecare 2002;8:20–1.

175. Pastuszak J, Rodowicz MO. Internal e-mail: an avenue of educational opportunity. J Contin Educ Nurs 2002;33:164–77.

176. Marshall JN, Stewart M, Ostbye T. Small-group CME using e-mail discussions. Can it work? Can Fam Physician 2001;47:557–63.

177. Haythornthwaite S. Videoconferencing training for those working with at-risk young people in rural areas of Western Australia. J Telemed Telecare 2002;8:29–33.

178. Davis P, McCraken P. Restructuring rural continuing medical education through videoconferencing. J Telemed Telecare 2002;8:108–9.

179. Allen M, Sargeant J, McDougall E, O'Brien B. Evaluation of videoconferencing grand rounds. J Telemed Telecare 2002;8:210–6.

180. Allen M. Sargeant J, McDougall E, Proctor-Simms M. Videoconferencing for continuing medical education: from pilot project to sustained programme. J Telemed Telecare 2002;8:131–7.

181. von Lubitz DKJE, Pletcher T, Treloar D, Wilkerson W, Wolf E. Immersive virtual reality platform for medical training: a "killer application." Abstract, proceedings of Medicine Meets Virtual Reality 2000: envisioning Healing—Interactive Technology and the Patient-Practitioner Dialogue. 2000.

182. von Lubitz DKJE, Levine H, Wolf E. The goose, the gander, or the Strasbourg paté for all: medical education, world, and the Internet. In: Chin W, Poatricelli F, Milutinovic V, editors. Electronic business and education: recent advances in Internet infrastructures. Boston: Kluwer Acad Pub 2002. p. 189–210.

183. Lamminen H, Niiranen S, Niemi K, Mattila H, Kalli S. Health-related services on the Internet. Med Inform Internet Med 2002;27:13–20.

184. Fay V, Feldt KS, Greenberg SA, Vezina M, Flaherty E, Ryan M, et al. Providing optimal hands-on experience. A guide for clinical preceptors. Adv Nurse Pract 2001;9:71–4, 110.

185. Hicks GD. An appeal for more "hands-on" surgical training and experience. Plast Reconstr Surg 2001;107:1612–3.

186. Gonzalez YM, Mohl ND. Care of patients with temporomandibular disorders: an educational challenge. J Orofac Pain 2002;16:200–6.

187. Robinson G. Do general practitioners' risk-taking propensities and learning styles influence their continuing medical education preferences? Med Tech 2002;24:71–8.

188. Girdler NM. Competency in sedation. Br Dent J 2001;191:119.

189. Mandavia DP, Argona J, Chan L, Chan D, Henderson SO. Ultrasound training for emergency physicians—a prospective study. Acad Emerg Med 2000;7:1008–14.

190. Haponik EF, Russell GB, Beamis JF Jr, Britt EJ, Kvale P, Mathur P, et al. Bronchoscopy training: current fellows' experiences and some concerns for the future. Chest 2000;118:625–30.

191. Friedrich MJ. Practice makes perfect: risk-free medical training with patient simulators. JAMA 2002;288:2811–2.

192. Knowles WB. Aerospace simulation and human performance research. Hum Factors 1967;9:149–59.

193. Krebs WK, McCarley JS, Bryant EV. Effects of mission rehearsal simulation on air-to-ground target acquisition. Hum Factors 1999;41: 553–8.

194. Ricard GL. Acquisition of control skill with delayed and compensated displays. Hum Factors 1995;37:652–8.

195. Brannick MT, Prince A, Prince C, Salas E. The measurement of team process. Hum Factors 1995;37:641–51.

196. Nagoshi MH. Role of standardized patients in medical education. Hawaii Med J 2001;60:323–4.

197. Vardi A, Levin I, Berkenstadt H, Hourvitz A, Eisenkraft A, Cohen A, et al. Simulation-based training of medical teams to manage chemical warfare casualties. Isr Med Assoc J 2002;4:540–4.

198. Greenberg R, Loyd G, Wesley G. Integrated simulation experiences to enhance clinical education. Med Educ 2002;36:1109–10.

199. Bond WF, Spillane L. The use of simulation for emergency medicine resident assessment. Acad Emerg Med 2002;9:1295–9.

200. Shapiro M, Morchi R. High-fidelity medical simulation and teamwork training to enhance medical student performance in cardiac resuscitation. Acad Emerg Med 2002;9:1055–6.

201. Pittini R, Oepkes D, Macrury K, Reznick R, Beyene J, Windrim R. Teaching invasive perinatal assessment of a high fidelity simulator-based curriculum. Ultrasound Obstet Gynecol 2002;19:478–83.

202. Weller JM, Bloch M, Young S, Maze M, Oyesolsa S, Wyner J, et al. Evaluation of high fidelity patient simulator in assessment of performance of anaesthetists. Br J Anaesth 2003;909:43–47.

203. Kanter RK, Fordyce WE, Tompkins JM. Evaluation of resuscitation proficiency in simulation: the impact of simultaneous cognitive task. Pediatr Emerg Care 1990;6:260–2.

204. Small SD, Wuertz RC, Simon R, Shapiro N, Conn A, Setnik G. Demonstration of high fidelity simulation team training for emergency medicine. Acad Emerg Med 1999;6:213–23.

205. Mackenzie CF, Jefferies NJ, Hunter WA, Nernhard WN, Xiao Y. Comparison of self-reporting of deficiencies in airway management with video analysis of actual performance. LOTAS group. Level one trauma anesthesia simulation. Hum Factors 1996;38:623–35.

206. Garden A, Robinson B, Weller J, Wilson L, Crone D. Education to address medical error—a role for high fidelity patient simulation. NZ Med J 2002;115:133–4.

207. Jeanguiot NP. Learning by mistake. The status of error in the initial education of nurses. Rech Soins Infirm 2000 Sep;62:36–78.

208. Graschew G. Roelofs TA, Rakowsky S, Schlag PM. Interactive telemedical applications in OP 2000 via satellite. BioMed Tech (Berl) 2002; 47:330–3.

209. Patterson PE. Development of a learning module using a virtual environment to demonstrate EMG and telerobotic control principles. Biomed Sci Instrum 2002;38:313–6.

210. Agazio JB, Pavlides CC, Lasome CE, Flaherty NJ, Torrance RJ. Evaluation of a virtual reality simulator in sustainment training. Mil Med 2002;167: 893–7.

211. Seymour NE, Gallagher AG, Roman SA, O'Brien MK, Bansal VK, Anderson DK, et al. Virtual reality training improves operating room performance: results of a randomized, double blinded study. Ann Surg 2002;236: 463–4.

212. Hotchkiss MA, Mendoza SN. Update for nurse anesthetists. Part 6. Full-body patient simulation technology: gaining experience using a malignant hyperthermia model. AANA J 2001;69:59–65.

213. Watterson L, Flanagan B, Donovan B, Robinson B. Anaesthetic simulators: training for the broader health-care profession. Aust NZ J Surg 2000;70:735–7.

214. Fletcher JL. AANA journal course: update for nurse anesthetists—anesthesia simulation: a tool for learning and research. AANA J 1995;63:61–7.

215. Issenberg SB, McGaghie WC, Hart IR, Mayer JW, Felner JM, Petrusa ER, et al. Simulation technology for health professional skills training and assessment. JAMA 1999;282:861–6.

216. Schwid HA, Rooke GA, Carline J, Steadman RH, Murray WB, Olympio M, et al. The Anesthesia Simulator Research Consortium. Evaluation of anesthesia residents using mannequin-based simulation: a multiinstitutional study. Anesthes 2002;97:1434–44.

217. Wong SH, Ng KF, Chen PP. The application of clinical simulation in crisis management training. Hong Kong Med J 2002;8:131–5.

218. Cosman PH, Cregan PC, Martin CJ, Cartmill JA. Virtual reality simulators: current status in acquisition and assessment of surgical skills. ANZ J Surg 2002;72:30–4.

219. Gaba DM, DeAnda A. A comprehensive anesthesia environment: re-creating the operating room for research and training. Anesthes 1988;69:387–94.

220. Byrne AJ, Jones JG. The expanding role of simulators in risk management. Br J Anaesth 1997;79:411.

221. Spence AA. The expanding role of simulators in risk management. Br J Anaesth 1997;78:633–4.

222. Devitt JH, Kurrek MM, Cohen MM, Cleave-Hogg D. The validity of performance assessments using simulation. Anesthes 2001;95:36–42.

223. DeAnda A, Gaba DM. Unplanned incidents during comprehensive anesthesia simulation. Anesth Analg 1990;71:77–82.

224. Schaefer JJ III, Grenvik A. Simulation-based training at the University of Pittsburgh. Ann Acad Med Singapore 2001;30:274–80.

225. Gordon JA, Pawlowski J. Education on demand: the development of a simulator-based medical education service. Acad Med 2002;77:751–21.

226. von Lubitz DKJE, Montgomery J, Russell W. Just in time training: emergency medicine training aboard a ship. Navy Med 2000: 24–8.

227. Treloar D, Beier KP, Freer J, Levine H, von Lubitz DKJE, Wilkerson W, et al. On site and distance education of emergency medicine personnel with a human patient simulator. J Mil Med 2001;166:1003–6.

228. von Lubitz DKJE, Beier KP, Freer J, Levine H, Pletcher T, Wilkerson W, et al. Simulation-based medical training: the medical readiness trainer concept and the preparation for military and civilian medical field operations. In: Richir S, Richard P, Taravel B, editors. Virtual Reality International Conference; 2001 May; ISTIA Innovation; 2001. p. 215–24.

229. von Lubitz DKJE, Carrasco B, Gabbrielli F, Ludwig T, et al. Transatlantic medical education: preliminary data on distance-based high fidelity human patient simulation training. In: Westwood JD, Hoffman MH, Mogul GT, et al., editors. Medicine Meets Virtual Reality 11 (Studies in Health Technology and Informatics, 94). Amsterdam: IOS Press; 2003. p. 379–85.

230. von Lubitz DKJE, Carrasco B, Levine H, Poirier C. High fidelity human patient simulation training in trauma and emergency medicine—distributed multiplatform environments in distance learning setting. Proc. VRIC 2003; ISTIA Innovation (University of Angers); 2003. p. 107–12 (ter).

231. Graschew G. Roelofs TA, Rakowsky S, Schlag PM. Interactive telemedical applications in OP 2000 via satellite. Biomed Tech (Berl) 2002;47: 330–3.

232. Holcomb G. Coherent medical informatics. 2002. Available from: www.som.tulane.edu/oit/documents/CMI.PDF. Accessed June 3, 2003.

233. von Lubitz DKJE, Carrasco B, Fausone CA, et al. Bioterrorism: development of large-scale medical readiness using multipoint distance-based simulation training. In: Westwood JD, Hoffman MH, Mogul GT, et al., editors. Medicine Meets Virtual Reality; 2004. Amsterdam: IOS Press. (In press).

234. von Lubitz DKJE. 2002, EMERGENCY! Medicine and modern education technology. In: Proceedings Intl Conf on Internet, Business, Science, and Medicine. L'Aquila; 2002 Aug [on CD-ROM]. SSGRR (L'Aquila).

235. MRT (Medical Readiness Trainer) Team. Immersive virtual reality platform for medical training: a "killer application." In: Williams J, et al., editors. Medicine Meets Virtual Reality; 2000. Amsterdam: IOS Press; 2000. p. 207–13.

236. von Lubitz DKJE, Freer J, French A, Hawayek J, Montgomery J, et al. Autostereoscopy in medical telepresence: the medical readiness trainer experience. In: Patricelli F, Ray PK, editors. Proceedings of HEALTHCOM 2001, 3rd Intl Workshop on Enterprise, Networking, and Computing in Healthcare Industry; June 29–July 10, 2001. L'Aquila, Italy: Scuola Superiore G. Reiss Romoli; 2001. p. 61–76.

237. Available from: www.ssgrr.it/en/ssgrr2003s/panel.htm. Accessed July 10, 2003.

238. Gordon JA, Pawlowski J. Education on-demand: the development of a simulator-based medical education service. Acad Med 2002 Jul;77:751–2.

239. Coram R. Boyd: the fighter pilot who changed the art of war. Boston: Little Brown; 2002. p. 1–484.

240. von Lubitz DKJE. OODA. In: Milutinovic V, editor. Proceedings IPSI 2003 Montenegro Conference, Sveti Stefan 2003 Oct. IPSI/Academic Mind. Belgrade; 2003.

241. von Lubitz DKJE and the MRT Team. Medicine in the village: technology, health, and the world. In: Vlasovic B, Cesar A, Meolic R, Balan FS, editors. IEEE Proc. "Conf on extra skills for young engineers" symposium. Maribor, Slovenia: Maribor Univ Press; 2000. p. 27–33.

242. See www.med-smart.org for details.

243. UK Department of Health Chief Medical Officer. Exercise Global Mercury: post exercise report. 2003. Available from: www.doh.gov.uk/cmo/exerciseglobalmercury/. Accessed September 2, 2004.

244. Trust for America's Health Report. Ready or not? Practicing the public health in the age of bioterrorism. 2003. Available from: healthyamericans.org/state/bioterror. Accessed September 11, 2003.

245. Office of Transitional Issues. The darker bioweapons future. Washington, DC: Central Intelligence Agency, Directorate of Intelligence; 2003.

246. von Clausewitz C. On war. London: Penguin Classics; 1982. p. 9–453.

247. Marcinko R. Rogue warrior. New York: Atria Books; 1992. p. 1–352.

248. Chamberlain D, Smith A, Woollard M, Colquhoun M, Handley AJ, Leaves S, et al. Trials of teaching methods in basic life support (3): comparison of simulated CPR performance after first training and at 6 months, with a note on the value of re-training. Resuscitation 2002;53:179–87.

249. Hammond F, Saba M, Simon T, Cross R. Advanced life support: retention of registered nurses' knowledge 18 months after initial training. Aust Crit Care 2000;13:99–104.

250. Su E, Schmidt TA, Mann NC, Zechnich AD. A randomized trial to assess decay in acquired knowledge among paramedics completing a pediatric resuscitation course. Acad Emerg Med 2000;7:779–86.

251. Young R, King L. An evaluation of knowledge and skill retention following an in-house advanced life support course. Nurs Crit Care 2000;5: 7–14.

17 The Role of Spirituality and Community

Kay Haw

Today, many factors have begun to influence us as individuals as well as collectively—as a whole nation that at times lives in fear. We have experienced the disaster of 9/11, and this event will have an everlasting effect on our lives and the lives of our children for generations to come. We live in a world of uncertainty and search for a place to feel safe and secure, protected from the dangers of the world. It is within times of chaos and turmoil that our fears seem to overtake us and we seek a place of rational peace, an inner peace. The spiritual dimension of our lives can provide us this assurance and guidance that we long for to bring some calm to our overwhelming emotions of despair.

Spirituality is an inner search for meaning in our lives. It provides us with mechanisms to relieve our fears, such as prayer for those whom we feel may be suffering, and for our own personal suffering. Our spirituality affords us the chance for healing through our faith in a higher power. It has been linked to our ability to cope with catastrophic events. Prayer can serve as a source of comfort to us if we choose to embrace and practice it. It is through the practice of prayer that our questions of meaning and purpose can evolve and answers can be found. Buddhist belief, for example, is that suffering can be overcome by living and thinking in the right ways. Christianity teaches us that if we live our lives according to the teachings of the Jesus Christ, we can find solitude and peace as we long for the answers to troublesome times. For Christians, it is in the church of worship that one can find fulfillment to alleviate one's worries, since worrying can fragment lives. Attending church services can fill a void for us—thus preventing the world from filling our lives—and instead allow us to choose richness and grace to fill our emptiness. It allows us to rid ourselves of the outside world. However, we need to set aside time and space for the spirit to give us this life of inner sanctity. The spiritual community allocates this special resource for us as believers, as we seek a place of comfort and security, offering us a place to truly be ourselves and to be unconditionally loved, as only in God's hands.

The spiritual community as a discipline is the effort to create free and empty space among people where together they can practice true obedience. In this community, we prevent ourselves from clinging to each other in fear and loneliness; we clear free space to listen to the liberating voice of God. It is where solitude meets solitude, the spirit speaks to the spirit, and one can hear the heart calling to another heart. The spiritual community is the place where God calls us together, to gather in the place where God embraces us all and allows for us to safely put away our differences and live and pray together as sisters and brothers in Christ. This same community allows us to be silent together and pay attention or shift our attention to the Lord who has called us here together. It is within this place that a common openness is created, and this allows us to recognize that we are safe together in that word, the word of God. The discipline of this community allows us to be free of the boundaries of race, age, and ethnicity, and it permits us to be one in the eyes of God and for each other.

Community is obedience practiced together, the practice of prayer collectively. The discipline of community frees us to go where the spirit guides us—it has no boundaries and no distance of time or place. It is within this safe haven that we are given a vision to serve as an avenue for hope, even in our moments of greatest despair. We become free to be with others in a new way, not seeing them as people but rather as fellow human beings creating a new space for God. The spirituality that lies within creates an openness to relationships at the deepest level, in the most elegant sense of the term. Through this personal accessibility, we may examine and safely explore the window to our souls. Our dreams and possibilities can manifest and be brought to life through our self-exploration. The spiritual community allows us to relieve our turmoil and be amid a field of peace. Through this nourishing of peacefulness, our senses are rekindled. We are then provided with a sense or feeling of acceptance, no matter who we are, because God's expectation is that we "love." Quietness and composure will prevail in a world full of turmoil and chaos.

Our spirituality is our personal quest as we search for something greater: the unknown. It can be simplistic and does not require a great deal of energy. Our level of commitment to this dimension of the human spirit is a very personal journey. However, in the face of threats and the distasteful seeds of terrorism, our spiritual life can bring us a peaceful heart, providing us escape from a troubled world.

Bibliography

Agency for Health Care Research and Quality. Bioterrorism and emerging infections site. Available from: www.bioterrorism.uab.edu/.

Benenson A. Control of communicable diseases manual. 16th ed. Washington, DC: American Public Health Association; 1995.

Bogue RJ, Antia M, Harmata R, Hall CH Jr. Community experiments in action: developing community-defined models for reconfiguring healthcare delivery. J Health Pol, Policy and Law 1997 Aug;22(4).

Bozeman B, Kingsley G. Risk culture in public and private organizations. Pub Admin.

Canter MS, Cole JB, Sandor RL. Insurance derivatives: a new asset class for the capital markets and a new hedging tool for the insurance industry. J Appl Corp Fin 1997 Autumn:69–83.

Carter AB. The architecture of government in the face of terrorism. International Security 2001;26(3):5–23.

Centers for Disease Control and Prevention. Emergency preparedness and response. Agents, diseases and other threats. Available from: www.bt.cdc.gov/agent/.

Choussudovsky M. Economic terrorism. Available from: emperors-clothes/articles/choss/econ2.htm.

Cole CR, McCullough KA. Excluding Terror, CPCU eJournal 2002 Aug: 1–7.

Cronin AK. Behind the curve: globalization and international terrorism. International Security 2003;27(3):30–58.

Cummins JD, Lalonde D, Phillips R. Basis risk of index-linked CAT risk securities. Meeting of Wharton Project on Managing Catastrophic Risks; June 14–15, 1999; Philadelphia, PA.

Emerson S. American jihad: The terrorists living among us. New York: Free Press; 2002.

Farberow, NL. Training Manual for Human Service Workers in Major Disasters (DHHS Publication No. ADM 83-538). Rockville, MD: NIMH; 1978d.

Foreman S. Social responsibility and the academic medical center: building community-based systems for the nation's health. Acad Med 1994 Feb;69(2).

Froot KA, Murphy BS, Stern B, Usher SE. The emerging asset class: insurance risk. Guy Carpenter and Co., Inc.; 1995 July.

Galbraith JK, Gamkhar S. Homeland security and the states: a policy perspective on intergovernmental sharing of funding responsibilities, in Security after 9/11: strategy choices and budget tradeoffs, produced by the Security Policy Workgroup. 2003. Available from www.cdi.org/spwg/. Accessed October 13, 2003.

Hartwig RP. September 11, 2001: the first year. One hundred minutes of terror that changed the global industry forever. Insurance Information Institute; 2002.

Howard R, Sawyer R. Terrorism and counterterrorism: understanding the new security environment. Guilford, CT: McGraw-Hill; 2002.

International Risk Management Institute (IRMI). Commercial property insurance. Dallas: IRMI; 2003.

Ledlow GR, Cwiek MA, Johnson JA. Business and terrorism: think globally, act locally. New York, NY: GBATA, St. Johns University Press; 2002.

Litzenberger RH, Beaglehole DR, Reynolds CE. Assessing catastrophe-reinsurance-linked securities as a new asset class. J Portfolio Management 1996 Winter:76–86.

Miami Medical School. Q fever. Available from: www.med.miami.edu/glossary/art.asp?articlekey=3430.

Miller CA, Moore KS, Richards TB, Kotelchuck M, Kaluzny AD. Longitudinal observations on a selected group of local health departments. J Pub Health Pol 1993;14:34–50.

100 attend USFA incident command course [press release]. 2003 May 7. Available from: www.fema.gov.

Pinkerton Consulting & Investigations, Inc. Top security threats and management issues facing corporate America. Rev 2000;58(2):109–18.

Robinson LG. 2003, Terrorism insurance: what risk and insurance professionals must know, (Dallas: International Risk Management Institute).

Roper WL, Baker EL, Dyal WW, Nicola RM. Strengthening the public health system. Pub Health Rep 1992;107:609–15.

St. Louis University School of Public Health. Center for the Study of Bioterrorism and Emerging Infections. Available from: www.bioterrorism.slu.edu/.

Sanctum Corporation Press Release. Sanctum Study Reveals 9–18 had stronger impact on IT security spending than 9–11. 2002 Aug 26.

Schlesinger M, Gray B. A broader vision for managed care, part I: measuring the benefit to communities. Health Affairs 1998 May/June;17(3).

Schwab M, Syme SL. On the other hand: on paradigms, community participation and the future of public health. Amer J Pub Health 1997 Dec; 87(12):2049–52.

Scott HD, Tierney JT, Waters WJ. The future of public health: a survey of the states. J Pub Health Pol 1990;11:296–304.

Social Science Research Council. After Sept. 11. Available from: www.ssrc.org/sept11/.

United Nations Action Against Terrorism. Available from: www.un.org/terrorism/.

U.S. Department of Health and Human Services. Healthy people 2010: understanding and improving health. 2nd ed. Washington, DC: U.S. Government Printing Office; 2000 Nov.

U.S. Department of Justice. Uniting and strengthening America by Providing Appropriate Tools Required to Intercept and Obstruct Terrorism Act of 2001 (USA Patriot Act). Pub. L 107-56. U.S. Department of Justice; 2001.

U.S. Department of Justice, Federal Bureau of Investigation. Terrorism in the United States. U.S. Department of Justice; 1999.

U.S. Department of State. Patterns of global terrorism 2001. 2002. Available from: www.state.gov/s/ct/rls/pgtrpt/.

Washington Business Group on Health (WBGH) prepared for the W. K. Kellogg Foundation. Available from: www.wbgh.org.

Index

Disaster medicine, 132
Disaster mental health, 181, 183, 184–87, 193, 196
Disaster mental health services, 183, 193
Disaster planning, 109, 130, 135
District of Columbia, 75
DNA, 111, 251
Dole, Senator Elizabeth, 179
Domestic terrorism, 20, 28, 152, 166
Doty, Byron, 208
Doxycycline, 2, 9–10, 138
Duke University, 77
Dulles International Airport, 68

Ebola, 10–11
Emergency Management Strategic Healthcare Group (EMSHG), 148, 150–51, 153–60
Emergency Manager, 132, 139, 213–14, 243–44; AEM and, 153, 155–56; performance of, 236; roles and, 218, 226; training and, 137, 214
Emergency medical services (EMS), 27, 118, 125, 138–39, 215
Emergency Mobilization Preparedness Board, 152
Emergency Operations Center, 24, 153, 214, 217, 219
Emergency preparedness, 73, 125–31, 133, 152, 218, 240; communities and, 142; coordinators and, 158, 215; plans for, 116; public health and, 259
Emergency Support Function (ESF), 149
EMT, 154, 270
Environmental Protection Agency, 12

Escherichia coli, 8
Eshoo, Senator Anna, 179
Etiological hazards, 34
Europe, 126
Evans, Deb, 207
Explosive device, 31–32, 37, 70
Export Administration Act, 127
Exposure, 111

Federal Bureau of Investigation (FBI), 41, 49; investigation by, 41, 107; JTTF and, 27; NIPC and, 51; terrorism and, 20, 66
Federal coordinating centers, 153–54, 174, 180
Federal Emergency Management Agency (FEMA), 139, 152, 164; B-NICE and, 30; creation of, 126–27; FRP and, 152; training and, 221; VAL and, 173
Federal Office of Emergency Preparedness, 110
Federal Radiological Emergency Response Plan, 152
Federal Response Plan (FRP), 147, 149, 152
Field, 68, 196
Filoviridae, 10
Firewalls 47, 52
Fitzgerald, Cantor, 192
Flaviviridae, 11
Florida, 149, 159, 175
Fluoroquinolone, 5
Fort Pitt, PA, 108
France, 62, 65, 289, 297
Future of Public Health Committee, 260

General Accounting Office, 49, 110, 174
Geneva, 127
Gentamycine, 4

Paradigm, 19, 100, 105, 140
Parma Community General Hospital, 117
Parma, OH, 117
Password, 46
Pataki, George, 20
Pearl Harbor, 42, 293
Pearl, MS, 201
Pennsylvania, 15, 108, 157, 163–66
Pentagon, 15, 181, 196
Pericardiocenthesis, 275
Personal protective equipment (PPE), 34–35
Philippines, 91
Pier 94, 188
Pimpernel Effect, 292, 294
Pinkerton survey of *Fortune*, 69–70, 78
Plague, 1, 4, 43, 108, 113, 126, 256
Pneumonic plague. *See* Plague
Port Huron, MI, 201
Potential Injury/Illness Creating Event (PICE), 132
Preparedness, 134
Primary receiving center (PRC), 151
Primer on 10 Classical Biological Agents, 116
Professional Emergency Manager (PEM), 231–38
Professional Emergency Manager Assessment Center (PEMAC), 230–38, 242–43
Project access, 261
Protection suite, 47–48
Protocol, 177
Ptosis, 3
Public Health Service (PHS), 149, 152
Puerto Rico, 75
Pustules, 5, 286

Q fever, 9–10
QAZ, 43
QUAD, 207

Radio Amateur Communications Emergency Services, 153
Radiological, 24, 34, 73, 129, 150, 152, 155, 160, 221
Radiological Weapons, 132
Red Cell Team, 294, 296
Red Cross, 125, 169, 181, 188–96, 222. *See also* American Red Cross
RedSiren Technologies, 48
Reign of Terror, 65
Religious terrorists, 67
Republican and Democratic National Conventions, 149
Responder Awareness and Planning Seminar, 117
Rhizobium melitoli, 12
Ribavirin, 11
Richmond Medical Center, 150
Ricin, 6, 30, 126
Rickettsia, 30
Rifampin, 9
Rift Valley fever virus, 10
Right wing terrorist, 67
Risk premium, 58
Risk transfer, 58, 60
Riverview Mall, 213
Role, 22
Roman, 67
Rudman, Senator Warren, 80
Rural, 194
Russia, 108

Safe Horizon, 188
Saginaw Chippewa Indian Tribal Reservation, 200
Saginaw Chippewa Indian Tribe, 199–200, 207
Saginaw, MI, 116, 199–200, 207

About the Editors and Contributors

LAURA K. ACTON, MA, RN, C, EMT, is the director of educational resources at Saint Mary's Medical Center in Saginaw, Michigan, and serves on the Breckenridge/Wheeler Rescue. She is also certified in nursing staff development and continuing education. Her MA is from Central Michigan University.

JOHN ANGELIDIS, DBA, is professor of management and chair of the Department of Management, St. John's University. He teaches courses in strategic management, business and society, and entrepreneurship. He has authored many articles in academic and practitioner journals. His doctorate is from Georgia State University.

JAMES BARRESE, PhD, is a professor in St. John's University's Department of Risk Management. He has published dozens of articles and served on the editorial boards of several industry and academic journals and as a board member of the federal Advisory Commission on Intergovernmental Relations Thinkers Group. He earned his PhD at Rutgers University.

SYLVIE BOURIAUX, PhD, is an assistant professor of finance at Illinois State University. Her research interests include insurance and credit securitization and derivative markets. She has previously published research papers on insurance-linked transactions. Before her current position with ISU, Bouriaux was director of research and product development at the Chicago Board of Trade in Chicago, Illinois. She also provided expert testimony to various Committees of the U.S. House of Representatives and to state legislatures on diverse industry issues, such as the National Disaster Legislation. She earned her PhD at University of Paris, France.

CHARLANE BROWN, JD, is an attorney, an eighteen-year veteran of the New York City Police Department, and a Fulbright Fellow in Police Studies. She is currently an assistant adjunct professor at St. John's University in New York. Charlane Brown received her JD degree from New York Law School.

NEJDET DELENER, PhD, is an associate dean for academic affairs and professor of marketing and international business at the Tobin College of Business, St. John's University. He is currently an executive editor for the *Journal of Global Business and Technology*. He received his PhD from the City University of New York, and he holds a diploma in economics from Oxford Polytechnic Institute, England.

WILLIAM L. FERGUSON, PhD, is the eminent chair of insurance and risk management at the University of Louisiana at Lafayette. He is a Fulbright lecturer, Institut für Versicherungswirtschaft/Wirtschaftsuniversität Wien (Austria). Ferguson is an active member of numerous academic and professional organizations, and he earned his PhD from the University of Georgia.

JONATHAN H. GARDNER, MPA, FACHE, is director, Southern Arizona Veterans Administration Healthcare System in Tucson, Arizona. In 2000, President Clinton awarded Gardner with the rank of Meritorious Executive in the Senior Executive Service of the U.S. Government. His MPA is from Brigham Young University.

KAY HAW, RN, DHS, is director of nursing at the Collington Lifecare Community in Maryland. She earned her doctorate in health sciences at Nova University.

CAROL L. HOLLAND, DrPH, LPC, NCC, is a licensed psychologist in the Student Counseling Center at Slippery Rock University and a Disaster Mental Health volunteer for the American Red Cross. Her DrPH is from the University of Pittsburgh.

NABIL A. IBRAHIM, PhD, is professor of business administration and holder of the Grover Maxwell Chair of Business Administration at Augusta State University. He teaches courses in strategic management and applied statistics. He has authored numerous articles in academic and practitioner journals. His PhD is from Georgia State University.

JOSEPH N. INUNGU, MD, DrPH, is an associate professor of health sciences at Central Michigan University. He specializes in infectious disease, biostatistics, and community health. He earned his MD in the Republic of Congo and his DrPH is from Tulane University.

SVETLANA V. IVANITSKAYA, PhD, is an assistant professor at the Herbert H. and Grace A. Dow College of Health Professions, Central Michigan University. Ivanitskaya has consulted with organizations directly related to personnel training and development, turnover, organizational behavior, executive coaching, organizational culture, and strategic planning. Her PhD is from Central Michigan University.

JAMES A. JOHNSON, PhD, is a professor of health sciences at Central Michigan University and Visiting Scholar at Medical University of South Carolina. He has published nine books on a wide range of health-related topics, has published over 100 articles, and serves as a health science columnist for newspapers. He is involved in international health development, which includes work with the World Health Organization in Geneva, Switzerland. His PhD is from Florida State University.

DAN L. JOHNSTON, MPA, is area emergency manager for the Department of Veterans Affairs and coordinator for the National Disaster Medical System. He is assigned to the Southern Arizona Veterans Administration Health Care System in Tucson, Arizona. His MPA is from Brigham Young University.

MICHAEL H. KENNEDY, PhD, FACHE, is an associate professor at Central Michigan University and director of the Doctor of Health Administration Program. He has twenty-eight years experience in health services administration, which has been divided between academic positions and operational assignments in the military health service system in the United States and Germany. His PhD is from Rensselaer Polytechnic Institute.

DIANE E. KNUDSEN, RN, MSA, MSN, ANP, Doctoral Candidate, is currently the director of emergency services and critical care in a Northeastern, Pennsylvania, hospital. She has extensive experience in emergency services and emergency preparedness. She is pursuing a doctoral degree in healthcare administration from Central Michigan University.

MARVIS J. LARY, PhD, is professor and dean of The Herbert H. and Grace A. Dow College of Health Professions, Central Michigan University. Prior to her appointment, Lary was the associate dean for academic affairs and research at Wichita State University. While at WSU, she served for thirteen years as the chair of the Physician Assistant Department. In this position, she gained national prominence as a leader in physician assistant education and professional issues. Lary earned her PhD from Kansas State University.

GERALD R. LEDLOW, PhD, CHE, is a vice president for Sisters of Mercy Health System in St. Louis, Missouri, and former U.S. Army Medical Logistics and Health Systems Development/Health Administration Officer in the Medical Service Corps. His PhD is from the University of Oklahoma.

KEVIN G. LOVE, PhD, is an industrial psychologist and professor of organizational behavior and human resource management at Central Michigan University. He has provided HRM consulting services to public safety agencies and private sector organizations for over 25 years. He received his PhD from the University of South Florida.

MICHIGAN ASSOCIATION OF UNITED WAYS (MAUW), formerly known as the United Way of Michigan, is a nonprofit agency. In order to simplify the gathering and distribution of funds that were received through charitable giving, a group of community and labor leaders founded the agency in 1947. MAUW is comprised of 87 local United Ways, which represent the largest network of nongovernmental service providers and service funders in Michigan that support local health and human service organizations.

IRENE O'BOYLE, PhD, CHES, is assistant professor in the School of Health Sciences at Central Michigan University. O'Boyle is the former director for community health and education at the Mid-Michigan District Health Department. She is a 2001–2002 Public Health Education Leadership Scholar. O'Boyle's PhD is from Union Graduate Institute.

JAMES O'KEEFE, PhD, is the retired director of training for the New York City Police Department. He is currently an associate professor and director of the undergraduate Criminal Justice Program at St. John's University in New York. O'Keefe teaches undergraduate and graduate level classes in police administration, criminological theory, public policy, and police leadership. He has published many scholarly articles and books and is internationally recognized as an expert in law enforcement training. O'Keefe received his PhD in criminal justice administration from Sam Houston State University.

RENA E. RICHTIG, PhD, is assistant professor in educational administration and community leadership at Central Michigan University and former public educator and administrator in Michigan and Wisconsin. Her PhD is from Michigan State University.

ANTOINETTE COLLARINI SCHLOSSBERG, PhD, is currently associate professor at the College of Professional Studies in the Division of Criminal Justice and Legal Studies, St. John's University. Collarini Schlossberg is the former executive director of the Westchester County, New York, Youth Bureau in the Office of the County Executive and has worked closely with her husband and coauthor since the mid-1970s developing concepts related to hostage negotiations. She earned her PhD from Columbia University.

HARVEY SCHLOSSBERG, PhD, is currently associate professor at the College of Professional Studies in the Division of Criminal Justice and Legal Studies, St. John's University. Schlossberg is a former police officer, detective, and former founder and director of psychological services for the New York City Police Department. He is also retired chief psychologist for the Port Authority of New York and New Jersey and considered the creator of police hostage negotiations response. Since 1972, Schlossberg has trained thousands of law enforcement and security personnel on the federal, state, and local levels as well as internationally in the theory and practice of hostage rescue and response techniques. He earned his PhD at Yeshiva University.

NICOS A. SCORDIS, PhD, is an associate professor at the Tobin College of Business of St. John's University, where he holds the John R. Cox/ACE Limited Chair of Risk and Insurance. Scordis has written for insurance industry publications and other journals. He earned his PhD at the University of South Carolina.

MICHELE SIMMS, PhD, is assistant professor of management at the Cameron School of Business, University of St. Thomas in Houston, Texas. She is a former faculty member and interim director for the Michigan Public Health Leadership Institute and was a research fellow at the UST Center for Business Ethics. Her PhD is from Wayne State University.

DAG K. J. E. VON LUBITZ, PhD, MD, serves as the chairman and chief scientist at MedSMART, Inc., a nonprofit company devoted to the research and use of advanced simulation and telecommunication technologies in medical training and research. Apart from several publications devoted to simulation in medicine and to its global application in education and training, von Lubitz is the author of numerous book chapters and research papers on the treatment of stroke. He received his education at the University of Copenhagen, Denmark.